IRISH FEVER

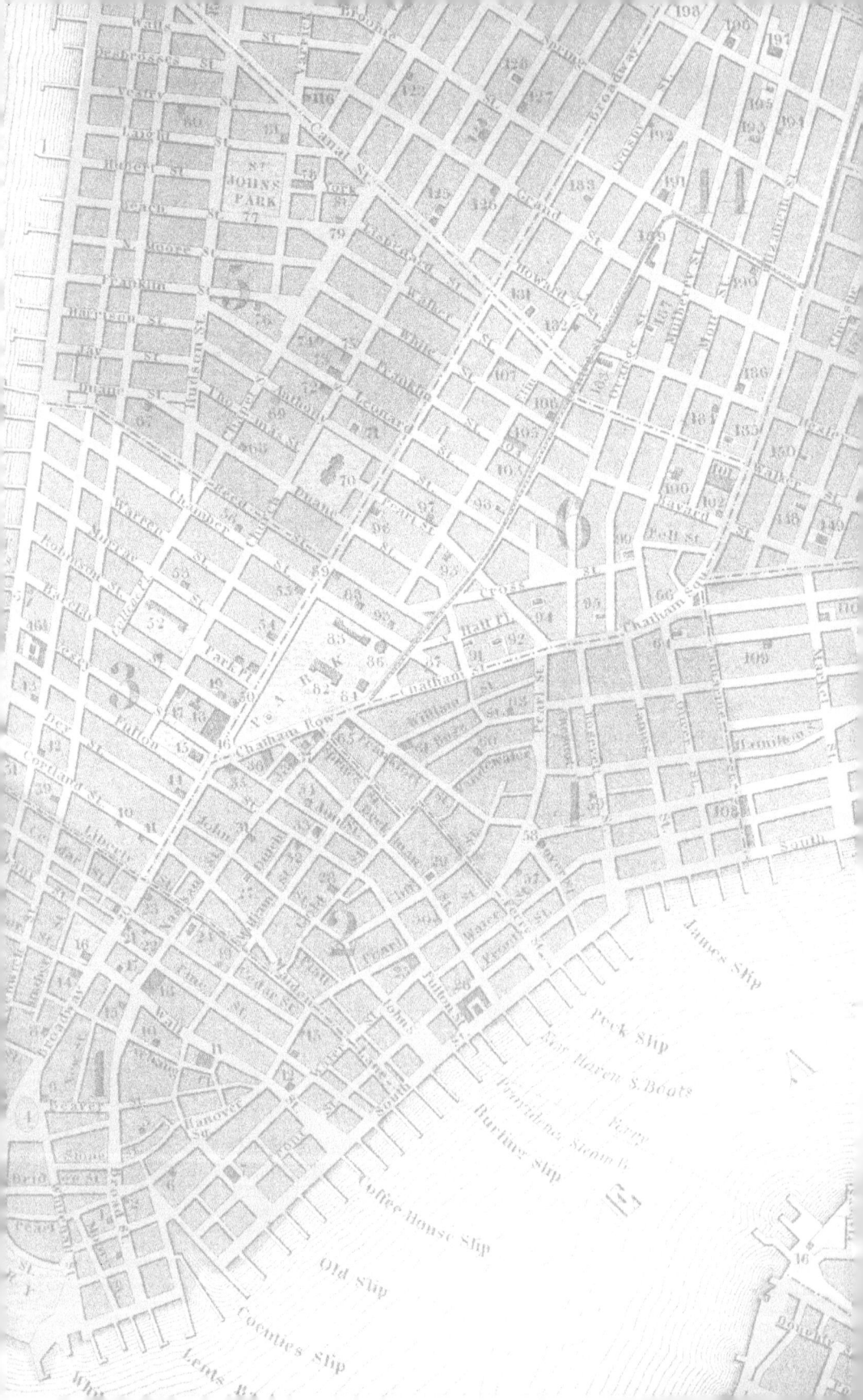

IRISH FEVER

An Archaeology of
Illness, Injury, and Healing
in New York City, 1845–1875

MEREDITH B. LINN

The University of Tennessee Press / Knoxville
and the Society for Historical Archaeology

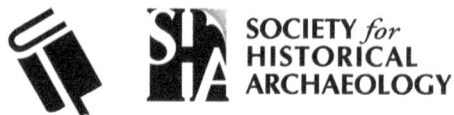

SOCIETY for HISTORICAL ARCHAEOLOGY

Copyright © 2024 by the Society for Historical Archaeology.
All Rights Reserved. Manufactured in the United States of America.
First Edition.

Library of Congress Cataloging-in-Publication Data

Names: Linn, Meredith B., 1975- author.
Title: Irish fever : an archaeology of illness, injury, and healing in New York City, 1845–1875 / Meredith B. Linn.
Description: First edition. | Knoxville : The University of Tennessee Press; [United States] : Society for Historical Archaeology, 2024. | Includes bibliographical references and index. | Summary: "This book builds upon the myriad of cultural-resource studies mining historic New York City and its Irish immigrant communities. Meredith B. Linn engages a number of primary sources from working-class Irish immigrants, focusing on illness, injury, and health care in the third quarter of the nineteenth century. She presents a 'visceral historical archaeology' using interdisciplinary methods and theories to examine how these newcomers to the United States experienced and reacted to three ailments that arguably were their leading causes of mortality and morbidity: typhus, tuberculosis, and work-related injuries. Because of how physicians and the American public understood these conditions, typhus exacerbated the stereotype of the Irish as sanguine, hot-headed, and animalistic, while tuberculosis, or the 'white death,' instead helped to 'whiten' and re-humanize the Irish. In using these ailments as a lens, this study also presents new perspectives about urban labor, housing, community building, and consumption of commodities in a context of Irish diaspora"—Provided by publisher.
Identifiers: LCCN 2023039421 (print) | LCCN 2023039422 (ebook) | ISBN 9781621908456 (hardcover) | ISBN 9781621908463 (pdf) | ISBN 9781621908913 (kindle edition)
Subjects: LCSH: Irish Americans—Health and hygiene—New York (State)—New York—History—19th century. | Irish Americans—New York (State)—New York—Social conditions—19th century. | Immigrants—Health and hygiene—New York (State)—New York—History—19th century. | Typhus fever—New York (State)—New York—History—19th century. | Tuberculosis—New York (State)—New York—History—19th century.
Classification: LCC RA448.5.I44 L56 2023 (print) | LCC RA448.5.I44 (ebook) | DDC 614/.30891620747—dc23/eng/20230925
LC record available at https://lccn.loc.gov/2023039421
LC ebook record available at https://lccn.loc.gov/2023039422

For Charlotte

CONTENTS

Acknowledgments — xiii

Introduction. Toward a Visceral Historical Archaeology of Irish Immigrant Life — 1

Chapter 1. The Case of Huxley McGuire: Irish and American Ethnomedicine Collide in a New York City Boardinghouse — 21

Chapter 2. "Irish Fever": Typhus Fever and an Epidemic of Anti-Irish Prejudice — 56

Chapter 3. Irish Immigrant Perspectives of and Remedies for Typhus Fever — 96

Chapter 4. Fractures: Work, Injuries, and Irish Difference — 131

Chapter 5. Irish Remedies for Relief: Old and New Recipes — 181

Chapter 6. A Phthisical Paradox: Tuberculosis and the Beginnings of Irish Immigrant Incorporation — 232

Chapter 7. Consumption and Community among the New York Irish — 279

Conclusion. Looking Backward to Move Forward — 328

Notes — 339
References Cited — 389
Index — 457

ILLUSTRATIONS

Figures

FIGURE 0.1. Painting of "The Bay and Harbor of New York" by Samuel Bell Waugh, ca. 1855	5
FIGURE 0.2. Photograph of Irish Folklore Commission Collector Recording Irish Women, County Kerry, 1942	14
FIGURE 0.3. Map Showing the Five Points Intersection and Excavation Site	16
FIGURE 0.4. Photograph of Five Points Excavation in Progress	17
FIGURE 0.5. Map Showing the Distribution of Irish Language Speakers in 1851	18
FIGURE 1.1. Portion of Samuel Augustus Mitchell's 1850 Map, "The City of New York," Showing Lower Manhattan	24
FIGURE 1.2. Photograph of "Aran Boy on a Rock, Insihmaan, Co. Galway," ca. 1930	43
FIGURE 2.1. "Destruction of the Quarantine Buildings near Tompkinsville, Staten Island," *Frank Leslie's Illustrated Newspaper*, 1858	64
FIGURE 2.2. Caricature of Irish "Bog Trotters" Attributed to William Elmes, 1812	66
FIGURE 2.3. New York Hospital Viewed from Broadway by Artist George Hayward and Lithographer Thomas Wood, ca. 1845	84
FIGURE 2.4. Cartoon Depicting Stereotypical Female Irish Domestic Servant by Frederick Burr Opper, *Puck*, 1883	92

FIGURE 3.1. Interior of an Emigrant Ship, *Illustrated London News*, 1851 — 98
FIGURE 3.2. Illustration of the Five Points in 1859 — 108
FIGURE 3.3. Plan Showing Features Identified by Archaeologists at the Five Points Site — 109
FIGURE 3.4. Clay Tobacco Pipe Unearthed in Feature J, Five Points — 110
FIGURE 3.5. Graph Showing Composition of Glass Bottle Assemblages at 472 and 474 Pearl Street — 111
FIGURE 3.6. Illustration of a Five Points Saloon Titled "The Voting-Place," *Harper's Weekly*, 1858 — 114
FIGURE 3.7. Locations of Porterhouses and Liquor Stores Near Five Points, ca. 1853 — 116
FIGURE 3.8. Graph Showing Types of Alcohol Bottles Found in Deposits at 472 and 474 Pearl Street — 118
FIGURE 3.9. Examples of 19th-Century Green Glass Bottles Used to Contain Wine and Champagne — 122
FIGURE 3.10. Photograph of Interior of House of M. Breathnach, Maam Cross, County Galway, 1935 — 124
FIGURE 4.1. Portion of Cartoon Titled "American Gold" Depicting Stereotypical Irish Laborers by Frederick Burr Opper, *Puck*, 1882 — 141
FIGURE 4.2. Early Photograph of Mill Worker at Jerpoint, County Kilkenny, ca. 1860 — 153
FIGURE 4.3. Sketch of a Ward in the New York Hospital, ca. 1871 — 157
FIGURE 4.4. Photograph of Women Scrubbing the Entry to City Home, Blackwell's Island, ca. 1895–1905 — 165
FIGURE 4.5. Advertisement for Pomeroy's "Wire Spring Truss" and "Elastic Rupture Belt," Two Braces for Supporting Hernias, *Harper's Weekly*, 1872 — 167
FIGURE 4.6. Daguerreotype Titled "Use of Ether for Anesthesia" by Albert Sands Southworth and Josiah Johnson Hawes, 1847 — 171
FIGURE 4.7. Illustration of St. Vincent's Hospital on the Corner of Eleventh Street and Seventh Avenue, ca. 1856–1870 — 178

FIGURE 5.1. Illustration of "St. Bridget's Chair" natural rock formation, 1840 — 186
FIGURE 5.2. Photograph of Common Chickweed Plant — 193
FIGURE 5.3. Nineteenth-Century Trade Card for Mexican Mustang Liniment — 199
FIGURE 5.4. Metal Syringes Discovered at the Five Points — 212
FIGURE 5.5. Advertisement for Radway's Ready Relief and Bottle of Radway's Unearthed from Feature O, Five Points — 216
FIGURE 5.6. Advertisement for Hyatt's Life Balsam, *New York Times* 1863 — 218
FIGURE 5.7. Lithograph Titled "Mose, Lize & Little Mose Going to California" by Henry R. Robinson, ca. 1849 — 227
FIGURE 5.8. Cartoon of a Young Irish Immigrant Conversing with an Older Irish Immigrant, *Harper's Weekly*, 1867 — 230
FIGURE 6.1. Typographic Facsimile of James McPeake's Obituary, *Irish American Weekly*, 1857 — 233
FIGURE 6.2. Plan of the Dispensary Districts of New York City in 1856 — 237
FIGURE 6.3. Graph of Patients Admitted to New York Hospital with Phthisis 1835 to 1865 — 238
FIGURE 6.4. Illustration of the New York Dispensary, 1860 — 240
FIGURE 6.5. A Section of the Perris Map of 1853 — 244
FIGURE 6.6. "A Saturday Night Scene in the Bowery, New York," *Harper's Weekly*, 1871 — 249
FIGURE 6.7. Illustration Titled "An Irish Wake—From a sketch by M. Woolf," *Harper's Weekly*, 1873 — 257
FIGURE 6.8. Map Showing Consumption Mortality by County in Ireland in 1840 — 265
FIGURE 6.9. Illustration Titled "He Giveth His Beloved Sleep," *Harper's Weekly*, 1868 — 273
FIGURE 6.10. Cartoon Titled "The Mortar of Assimilation—and the One Element That Won't Mix" by Charles Jay Taylor, *Puck*, 1889 — 276
FIGURE 7.1. "The Fairy Doctor" by E. Fitzpatrick, *Illustrated London News*, 1859 — 283
FIGURE 7.2. Cartoon Titled "What's Next," *Harper's Weekly*, 1874 — 295

FIGURE 7.3. Advertisement for J. R. Stafford's Olive Tar, *Harper's Weekly*, 1867 and J. R. Stafford's Olive Tar Bottle Recovered from Feature J, Five Points   299

FIGURE 7.4. Photograph of of Soda Water Bottles from Feature J, Five Points   306

FIGURE 7.5. Illustration of a Soda Water Fountain, *Harper's New Monthly Magazine*, 1872   308

FIGURE 7.6. Etching of Patron's Day at Ronogue's Well Near Cork by Daniel Maclise, 1836   311

FIGURE 7.7. Clarke & White Mineral Water Bottle, ca. 1856 to 1866   316

FIGURE C.1. Cartoon Titled "Looking Backward" by Joseph Keppler, *Puck*, 1893   338

Tables

TABLE 1.1. Associations of Humors, Qualities, and Illnesses	27
TABLE 2.1. Humoral Temperaments and Their Associations	73
TABLE 2.2. Percentage of Deaths of Typhus Fever Patients at New York Hospital (1845–1852)	89
TABLE 4.1. Percentage of Patients Admitted to New York Hospital for the Listed Ailments Who Were Irish Born (1845–1852)	147
TABLE 4.2. Sample of Work-Related Injuries among Irish Immigrants at New York City Hospitals (1847–1874)	149
TABLE 5.1. Patent Medicine Containers: Numbers, Types, and Brands Identified at the Five Points, Paterson, and Greenwich Village—in Irish, German, and American Contexts	203
TABLE 5.2. Full Names of Patent Medicine and Cosmetic Brands Referenced in TABLE 5.1	206

ACKNOWLEDGMENTS

THIS BOOK was a very long time in the making and possible only because of the assistance of many people—advisors, fellow scholars, archivists, family, and friends. First and foremost, I thank Nan A. Rothschild, my dissertation advisor, teacher, mentor, and friend. It was upon her suggestion that I first looked into the Five Points site, when I was searching for a research paper topic for a course she co-taught with Diana diZerega Wall during my first year of doctoral studies. Nan has supported me and the development of this project from its origin in that paper through conference presentations, the dissertation, journal articles, and drafts of this book. Her steadfast encouragement, willingness to read draft after draft, unrivaled ability to see the larger view, sound advice, and endless energy and generosity have been a constant source of help and inspiration, without which I could not have written this book and would not have become the scholar and teacher I am today. I cannot thank Nan enough.

I am also deeply grateful to Diana diZerega Wall for her unwavering support since that first historical archaeology course. Soon afterwards, Diana invited me to be a part of her weekly archaeology lab day at City College. Analyzing artifacts and conversing with Diana, Arnold Pickman, and the group of graduate students who regularly met there—Felipe Gaitan-Ammann, Jessica Striebel MacLean, and Lizzie Martin—greatly influenced how I interpret archaeological remains and reports. Diana has also always been willing to share her expert knowledge and advice on drafts of this project, as well as kind words of encouragement, especially when they were most needed. It is an ongoing honor and privilege to work with Nan and Diana on the Seneca Village Project, investigating the 19th-century majority African American and minority Irish community of Seneca Village for the past many years. Investigating and writing about Seneca Village with both of them has made me a better thinker and writer, which I hope is reflected in this book.

I am also very appreciative of other Columbia University faculty members who were on my dissertation committee along with Nan and Diana: Lesley Sharp, Lynn Meskell, and Elizabeth Blackmar. Lesley introduced me to medical anthropology and inspired my great interest in the discipline; I am grateful for her insightful comments on my dissertation chapters. Lynn's classes about objects and materiality were formative in my approach to thinking about and studying objects. Elizabeth's publications about the social history of New York City remain an inspiration. I also thank Terry D'Altroy and Robert Scally (of New York University) who provided thoughtful suggestions in the early phases of the project. My graduate work was funded by a Columbia University Graduate Fellowship, and much of my initial archival research was made possible by the Sheldon Scheps Memorial Fellowship for Summer Research and the Robert Stigler Fund for Archaeological Fieldwork. I am thankful for this essential early financial support.

Archivists at a number of institutions aided me as I conducted research and kindly shared their expert advice about relevant sources. I wish to extend special thanks to Steven Novak at Columbia University's Health Sciences Library; James Gehrlich and Elizabeth Shepard at the Weill Cornell Medicine Medical Center Archives; Sisters Rita King and Constance Brennan at the Archives of the Sisters of Charity at Mount St. Vincent; Colleen Bradley-Sanders at New York University's Medical Archives; James Leach at St. Vincent's Hospital Archives; Joseph Coen at the Archives of the Archdiocese of Brooklyn; Mary Cargill at Columbia University's Butler Library; Emer Ní Cheallaigh and Jonny Dillon at the National Folklore Collection, University College Dublin; Marie Boran at the James Hardiman Library, the National University of Ireland in Galway; and Mary O'Doherty at the Mercer Library, Royal College of Surgeons in Ireland. I also greatly appreciate the assistance offered to me by the staff at the National Library of Ireland, the Manuscripts Reading Room at Trinity College in Dublin, the New-York Historical Society Library, the New York Public Library, and the Rare Book and Manuscript Library at Columbia University.

Several scholars shared important ideas and resources with me that were essential for completing this project; I am so thankful for their generosity. Barbara Ní Fhloinn and Crístóir Mac Cárthaigh from the Department of Irish, Celtic Studies, and Folklore at University College Dublin helped me to decipher some unfamiliar Irish folk practices and made invaluable suggestions about sources for the study of Irish folk medicine and fairy lore. Adrian Praetzellis and Jack McIlroy shared information about and images from their excavations of Irish households in San Francisco. Rebecca Yamin mailed me a copy of her multi-volume site report of the Dublin Neighborhood of Paterson, NJ and donated photographic slides of the Five Points excavation and associated artifacts to the New York City Archaeological Repository, where they are now available to researchers. Diana diZerega Wall shared notes she took about the Five Points archaeological collection before it was destroyed on September 11, 2001.

The 2010 Society for Historical Archaeology (SHA) Dissertation Award aided the long transformation of this project from dissertation to book. For the support from the SHA, including advice from Terry Majewski, Annalies Corbin, and Ben Ford and their assistance securing University of Tennessee Press as the publisher, I am most appreciative. I am also extremely grateful to the University of Tennessee Press, especially to editor Thomas Wells for his patience and excellent counsel, Mary Ann Simek for her expert copy editing, Linsey Perry for her marketing assistance, Jon Boggs for his help with page proofs, and the book design team for making the book look so beautiful. Thank you also to Joe Pellrine for making the index so quickly.

Peter Miller, former dean of Bard Graduate Center, suggested and sponsored convening a group of scholars to informally review my book manuscript. For this and his support of my work at BGC, I am very grateful. That group—Jeffrey Collins, Kevin Kenny, Cian McMahon, Matt Reilly, and Nan Rothschild—gave me crucial feedback and guidance for final revisions. This book is much improved because of their counsel. I am especially appreciative of Kevin's and Cian's important comments, which they so generously offered to someone outside of their field. Jeffrey's writing advice was also invaluable, and his writing skills are an inspiration. Stephen Brighton reviewed the subsequent draft of the manuscript for University of Tennessee Press, and I cannot adequately express how truly I appreciate his helpful and positive review.

Many other brilliant friends and colleagues also offered important suggestions and encouragement on portions of this project at various stages of development, including Heather Atherton, Gergely Baics, Kelly Britt, Hannah Chazin, Zoe Crossland, Christopher Fennell, Severin Fowles, Felipe Gaitan-Ammann, Diane George, Erin Hasinoff, Bernice Kurchin, Jessica Striebel MacLean, Lizzie Martin, Elizabeth Meade, and Lindsay Weiss. I am very thankful for their help and honored to know so many talented and kind people. Likewise, it is my ongoing pleasure to be a member of the faculty of Bard Graduate Center (BGC) and to be surrounded and supported by so many exceptional scholars and students. I extend special thanks to BGC's founder and director, Susan Weber, for her support of me and the institution and to doctoral student Michael Assis, who assisted in the preparation of the references cited section.

Last, but principally, without the consistent support and endurance of my family, who had almost given up asking me when the book would be finished, I could have neither started nor completed this project. Thank you, Mom, Dad, Graig, Uncle Greg, Mom and Dad J, and especially Matt and Charlotte, for teaching me so much, putting up with my book-related absences, and always having faith in me.

INTRODUCTION

Toward a Visceral Historical Archaeology of Irish Immigrant Life

AFTER ENDURING nearly a month of constant seasickness, sixteen-year-old Mary MacLean was thankful to finally step onto solid ground. In May of 1832, Mary and her parents and siblings landed in Quebec City, far from County Leitrim in Ireland where they had begun their journey (MacLean [1886–1900]). Mary's family, like the hundreds of thousands of Irish before them and the millions after, courageously left their home and crossed the Atlantic Ocean seeking to build an adequate life. This modest aspiration was no longer possible for them in Ireland. In the 1830s, the mechanization of the linen industry had ravaged the local economy in Leitrim, leaving families like Mary's with few options (Kenny 1998:27–28). Other Irish families had different reasons for emigration, including eviction resulting from the consolidation of farmland; periodic food shortages and, later, the Great Famine; and political and religious oppression propagated by the British government and colonial settlers. For much of the 19th century, Irish people departed their homeland in vast numbers and encountered previously unimagined challenges to body, spirit, and community.

In a document she wrote more than half a century later, for example, Mary explained how her initial joy at having finally arrived in the New World was short-lived. Painful experiences soon followed that were permanently etched into her memory and that irrevocably changed her family's plans. The morning after her arrival in Quebec, Mary became critically ill. She had been struck down by cholera, a deadly and misunderstood epidemic disease, which had just arrived in North America for the first time. The ship captain took Mary to a makeshift hospital on the edge of town, past city dwellers holding burning tar on sticks between their teeth for protection, reminiscent of medieval efforts to drive away the Black Death.[1] Within a few days, three of her siblings followed her to the hospital (MacLean [1886–1900]). There, along with hundreds of others, Mary "suffer[ed] indescribable torments from the deadly cramps of Asiatic cholera." It was a dreadful place, "a veritable house of torture; where the most appalling shrieks, groans, prayers, and curses filled the air continually, and as if, in answer to this day and night, from the sheds outside came the tap tap tap of the workmen's hammers as they drove the nails into the rough coffins, which could not be put together hastily enough" (MacLean [1886–1900]).

Mary's physicians applied the latest medical knowledge and prescribed a diet of "brandy and water, lemon juice and water without sugar and very thin gruel without salt. . . . None of these satisfied [her]," however, "for [her] bed was near a window, through which could be seen a well and this sent [her] dreaming." She persuaded an Irish nurse to get her a glass of plain water and some broth. When physicians discovered that "someone had tampered with her," they were furious. Mary, nevertheless, recovered and refused to incriminate her nurse. "The nurse, a big jolly Irishwoman[,] declared, when we were alone, that I was a 'little brick' and that she was proud of her countrywoman" for surviving the disease and the doctors' interrogation (MacLean [1886–1900]). Her siblings were not as fortunate.

The particulars of Mary's account are unique, but elements of her experience have been shared by many immigrants around the globe, namely suffering significant illness and/or injury that brought them into contact, and often conflict, with physicians and other locals and altered their plans for a better life. This book is about how these issues affected Mary MacLean's countrymen and women, focusing on those who began to arrive in New York City about a decade and a half later, fleeing the Great Famine in Ireland (1845 to 1852), and their lives in New York City into the 1870s.

This book explores the effects of three kinds of afflictions—typhus fever, injuries, and tuberculosis—that disproportionately affected Irish immigrants. It traces how the medical ideas of the era, combined with preexisting prejudice, led many native-born Americans to have strongly negative visceral responses to this culturally distinct and largely impoverished group, which further added to their struggles.² More specifically, I argue that in the 1840s and 1850s, many native-born Americans read high incidence of typhus fever and injuries among Irish immigrants, as well as their symptoms and scars upon Irish bodies, as evidence supporting tropes of Irish incivility and poverty, bolstering claims of natural differences between the Irish and the English (and Anglo-Americans). These interpretations of medical conditions contributed to essentializing and dehumanizing views of the Irish as a group of lesser humans who were suited to manual labor. Beginning in the mid-1850s, tuberculosis skyrocketed among Irish immigrants, threatening to further intensify anti-Irish prejudice. Surprisingly, it did not, and instead, appears to have contributed to softening views of the Irish, even while it ravaged Irish immigrant communities. I suggest that the ways Americans understood tuberculosis at this moment before the discovery of the germ theory encouraged them to recognize the equal humanity of Irish individuals who suffered from this terrible illness. This book thus illustrates how etiological theories and social meanings of particular ailments at specific points in time have deeply affected the reception of immigrants to the U.S. Core ideas about the body and health had tremendous authority because of their presumed natural origins, stability, and perceptible signs, despite the reality that ideas and interpretations varied by culture and changed over time.

This book does not focus solely upon the perspectives of native-born Americans, however. It also investigates how Irish newcomers themselves experienced and responded to illness, injury, and prejudice. Drawing upon archaeological and folkloric sources, as well as documents, this study focuses primarily upon working-class Irish immigrants, who are underrepresented in textual sources. It examines how they suffered from these ailments but also resourcefully utilized healing strategies from both their old and new homes to build and sustain their families and communities. In viewing mid-19th-century working-class Irish immigrant life in New York City through the lens of health and employing a combination of novel sources, this book excavates previously unexplored aspects of experience and agency that were significant for individuals and communities and that had lasting impacts on American society and culture.

Illness, Injury, and Irish Immigration to New York City

Just over a decade after the departure of Mary MacLean's family, emigration from Ireland dramatically increased as a result of the Great Famine (*An Gorta Mór*) (1845 to 1852), a watershed event in Irish and global history.[3] Also known as the Irish Potato Famine and the Great Hunger, the famine resulted from a devastating multi-year potato blight combined with mismanagement of the country's resources and centuries of economic and social oppression of Roman Catholics and nonconforming Protestants.[4] About a million people perished from starvation and disease, while approximately 2.1 million, nearly a quarter of the pre-famine population of Ireland, were forced to emigrate.[5] "An entire generation virtually disappeared from the land" (Miller 1985:291). The Great Famine and other chapters in the longer history of the Irish diaspora scattered Irish-born people throughout the globe, but chiefly to Canada, England, Australia, and the U.S., especially (Kenny 2003; McMahon 2015a).[6] Between the years of 1847 and 1851 alone, nearly 850,000 Irish men, women, and children disembarked in New York City, which by the 1830s had become the U.S.'s preeminent immigrant port (Figure 0.1). New York City became "the most Irish city in the Union" as it became the "Empire City," the nation's most commercial and cosmopolitan urban center. By 1860, 25% of the city's population had been born in Ireland, and by 1880 more than 33% of New Yorkers had been born in Ireland or were of Irish parentage (Diner 1996:87, 91, 93, 94).

Despite the large number who settled in and greatly contributed to New York City, famine-era Irish immigrants encountered tremendous difficulties—physical, emotional, social, economic, and political—including anti-Irish prejudice that reached a fever pitch during the 1840s and 1850s. Historians of medicine have noted that Irish immigrants experienced a great deal of illness and injury and that Americans stigmatized them as carriers of disease, but they have not fully examined how perceptions of these immigrants' bodies profoundly influenced their encounters with Americans, nor immigrants' own health-related ideas, experiences, practices, and decisions (Ernst 1949; Rosenberg 1987a; Kraut 1994, 1995, 1996). Historians of the Irish in the U.S., meanwhile, have produced wonderfully rich studies

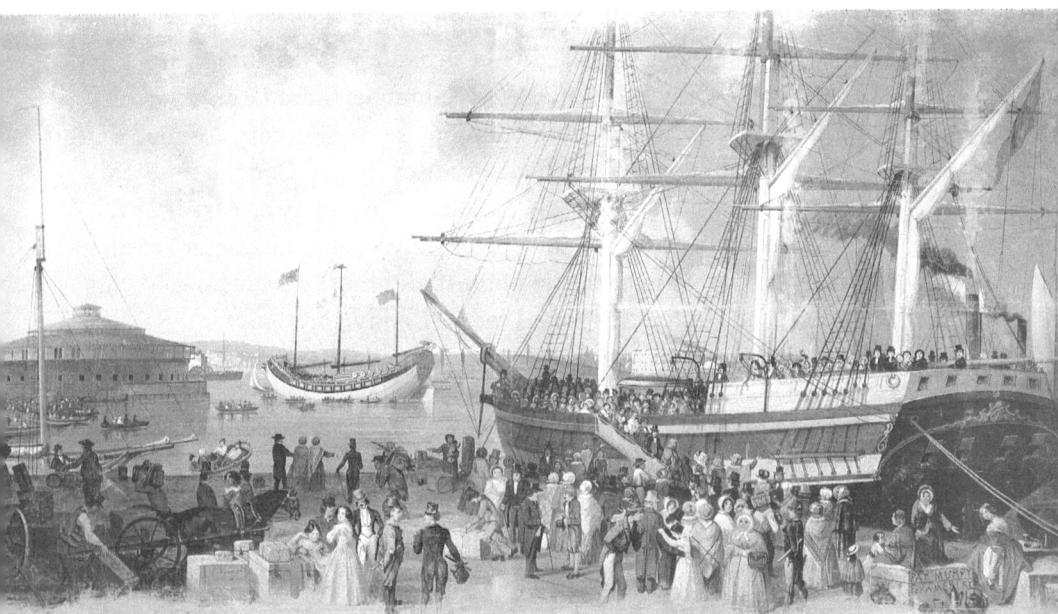

FIGURE 0.1. "The Bay and Harbor of New York" (ca. 1855) by Samuel Bell Waugh. This oil painting shows Irish immigrants disembarking from a crowded immigrant ship at the Port of New York in 1847. Castle Garden, which became the U.S.'s first official immigration center in 1855, is the round structure in the background. Courtesy of the Museum of the City of New York, Gift of Mrs. Robert M. Littlejohn, 1933. 33.169.1.

of a variety of Irish experiences in the U.S., and in New York City especially, but the impacts of illness and injury have not yet been a major focus (Miller 1985; Knobel 1986, 2001; Bayor and Meagher 1996; Kenny 2000; Kelly 2005; Lee and Casey 2007; Barrett 2012). Historians have detailed the important differences in class, culture, religion, and skills that made it more difficult for the famine Irish, especially those who settled in urban areas, to adapt to life in America than immigrants from some other locations and other Irish who arrived before them. A greater number of the earlier Irish arrivals had been skilled Protestant English speakers from more Anglicized and urbanized northern and eastern regions of Ulster and Leinster. In contrast, the vast majority of famine-era arrivals were small or tenant farmers and laborers from rural areas, although some middling farmers, craftsmen, and small entrepreneurs some with origins in urban areas (including Ireland's two largest, Dublin and Belfast) were among them (Anbinder et al. 2019a:1607). At least half of the famine-era immigrants originated in the western and southern regions of Munster and Connaught, nearly nine-tenths were Catholic, and about a quarter were Irish speakers. "The Famine exodus had a decidedly Gaelic character" (Miller 1985:297). They were also "the poorest and most disadvantaged [immigrants] the United States had seen" (Kenny 2006:367).

Historians have shown that many native-born Americans were concerned that this group's foreign ways, especially their Catholicism and supposed blind loyalty to priests and the Pope, were dangers to the nation; how they feared that Irish immigrants' supposed lack of skills, capital, ambition, and self-discipline would mire them in perpetual poverty and dependency upon public support; and how they condemned collective violence and violent Irish nationalism in which some Irish immigrants engaged. Some Americans believed these qualities were shared by virtually all Irish newcomers, and thus the Irish as a people were unfit for full U.S. citizenship. Many historians have also noted that the haggard appearances of famine-era immigrants upon arrival did not make a favorable impression. The conditions of poor Irish men, women, and children, whose emigration was aided by landlords and poorhouses, had an outsized impact on Americans' views of all Irish famine refugees. "Witnesses in North America frequently described all Famine emigrants as the dregs of humanity" with "universally wretched appearances" (Miller 1985:293; Knobel 1986, 2001; Kenny 2006; Hirota 2017). This book augments previous studies by delving more deeply into the physical experiences and appearances of Irish immigrants of this period and showing how gut-level—or visceral—reactions and prevailing medical ideas both affected native-born New Yorkers' reception of these newcomers, which, in turn, further shaped immigrants' lives.

A variety of documentary sources suggest that there was some truth to some observers' descriptions. Many famine-era Irish arrived in New York in terrible condition after the ordeals of their passage, exhibiting some combination of illness, undernourishment, and inadequate or unfashionable clothing, despite reported efforts to spruce themselves up for arrival (McMahon 2021:196). More than a few were traumatized, and an unknown number were permanently injured by physical or mental disabilities caused by famine-related malnutrition, disease, anguish, and/or shipboard incidents (see Chapter 2). The Irish writer and politician John Francis Maguire (1868:181), who traveled through the U.S. collecting information about Irish immigrants, asserted that "it was no unusual occurrence for the survivor of a family of ten or twelve to land alone, bewildered and broken-hearted, on the wharf at New York; the rest—the family— parents and children, had been swallowed in the sea."

Most immigrants' travails did not end once they stepped foot onto American soil. A variety of sources, including hospital, dispensary, and city mortality records, attest that Irish immigrants of this period experienced much higher rates of illness, injury, and death than other immigrant groups and native-born Americans (Kraut 1996:159; see also Chapters 2, 4, and 6). This immense suffering left visible marks on Irish bodies and was, of course, recognized by Irish immigrants themselves. In a letter published in the *Cork Examiner*, for example, one remarked: it was a "well established fact" that "the average length of life of the [Irish] emigrant after landing here is six years; and many insist it is much less" (Miller 1985:319). Poverty, famine, and oppression in their homeland, difficult immigration journeys, and then dangerous jobs and miserable living conditions in places of resettlement were all factors that from a present-day perspective caused famine-era Irish immigrants to experience disproportionate rates of illness, injury, and death. The timing of their arrival also coincided with a period in which New York City was rapidly expanding and struggling with poor sanitation, deteriorating housing, and recurrent outbreaks of a variety of epidemic and endemic diseases (Rosner 1995). Both the public and physicians in New York were aware of these homegrown problems and of the emigration difficulties Irish immigrants had experienced. Nevertheless, many blamed immigrants, and Irish immigrants especially, for exacerbating conditions by bringing disease and unhealthy, foreign practices to American shores that mired them in poverty and encouraged dependency on public charity (Kraut 1994, 1995, 1996; Hirota 2017). Personal and public health were high on the list of New Yorkers' concerns and were intertwined with their economic, religious, and nationalist apprehensions of Irish immigrants.

Thus, although some New Yorkers responded to the poor conditions of these newcomers with sympathy and generosity, many others—including some physicians, scientists, reformers, labor leaders, and politicians—expressed fear and animosity. In addition to quarantine, restricting immigration, and even deportation, a proposed cure was to "Americanize" the Irish, to encourage greater self-sufficiency, thriftiness, restrained behavior, etc. Many hoped this could be quickly accomplished by the positive influences of democracy, the natural environment of North America, and the guidance of native-born, and largely Protestant, reformers. Local Catholic leadership and some Irish-born elites also encouraged acculturation. The continued suffering of many famine-era Irish immigrants for years after their arrival as well as the reluctance of many to abandon Irish cultural practices alarmed critics, however. To them, these patterns attested to the inability or unwillingness of the Irish to assimilate. In this context, illness and injury among Irish immigrants did not just affect Irish individuals personally; they were also social liabilities that exacerbated prejudice against nearly all Irish-born people and thus could have drastic effects upon their abilities to gain good jobs and housing, to get equal treatment in hospitals, and to form relationships and alliances with other New Yorkers. Illness and injury deeply affected Irish immigrant life in the U.S. in multiple and complicated ways that require closer examination.

This book is a first step in that direction. It investigates how Irish newcomers to New York City experienced three leading causes of mortality and morbidity during the from the mid-1840s through the early 1870s: epidemic typhus fever, work-related injuries, and tuberculosis. It also probes how American physicians and the American public understood illness and health in ways quite different from today. The third quarter of the 19th century was a critical period in the development of modern medicine, before the acceptance of the germ theory of disease. Depending on the particular symptoms, medical practitioner, and moment in time, illnesses were usually understood to be caused by divine punishment, "bad air" (miasma), poisoned blood, or vague forms of human-to-human contagion, in combination with individuals' underlying temperament, formed by the relative balance of bodily humors. Centuries-old ideas about humoralism underlay explanations for illness, and they informed new "scientific" ideas about the nature of human variation.

As I will detail in Chapter 2, understanding these 19th-century views about bodies helps to explain why Americans associated typhus fever, a disease common on ships transporting immigrants from many places, with Irish immigrants particularly. So strong was the connection that in 1847 health officials referred to the disease as the "Irish fever" (Scally 1995:206; Hardy 1988:405; Gallman 2000:87; Darwen et al. 2020). The classic symptoms of typhus fever—high body temperature, delirium, and red rash—displayed by afflicted Irish immigrants were interpreted as confirming their sanguine humoral temperament, which was construed as different and lesser than the supposed phlegmatic temperament of the English, the Germans, and Americans of English descent. The supposed prevalence of the sanguine temperament among the Irish bolstered negative stereotypes inherited from the British and subsequently amplified in the U.S., often in dehumanizing and/or racializing terms.

In the months and years after their arrival, Irish immigrants sustained injuries, such as fractures, burns, wounds, and sunstroke, at much higher rates than non-Irish-born New Yorkers. These injuries caused many individuals and families to experience extreme financial hardship. Scars from injuries and robust muscle development from hard work also marked them as manual laborers. In Chapter 4, I contend that New Yorkers interpreted these bodily features as evidence that Irish immigrants were naturally suitable for work requiring brawn and unsuitable for work requiring brains.

Beginning in the 1850s, tuberculosis afflicted Irish immigrants in New York City at epidemic levels, but New Yorkers did not similarly stigmatize the Irish as naturally susceptible to this disease. Instead, as I suggest in Chapter 6, tuberculosis among the Irish, and especially among their American-born children, often elicited sympathy and recognition of shared humanity, in part because many native-born Americans and their loved ones suffered from this disease. At the time, many Americans understood tuberculosis to be a hereditary illness affecting sensitive individuals, especially those with phlegmatic temperaments. The classic symptoms of pulmonary tuberculosis—fatigue, pallor, and emaciation—produced bodies with appearances that did not conform to Irish stereotypes. Over several decades, prevailing views of Irish immigrants in the U.S. improved. As many historians have shown, this was a slow process that involved many factors.[7] In Chapters 6 and 7, I propose that tuberculosis was one of them.

This book is innovative in combining evidence from archaeological excavations and folklore/oral histories with documents to uncover previously unknown or underexamined Irish immigrant reactions and agency with regard to health. Together, these sources indicate that Irish immigrants in New York City attempted to maintain health and treat ailments at home with popular Irish remedies and English and American patent medicines and soda water; they sought care from healers and medical practitioners and institutions of many kinds; and they altered their appearances via clothing, cosmetics, and braces. Some became healers, nurses, physicians, or pharmacists themselves, and Irish Catholic elites even established their own hospital, St. Vincent's. This study thus also presents new insights about Irish involvement in urban healthcare institutions, consumption of commodities, and community building, issues critical to the study of the modern city (see Chapters 3, 5, and 7).

As the Irish were the first large wave of immigrants to New York City who were perceived to be foreign, their interactions with New Yorkers set precedents for subsequent immigrant groups. New York City "was a historical stage writ large for encounters that reverberated across the rest of the nation" (Stansell 1986:xiv). Many policies the city put into place later shaped federal immigration policy, for example (Fairchild 2003:14; Hirota 2017). Meanwhile, medical advances developed in the city's hospitals—many of which were pioneered on the bodies of Irish immigrants, in institutions founded and run by Irish immigrants, and/or by Irish physicians and nurses—spread throughout the country (Walsh 1965; Larrabee 1971; Leitman 1991).

This book thus presents ideas that are relevant to American history, as well as to the history of medicine and the histories of other immigrant groups. Compared with native-born Americans, immigrants to the U.S. historically have suffered disproportionately from illness and injury for many of the same reasons as the famine-era Irish, although the particulars of each case are unique. Stigmatizing newcomers as dirty and diseased is an age-old trope that insiders have repeatedly used to mark outsiders as different and lesser (Douglas 1966). Since at least the 19th century, native-born Americans have linked specific groups to particular diseases. In addition to connecting the Irish to typhus fever, for example, Americans have branded Jews as tubercular, Italians as carriers of polio, the Chinese as spreaders of bubonic plague, Haitians as transmitters of HIV, and most recently, in the 21st century, the Chinese as vectors of COVID-19 (Farmer 1993; Kraut 1994, 1995). As this study will explore in the case of the famine-era Irish, these linkages arose not only because of the timing of disease outbreaks and the groups' arrivals but also because of Americans' beliefs in a causal connection between the particular pathology and a group's practices and/or physical appearance. These perceived correspondences were based on then-current medical ideas, which were (and still are) unstable and influenced by social and cultural prejudices. Not surprisingly, these ideas often conflicted with immigrant groups' own understandings of illness and healing, which each group brought to the U.S. Newcomers have not and do not discard fundamental conceptions about their bodies and practices of healing when they cross into U.S. territory. Such practices have often brought significant positive health impacts and some, such as acupuncture, have been widely embraced by a broader American public (Chavez 2003).

A Visceral Historical Archaeology: Approach and Sources

In Mary MacLean's recounting of her experience in a Quebec hospital, she noted that she saw a well outside her window and then persuaded a nurse to bring her a cup of water. The way Mary noted that the well "sent [her] dreaming" hints that her reaction was more complex than a simple desire for a drink. In Ireland, wells were and still are special places, associated with healing and pilgrimage, as well as more ordinary activities (see Chapter 7). Making Irish immigrants' accounts and experiences central, focusing on material and sensory conditions and "gut-level" reactions, and trying to read evidence from 19th-century Irish cultural perspectives are elements critical to the approach of this study, a visceral historical archaeology.

By this term, I mean a perspective that is rooted first and foremost in historical archaeology and medical anthropology. Historical archaeology is a multidisciplinary field that investigates the history of the modern world primarily using material remains—usually from archaeological excavations—and written records (Majewski and Gaimster 2009:xvii–xx; Hall and Silliman 2006:1–2; Orser 1996:17, 23–28). Historical archaeologists are not limited to these sources, however, and draw upon oral histories, ethnographic comparisons, museum collections, and any other relevant evidence, as well as method and theory from anthropology, sociology, and history, among other fields. We are omnivorous in our approach to investigating the past. Material remains are still critical to our studies, however, because they are tangible traces of people's activities and the real things they used to construct their lives and identities. They can shed light on lives of people not well represented in written records and prompt us, in our own sensory engagement with them, to ask different questions than those provoked by documents or other sources (Wilkie 2009). Several recent historical archaeological projects have successfully complicated dominant narratives, based largely on written records, of life in working-class neighborhoods, including New York City's Five Points, Sydney's Rocks, Melbourne's Little Lon, and San Francisco's Chinatown (Greenwood 1996; Yamin 1998, 1999, 2000[1–6]; Reckner 2002; Mayne and Murray 2001; Praetzellis and Praetzellis 2004; Rothschild and Wall 2014). This study aims to expand upon this work, especially about the Five Points (see more below), a site which provides valuable evidence of Irish immigrant healing practices. I interpret the remains unearthed at the Five Points as well as documentary and folklore/oral history sources with methods and insights from medical anthropology.

Medical anthropology, an anthropological subfield that studies health, illness, injury, and healing within cultural and social contexts, is thus also central to my visceral approach. Medical anthropologists use interviews and participant observation to obtain a "thick" understanding of insiders' perspectives, their ethnomedical views and practices (Geertz 1973; Quinlan 2004; Singer et al. 2020). Although these ethnographic methods are not possible for this study, histories of medicine provide information about the perspectives and practices of professional physicians and medical scientists in 19th-century Ireland and the U.S. The perspectives of the Irish farmers, laborers, and artisans who composed the majority of famine-era immigrants to New York City are not well represented in these sources, however.[8] In order to discover their views and practices, I have mined immigrant letters and diaries as well as information collected by 19th- and early 20th-century folklorists and ethnographers, especially records housed in the Republic of Ireland's government-sponsored National Folklore Collection (NFC) (Figure 0.2).[9] From these sources, I compiled a database of approximately 3,500

Irish popular remedies and hundreds of statements relevant to health and healing.[10] I then analyzed them, borrowing the techniques of medical anthropologists and historians of medicine in looking for patterns to discern: how particular ailments were treated, which ailments were considered more serious than others and why, which ailments were considered to be related and why, how specific ailments were thought to originate and to be transmitted, the frequency with which particular cures were mentioned, variations in cures, consistency in cures over time and region, how and for which conditions certain healing substances were used, and the incorporation of new substances and approaches (Crandon-Malamud 1991; Duden 1991; Quinlan 2004). In Chapter 1, I present an overview of my resulting understanding of the major principles of 19th-century popular Irish medicine.[11]

I also call my approach "visceral" because it is attentive to unconscious or unexamined "gut-level" reactions. It incorporates a major principle of medical anthropology: health-related ideas and practices that appear to be natural, visceral responses are culturally constructed and intertwined with other cultural assumptions about the world. I have discovered how many mid-19th-century Irish immigrants reacted to illness and injury in New York City by turning to familiar remedies and explanations that were integral to their identities and cultural perspectives. Americans also initially reacted to sick Irish newcomers, judging them by their outward appearances, and resorting to customary American medical ideas about fever and unquestioned assumptions about Irish people. Medical anthropologists also appreciate how health-related issues are biosocial, in addition to cultural, and influenced by social, political, economic, and environmental contexts (Farmer 1993, 1996, 1999; Singer et al. 2020). This study investigates the biosocial aspects of Irish immigrants' experiences and examines these contexts in assessing their health-related strategies. Primary documents that inform my understanding of the differing—and often conflicting—views and practices of Irish immigrants and native-born Americans include mainstream New York City and Irish immigrant newspapers and magazines (both text and illustrations), a private physician's casebook (Townsend 1847), and case records and annual reports from several city hospitals and dispensaries (Bellevue Hospital, New York Hospital, St. Vincent's Hospital, the New York Dispensary, and the New York Orthopaedic Hospital and Dispensary). These and other

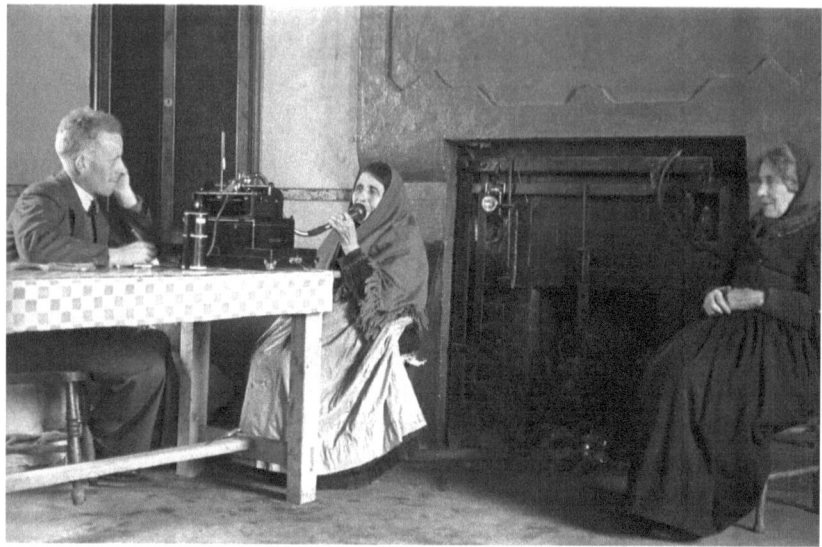

FIGURE 0.2. Photograph of Irish Folklore Commission collector Seosamh Ó Dálaigh recording information from Máire and Cáit Ruiséal on an Ediphone in Dunquin, County Kerry, in 1942 (National Folklore Collection 1942). Courtesy of the School of Irish, Celtic Studies, Irish Folklore and Linguistics, University College Dublin and the National Folklore Collection.

sources, such as censuses and maps, are also important for reconstructing the city's health-related landscape and the material conditions of Irish immigrants' lives.

Like medical anthropologists, in my visceral approach to interpreting these written records and archaeological materials, I pay close attention to sensory details and material qualities that provide insight into embodied experiences.[12] Material qualities of healing substances are important. As medical anthropologists Sjaak van der Geest, Susan Reynolds Whyte, and Anita Hardon (1996:154) explain, medicines are powerful because of "their concreteness. Their 'thingness' provides patients and healers with a means to deal with the problem at hand." How the "thingness" of healing substances was interpreted from the different perspectives of Irish immigrants and native-born Americans is a major concern of this study (see Chapters 3, 5, and 7). I also draw from Alana

Warner-Smith's (2022) recent bioarchaeological study that reveals new insights about how labor and (mal)nutrition affected the lives of hundreds of Irish-born individuals who passed away in New York City institutions, leaving traces on their bones. This book aims to bring embodied experiences into sharper focus.

The Five Points: A Critical Archaeological Site

The Five Points excavation provided invaluable material evidence for this study. The archaeological site encompassed more than a full city block in Lower Manhattan that had been part of the 19th-century Five Points neighborhood, named for the intersection of Anthony (later Worth), Orange (later Baxter), and Cross (later Park) Streets (Figure 0.3). Writers such as Charles Dickens, George Foster, and Herbert Asbury made the neighborhood infamous, depicting it as a hive of crime, debauchery, miscegenation, filth, disease, and poverty (Reckner 2002). From 1991 to 1993, Historic Conservation and Interpretation excavated the site in compliance with federal laws requiring investigation of cultural resources in advance of federal building projects, in this case the construction of a new courthouse. Archaeologists unearthed nearly one million artifacts from 22 features—including cisterns, drainage ditches, and privies—on 14 historic properties (Figure 0.4). John Milner Associates conducted extensive documentary investigation of the neighborhood and its residents, performed the analysis of the site and the artifacts, and published an extensive six-volume report (Yamin 2000[1]:1). The artifacts were subsequently stored in the World Trade Center. All but a few on loan were destroyed in the terrorist attack on September 11, 2001.

The team's results suggested that life in the Five Points was challenging but more complicated than the dominant slum narratives (Yamin 2000[1-6]). Housing and sanitation were generally poor, but there was some variability. Food remains and material culture, such as ceramics, suggested residents were not destitute. The neighborhood was working-class and ethnically diverse, including native-born White and Black Americans and immigrants from England, Scotland, Wales, France, Russia, Poland, Germany, Italy, and Ireland. Native-born White and Black Americans predominated during the first third of the century, Italians and Poles during the last quarter of the century. During

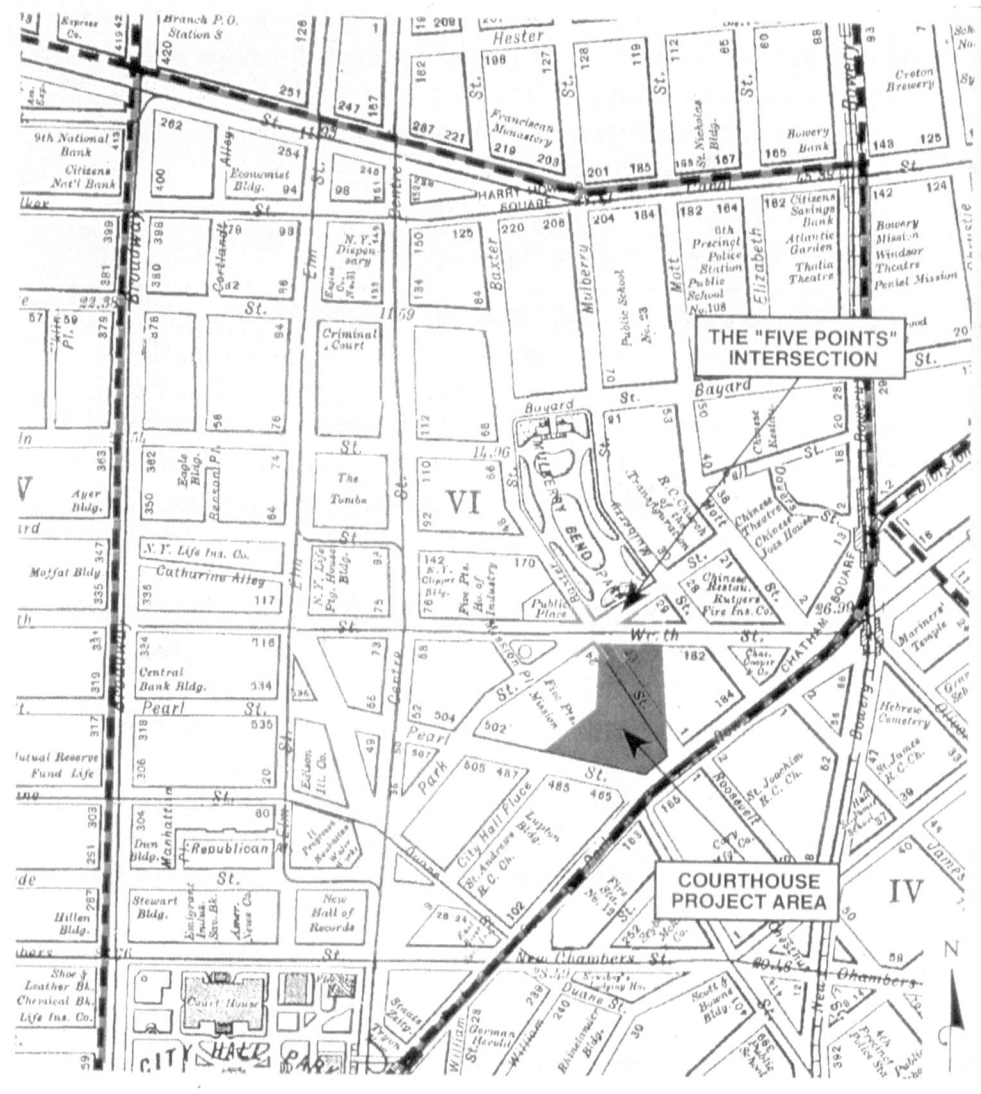

FIGURE 0.3. Map showing the location of the Five Points intersection and the site of the Five Points excavation (Yamin 2000[1]:3). Courtesy of Rebecca Yamin and the New York City Archaeological Repository: The Nan A. Rothschild Research Center.

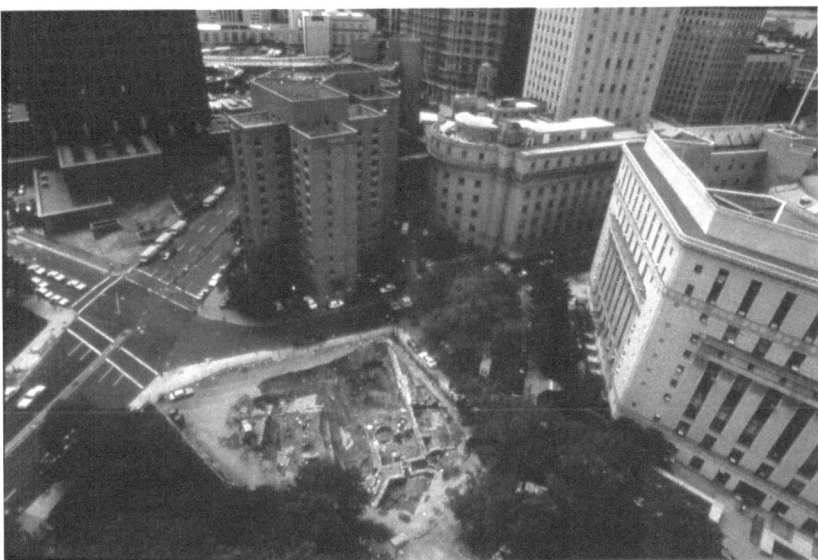

FIGURE 0.4. Photograph showing the Five Points excavation in progress. Courtesy of Rebecca Yamin and the New York City Archaeological Repository: The Nan A. Rothschild Research Center.

the middle of the century, the Irish were most numerous. More than 70% of people who lived on the excavated block between 1850 and 1870 were Irish or Irish American. The majority of the Five Points Irish came from the western counties of Kerry, Sligo, Tipperary, Cork, Galway, Mayo, Roscommon, and Clare, which were largely rural strongholds of Irish culture and language (Figure 0.5) (Anbinder 2002:356; Brighton 2011:36; Anbinder et al. 2019a).

Backyard features associated with tenements at 472 and 474 Pearl Street were particularly informative about the lives of mid-century Irish Five Pointers. Nearly all the residents of the two addresses between 1850 and 1870 were Irish born or born to Irish parents. Those whose places of origin could be identified from the records of the Emigrant Savings Bank and Transfiguration Church came mostly from the southern and western counties of Cork, Sligo, Galway, Kerry, and Clare, and the eastern county of Kildare (United States Bureau of the Census [USBC] 1850, 1870; New York State Census [NYSC] 1855; Yamin 2000[3]).[13] In the backyard features, archaeologists discovered a large number of

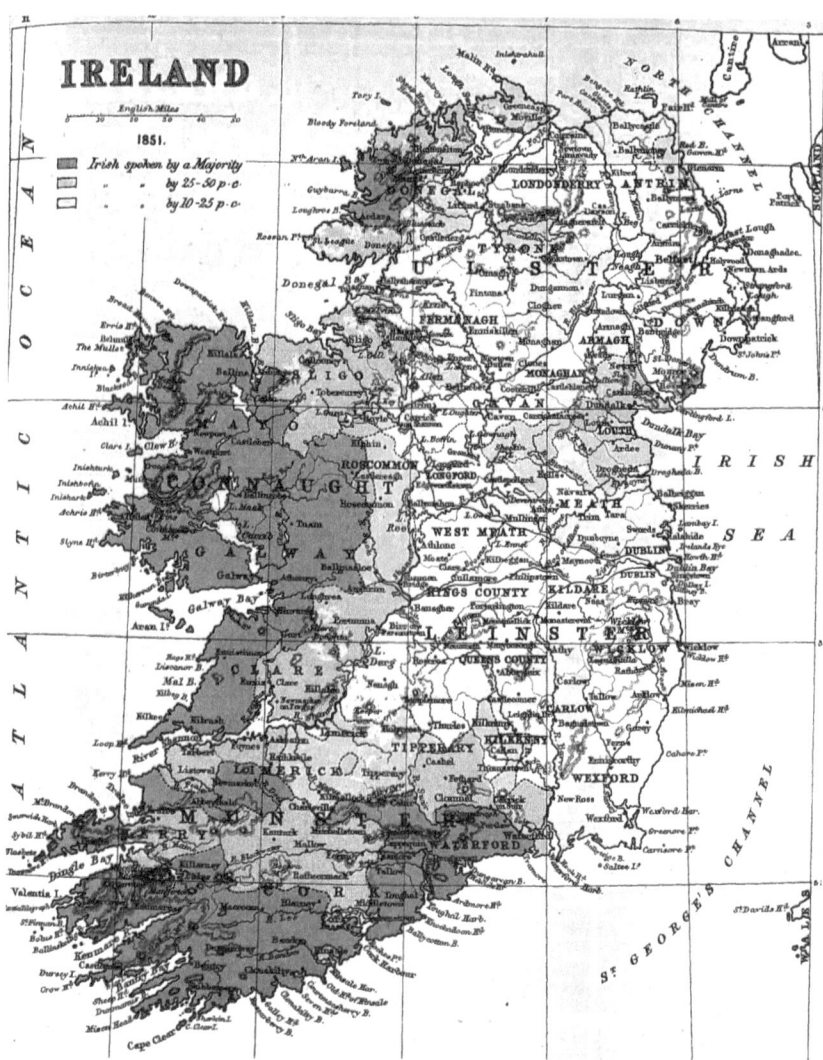

FIGURE 0.5. Map showing the distribution of Irish language speakers in 1851, based on the 1851 Irish Census (Ravenstein 1879:plate 1). The darkest shade indicates Irish was regularly spoken by the majority of the population, the middle shade by 25%–50%, the lightest by 10%–25%, and no shading by less than 10%.

health-related items, such as patent medicine and soda water bottles, compared with non-Irish residences in the Five Points and previously excavated native-born American residences elsewhere in New York City (Bonasera 2000a; Bonasera and Raymer 2001; Brighton 2008; Linn 2010). I will interpret these and other traces of Irish immigrant healing practices, including faunal and floral remains, as evidence of both challenging conditions and immigrants' creative agency in Chapters 3, 5, and 7.

The Organization of the Book

This book is organized into eight chapters. Chapter 1 presents more background about the context of immigrant life in New York City and the differences between the medical perspectives of 19th-century American medical professionals and Irish immigrants. The next six chapters are paired: Chapters 2 and 3 focus on typhus fever, Chapters 4 and 5 on injuries, and Chapters 6 and 7 on tuberculosis. The first chapter in each pair examines the extent of each ailment among Irish immigrants, how material conditions were involved from a present-day perspective, and how the ailment figured in Irish immigrant and native-born American interactions from the perspective of the latter. Chapter 2 examines the relationship between typhus fever, conditions on ships and in boardinghouses, and essentializing ideas about the supposed sanguine Irish temperament. Chapter 4 focuses on injuries and their relationship with working conditions and assumptions that the Irish were natural manual laborers. Chapter 6 centers on tuberculosis, living conditions, and growing acceptance of the Irish in New York. Each chapter also begins with a vignette focusing on the experiences of one or a few individuals, as I began this introduction with Mary MacLean's account of her illness.

The second chapter in each pair shifts to the perspectives and strategies of Irish immigrants with respect to each affliction, using insights from my study of Irish popular medicine to interpret hospital records, other written sources, and material remains from the Five Points for evidence of Irish immigrant healing agency. Chapter 3 highlights wine bottles, Chapter 5 patent medicine liniments and cosmetics, and Chapter 7 patent medicine balsams, cod liver oil, and soda water.

Each of these chapters also examines Irish immigrant uses of floral and faunal substances as well as the importance of a variety of healers in New York City, including Irish popular/folk healers—older women and bonesetters, for example—and professional physicians and druggists. These chapters reveal how Irish immigrants continued to utilize Irish remedies while also incorporating new medicinal substances to address new needs in New York. The last chapter, the Conclusion, includes a discussion of the broader relevance of illness, injury, and immigration in the present.

This project began many years ago in a graduate school course as a research paper endeavoring to explain why there were so many soda water and patent medicine bottles in the archaeological deposits associated with the Irish immigrant tenements at 472 and 474 Pearl Street in the Five Points. In order to answer that question, I soon realized I needed to research not only soda water and patent medicine (to answer questions such as: of what were they composed, how were they acquired, how much did they cost, what did their makers claim they could do, what could they do, what was their social and symbolic relevance, etc.) but also the other objects found in the same deposits, the historical context of 19th-century New York City and Ireland, and Irish immigrants' own perspectives, experiences, needs, and desires. Starting with these archaeological artifacts led me quickly to questions about health, healing, and differing perspectives, which, in turn, catalyzed my omnivorous search for any kinds of sources that might provide clues. In this resulting study, I hope that readers will find a "thick," materially anchored, and human-centered account of Irish immigrant life in New York City in the mid-19th century that brings greater insight into the experiences and perspectives of working-class Irish New Yorkers.[14] I also hope to impress upon readers how medical assumptions and social prejudices have long been intertwined, and how the health-related perspectives and practices of Irish immigrants and native-born Americans played important, previously underappreciated roles in their interactions as well as in immigrants' strategies to adjust to challenges in their new homes. The next chapter begins to examine this encounter on an individual scale, centering on a conflict between an American physician and an Irish grandmother in a lower Manhattan boardinghouse in December of 1847.

CHAPTER 1

The Case of Huxley McGuire

Irish and American Ethnomedicine Collide in a New York City Boardinghouse

About a decade and a half after Mary MacLean's ordeal in a Quebec City cholera hospital, another set of revealing doctor-patient interactions took place between an American physician and his patient's Irish grandmother in a New York City boardinghouse. In early December of 1847, Mrs. Huxley, an Irish woman who ran a boardinghouse on Church Street between Vesey and Barclay Streets (Figure 1.1), summoned Dr. Peter S. Townsend to attend to her three-year-old grandson, Huxley McGuire. Dr. Townsend (1796–1849), who had received his medical degree from the College of Physicians and Surgeons in 1816 and lived "a few doors down" from the Huxleys, was among the founders of the New York Academy of Medicine and had made a name for himself as a yellow fever expert (*New-York Evening Post* 1844:3; Townsend 1847:1).[1] In a handwritten book, Dr. Townsend recorded Huxley's case, along with those of other private patients, mostly workers and guests at the famous Astor House hotel. The doctor's notes about Huxley's case detail his increasing frustration over the course of a month with Mrs. Huxley and her boarders. Not only did they disobey his restrictive dietary orders for the child but also "decline[d] to look upon [his] prescription as one of almost marvelous character" (Townsend 1847:14). Dr. Townsend attributed their disobedience to tenderheartedness and ignorance, and he tried to retain his composure. By the end of the month, little Huxley's condition had improved, but the doctor was so aggravated by Mrs. Huxley that he absolved himself of further responsibility for the child's well-being.

This case exemplifies the private conflicts that occurred between American physicians and Irish immigrant patients and their families in mid-19th-century New York City. As I will show, these kinds of disagreements resulted not from ignorance, as Dr. Townsend and many other native-born Americans supposed, but from the meeting of two different cultural perspectives of health and healing, one professional American and the other popular Irish. This chapter will present a close analysis of Huxley's case, from Dr. Townsend's and Mrs. Huxley's views, as a means of outlining key principles of the conflicting ethnomedical perspectives. It will also analyze several of Dr. Townsend's other observations about the Huxley family's life that highlight important contextual information about Irish life in Lower Manhattan. This chapter will thus provide the background critical for understanding the health-related experiences of 19th-century Irish immigrants in New York City. Small-scale and private misunderstandings about health between people like Mrs. Huxley and Dr. Townsend were not isolated from larger public conflicts between Irish newcomers and native-born Americans. Both types of interactions influenced one another and Americans' views of Irish immigrants.

Dr. Townsend's Perspective: An Introduction to 19th-Century American Professional Medicine

Upon first arriving at Mrs. Huxley's house on December 2, 1847, Dr. Townsend noted in his casebook that he encountered a "restless, cross, and pale" little boy with "hot dry skin ... bright clear eyes, [and] a healthy expression." Huxley had a high fever, the doctor determined, and his most prominent symptom was "snuffles, . . . extreme stoppage and difficulty breathing through the nasal passages." Mrs. Huxley told the doctor that her grandson had "for two or three days been literally starving, having scarcely taken a sip of tea," and he had neither passed any urine nor moved his bowels. She also mentioned that he had recently suffered from whooping cough, which the doctor recorded would predispose him to "bronchitis, catarrh, pneumonia, pleurisy, etc., because it left the lining membranes of his bronchial tubes and cells irritable and engorged" (Townsend 1847:1–3).

Huxley's medical history and a physical examination led Dr. Townsend to diagnose the child with a fever and a "catarrhal case of bronchitis," an inflammation of the chest accompanied by the secretion of an abundance of mucus (Stewart 1846:40). He promptly prescribed his "usual" remedy, a powerful emetic and purgative containing antimony [now known to be toxic (Sundar and Chakravarty 2010)] to remove excess phlegm and restore Huxley's health (Townsend 1847:3, 7). Dr. Townsend noticed that Mrs. Huxley was worried about his prescriptions harming her grandson. As an "example to the too tender grandma," he force-fed a large tablespoon to Huxley six times, until it produced "full copious vomiting" and a bowel movement. Dr. Townsend was quite pleased with his work, noting that the boy looked "better" and gloating to his reader, "you see what a fine purgative it is." Before departing, he ordered Mrs. Huxley to restrict Huxley's diet to watered-down boiled milk, the juice of a "sweet orange or two," a little tea, and "a mouthful or two of cold water, if thirsty." The doctor planned to check on Huxley again the following day and expected a full recovery in a few days (Townsend 1847:7–10).

If Dr. Townsend administered these same prescriptions to a sick child today—a poison and severely restricted diet—he would likely face criminal charges. His diagnosis and prescriptions were consistent with the routine practices of professional American physicians at the time, however (Stewart 1846:40–49).[2] To understand how Dr. Townsend and his fellow physicians could prescribe such remedies in good faith requires recognizing that they were part of an ethnomedical system (the system of medical beliefs and practices embedded within a society and culture) that differs from ours of the present-day (Singer et al. 2020:161). American medicine 150 years ago was in many ways closer to that practiced in Ancient Rome than it is to contemporary American biomedicine.[3]

The renowned historian of medicine Charles Rosenberg (1977) has described how, during the 19th century, American physicians and the American public alike clung to an antiquated understanding of the body rooted in humoral theory. Central to this understanding was the idea that bodily equilibrium was necessary for good health. They perceived the body as "a kind of stew pot, or chemico-vital reaction, proceeding calmly only if all of its elements remained appropriately balanced" (Rosenberg 1977:488). This balance was easily upset, however, by any number of factors, such as environmental conditions—including weather, miasmas ("noxious vapour rising from putrescent organic matter" [OED 2001a]),

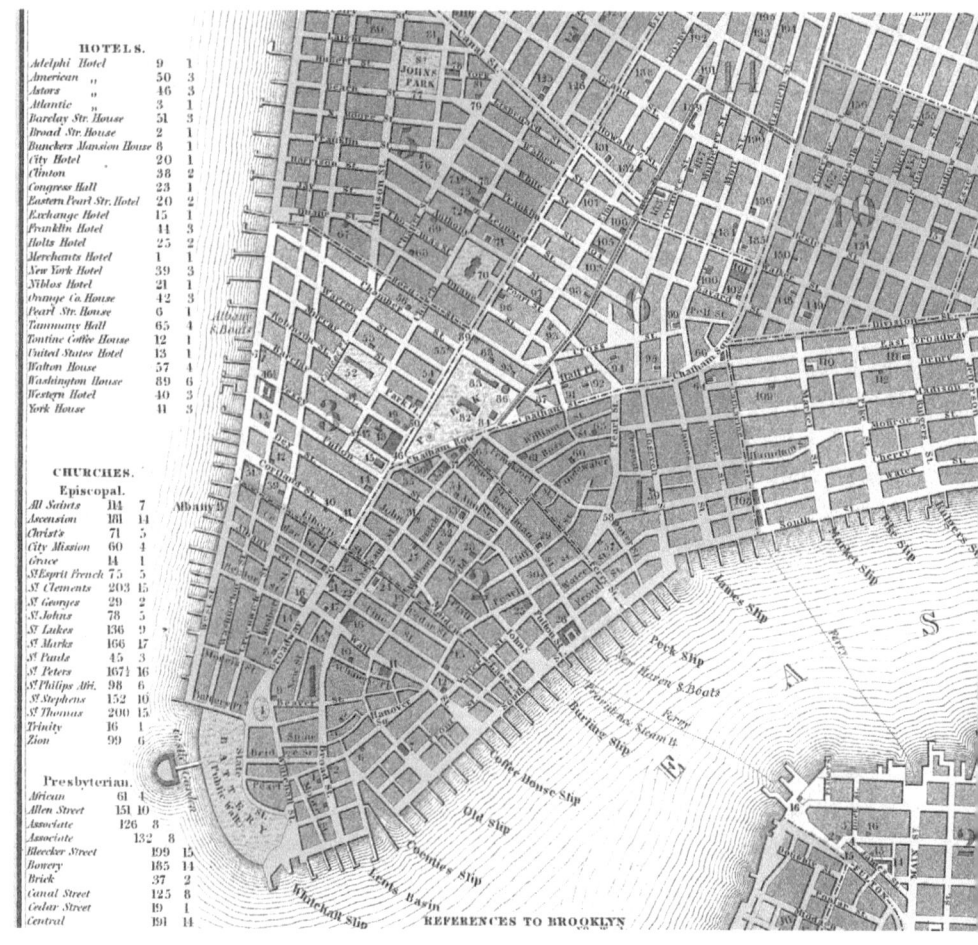

FIGURE 1.1. Portion of Samuel Augustus Mitchell's (1850) map of "The City of New York," showing Lower Manhattan. Wards are shaded and indicated by the large numbers. Institutions are indicated by smaller numbers corresponding to the key. Mrs. Huxley's boardinghouse was located on Church Street between Vesey and Barclay Streets, to the right of the large number 3. The triangular-shaped area just below the large 6 is the Five Points intersection. Courtesy of David Rumsey Map Collection, David Rumsey Map Center, Stanford Libraries, Creative Commons License 3.0, https://creativecommons.org/licenses/by-nc-sa/3.0/.

food, habits, work—and internal character or state of mind. American physicians and the public shared this holistic model of the body and its surroundings, believing that each part of the body could affect any other part, such that "a distracted mind could curdle the stomach, a dyspeptic stomach could agitate the mind" (Rosenberg 1977:488).

While these ideas might sound pleasantly holistic from a 21st-century point of view, they sharply diverge from a present-day biomedical perspective in the details of how physicians imagined the body's composition and how they understood, diagnosed, and treated illnesses. First, it is important to remember that not until after the 1870s did physicians understand that microscopic organisms ("germs") caused specific diseases. Prior to that, they believed bodily disequilibrium was ultimately either the cause of or a major contributing factor in all illnesses. Second, they believed that the same illness or the same medicine could have radically different effects on different people because of each person's own particular constitution (Rosenberg 1977:501-502). Thus, part of the physician's art was to be able to detect his or her (but mostly his, since an overwhelming majority of professional physicians were male) patients' constitutional proclivities, which they believed were influenced not only by the factors mentioned above, but also by heredity, race, and culture (Haller 1981a; Puckrein 1981; Harris and Ernst 1999). Third, physicians had few diagnostic tools and typically identified diseases on the basis of symptoms they could detect or intuit with their own senses. Particularly important were the pulse, color and condition of skin, eyes, and tongue, and the quality and quantity of bodily secretions. Last, they did not use specific drugs to target specific diseases. In fact, "advocacy of a specific drug in treating a specific ill was ordinarily viewed by regular physicians as a symptom of quackery" (Rosenberg 1977:490).

Physicians instead categorized drugs by their physiological effects, such as diuretics, cathartics, emetics, and diaphoretics. They used them to try to reestablish bodily equilibrium by aiding what they believed were the body's natural reactions to illness: urination, defecation, vomiting, and perspiration (Rosenberg 1977:489). Physicians also frequently administered opiates to relieve pain, especially to patients who they believed were particularly sensitive and not easily able to bear it. How they determined who was sensitive and who was not was profoundly influenced by their own culturally influenced interpretations of the appearance, gender, age, class, and race of the patient, as I will show in Chapters 2, 4, and 6.

Most drugs in the 19th-century professional physician's toolkit were, therefore, those that visibly, and sometimes violently, regulated bodily secretions and/or altered mental states. The more severe the illness, the stronger both physicians and their American patients, who shared the same worldview, believed a drug's action needed to be. This principle softened over the course of the 19th century as such so-called "heroic" practices were critiqued from multiple angles, including from physicians themselves (many at what we would today call research hospitals), sectarian doctors (such as homeopathists or hydropathists), and the American public (including Irish immigrants). By the middle of the 19th century, some professional physicians, who were all too aware of the limits of their conventional therapies, embraced some new alternatives. As medical historian John Haller (1981a:vii) describes, "new theories and old habits jostled uncomfortably in the same medical handbags."

The most infamous "heroic" practice of American professional medicine was bleeding a patient, in some cases removing up to several pints of blood. Physicians continued to bleed patients throughout the 19th century. By the middle of the century, however, most physicians in urban areas exposed to newer ideas typically extracted only a few ounces, using gentler cupping and leeching techniques instead of the lancet. Yet, as Rosenberg writes, "no mid-century American practitioner rejected conventional therapeutics [e.g., bleeding, purging, etc.] with a ruthless consistency. The self-confident empiricism which denied the utility of any therapeutic measure not proven efficacious in clinical trials seemed an ideological excess suited to a handful of European academics, not to the realities of practice" (Rosenberg 1977:498). American physicians, not unlike Irish healers, held fast to the techniques that had been passed down to them by previous generations, and, at times, also selectively embraced new practices, some pioneered by European physicians. The result of adherence to "heroic" practices is summed up by medical historian Eric Larrabee (1971:120): "In the famous phrase of Professor Henderson of Harvard, not until 1900 would the average patient, treated by the average physician, stand a better than fifty-fifty chance of benefiting from the encounter."

The reason physicians and their patients considered regulating bodily secretions to be so important is because humoral theory still deeply influenced their understanding of the body. This theory, first described by ancient Greek writers, notably Hippocrates, and later refined by the ancient Roman physician Galen, proposed that all things were composed of four elements—fire, air, water, and earth—that each had their own quality, hot, cold, wet, and dry, respectively. Through eating and digesting food, the body converted these elements into humors, namely blood, phlegm, yellow bile, and black bile, which each partook of two qualities. Blood was hot and wet, yellow bile was hot and dry, black bile was cold and dry, and phlegm was cold and wet. Proper balance of humors, which was specific to each individual, was necessary to maintain proper organ function and health. Imbalance caused illness as well as humoral temperament: sanguinous, phlegmatic, choleric, or melancholic (see Chapter 2 and Table 2.1). The particular symptoms of the illness indicated the humor in excess or in scarcity (Table 1.1). For example, fever (elevated body temperature) suggested an excess of a hot humor, such as blood, which bloodletting would relieve. A stuffy or runny nose, like Huxley's, indicated an excess of phlegm that required removal. Secondary to depleting the offending humor, physicians prescribed substances with the opposite characteristics, such as cool beverages to a fever patient or warming compresses to a patient with a "cold." Environmental conditions, substances applied to or ingested into the body, and emotional states could restore or impair humoral balance (Puckrein 1981; Stelmack and Stalikas 1991).

TABLE 1.1. Associations of Humors, Qualities, and Illnesses.

Humor	Qualities	Examples of Associated Illness
Blood	Hot & wet	Rash, fever, nosebleeds
Yellow bile	Hot & dry	Jaundice, headaches
Black bile	Cold & dry	Dysentery, cholera, and intestinal disorders
Phlegm	Cold & wet	Respiratory diseases, such as pneumonia, pleurisy, pulmonary tuberculosis

Note: This table outlines associations between humors, their qualities, and certain illnesses as generally understood from Classical period Greece through the 19th century.

Sources: Puckrein (1981); Stelmack and Stalikas (1991).

Despite the fact that physicians and scientists had developed a number of competing models, humoral theory still held considerable influence in the 19th century in patient treatment and medical research, homeopathic medicine, phrenology, and the life insurance business.[4] Medical textbooks steeped in the humoralist tradition continued to be published into the 1870s, and the theory's nearly 2,000 years of predominance had infused it into European and European American cultures (Haller 1981a:3; Puckrein 1981:1755). Over the course of the 19th century, physicians came to treat humoral imbalance as a factor that did not necessarily directly cause all illnesses, but instead made the body more susceptible, or predisposed, to illnesses caused by other factors, such as miasmas (Stewart 1846; Rosenberg 1977). Until the 1850s, for example, physicians believed that airborne miasmas caused cholera, the pandemic illness that afflicted millions in the 19th century, including Mary MacLean and her siblings, described in the previous chapter (Rosenberg 1987a:193–196).[5] Dr. Townsend's (1847:17) remark about another patient, an Irish-born young man and servant at the Astor Hotel, made clear that he considered humoral temperament in patient care. Townsend recorded that the patient had a "rosy complexion" and was "a perfect specimen of sanguinous temperament."

Because there were no specific drugs to target diseases, physicians continued to follow ancient practices of reestablishing bodily equilibrium by removing the excessive humor(s) indicated by the patient's symptoms and then prescribing food, medicine, or other treatments with the opposite qualities. At the time Dr. Townsend attended to Huxley, physicians' methods of treating children's fevers tended toward purgatives and emetics to cleanse the digestive system rather than toward bleeding, which some had come to view as dangerous for children (Stewart 1846:78–79). Depleting a patient with purgatives and emetics was so popular that it was most physicians' first approach to treating most afflictions. Medical casebooks from New York Hospital suggest that this was the standard practice of physicians there throughout the 1840s and 1850s (New York Hospital Medical Casebooks [NYHMCB] 1847–1853). Stewart (1846:78–79) also noted that physicians believed that fevers in children could be brought on by the overheating effects of partially digested food rotting in their digestive systems, another reason to evacuate their systems.

From a 19th-century American professional medical perspective, Dr. Townsend's administration of a powerful emetic and purgative to Huxley was appropriate. Dr. Townsend recorded that he ruled out using cups or leeches to bleed the child, despite his fever, because he observed "little difficulty of the chest proper." Instead, he addressed the child's "most prominent symptom . . . extreme stoppage and difficulty breathing through the nasal passages [because of] accumulated mucus" with a strong emetic. Dr. Townsend's initial recommendation to Mrs. Huxley to keep her grandson "well clad" (Townsend 1847:10) also shows that he tried to counteract the cold and wet qualities of Huxley's most prominent symptom to prevent him from relapsing. After removing Huxley's excess phlegm, the doctor followed a standard procedure, gentler than bleeding, to remedy Huxley's second symptom of fever by prescribing a restricted diet of cooling and easily digestible foods (Townsend 1847:1, 10).

Rosenberg (1977:492, 497–498) explains that the dramatic effects of the powerful drugs, such as antimony, that 19th century-physicians used played a vital role in the doctor-patient relationship, a principle also supported by medical anthropologists who study healing in more recent times (Van der Geest and Whyte 1989; Moerman 2002). Rosenberg writes that "on the emotional level, the very severity of the drug action assured the patient and his family that something was indeed being done." With so few medicines having verifiable beneficial effects on particular diseases, the placebo effect, or what Daniel Moerman (2002:10–19) argues should more accurately be called the "meaning response," played an even more important role in healing than it does today.[6] A large portion of the 19th-century physician's role was akin to that of a folk healer in that the confidence he projected in his treatment often had an even greater impact on the patient's outcome than the treatment itself.

Dr. Townsend seems to have understood the importance of creating the appearance of a skillful and confident healer. In the case record of another patient, a worker at the Astor House, he wrote that his fear that the patient might die is "anguish of heart and a thought that you must endure . . . in secret and not show . . . and not let them know . . . what tortures are agonizing you [otherwise] . . . you would lower yourself in their estimation. No[,] keep firm in step and a stiff upper lip, so long as you have amounted to no actual blunder or malpractice"

(Townsend 1847:38). In his view, a skillful healer does not reveal his own apprehension about a patient's condition, but instead remains in character, and thus communicates to his anxious patient that he has power over illness and injury.

Dr. Townsend's composure was tested, however, when he returned to check on Huxley on December 12th, just over a week after his initial visit. He found that Huxley was still running a fever and that Huxley had been sleeping on a feather mattress with Mrs. Huxley and her niece, Mary Ann. This sleeping arrangement, the doctor believed, was overheating the child and prolonging his fever (Townsend 1847:42).[7] What made Dr. Townsend even more upset, however, was that the grandmother had fed Huxley "a meal of potatoes besides a little brandy." This information led the doctor to write a paragraph-long diatribe about the inability of convalescing patients, especially children, to digest "such crudities as . . . potatoes however well-greased they are with butter" (Townsend 1847:42). He did not comment about the brandy, but as I will demonstrate in Chapter 2, physicians at this time generally thought liquor to be stimulating and warming (Rosenberg 1987b:42; Bowditch 1994a:84).

A few days after the initial potato incident, the doctor visited the child and found that Mrs. Huxley continued to ignore his advice. According to the then-livid Dr. Townsend, Mrs. Huxley gave into the boy's cries for codfish and potatoes, and her boarders, "being of a coarse description[,] have been in the habit of feeding him at dinner with meats of all kinds in fact stuffing and gorging him daily." The only positive change in Huxley's environment, in the doctor's opinion, was that the weather had cooled about 20 degrees. Dr. Townsend warned Mrs. Huxley again about the importance of his dietary advice and the "drying heating nature of too much animal food," which he felt was prolonging the child's fever. At this point, Dr. Townsend absolved himself of responsibility for Huxley's health, telling the grandmother that if the child became feverish again, "the whole blame would be on her" (Townsend 1847:47).

This close reading of Dr. Townsend's notes indicates that he was well aware of the importance of the doctor-patient relationship in healing and was a well-respected physician who used the best professional American medical practices of the day. Why did he lose his composure? Was Mrs. Huxley, who Dr. Townsend observed to be "obedient" while in his presence and genuinely concerned with her grandson's health, truly an ignorant and "too tender" woman, as the doctor believed (Townsend 1847:7, 42)? Details of this case, when read through a 19th-century Irish lens, reveal that the grandmother had good reasons for disregarding some of Dr. Townsend's orders, reasons that even the skillful and self-reflective doctor could not and/or did not want to understand. Many of Dr. Townsend's orders directly conflicted with her own Irish understanding of her grandson's illness and the appropriate ways to heal him. Two different systems of healing met awkwardly in Mrs. Huxley's boardinghouse.

Mrs. Huxley's Perspective: An Introduction to 19th-Century Irish Popular Medicine

Dr. Townsend's notes provide a detailed account of his own point of view of Huxley's case, but they only hint at Mrs. Huxley's perspective. The following fictional narrative attempts to reconstruct her position. Creating such a narrative follows the example of other archaeologists who have used this method to interpret perspectives of people who are not well represented in historical records (Schrire 1995; Beaudry 1998, 2013; Praetzellis and Praetzellis 1998; Yamin 1998; Janowitz and Dallal 2013). In order to make good narratives for this purpose, Mary Beaudry (2013:ix) explains that both "close readings of data drawn from multiple lines of evidence" and an "informed imagination that situates people within their time" are necessary. I would also add that situating people within their own cultural context is essential. Thus, I have based the following narrative upon a combination of information from Dr. Townsend's notes and research about 19th-century Irish popular medicine and immigrant life. The narrative is then followed by an overview of Irish popular medicine and a more detailed analysis of the conflicts between Dr. Townsend and Mrs. Huxley, from her point of view.

Mrs. Huxley's Narrative

Mrs. Huxley was very worried about her little boy. As she told the doctor, Huxley was not only her grandson by blood, but also her and her second husband's (Mr. Huxley) son by law, because her son from her first marriage (to Mr. McGuire) could no longer be his father.[8] Little Huxley had recently recovered from a frightful case of whooping cough, and he had just fallen ill again. He had not eaten or drunk more than a sip of tea for two days, or was it three? He was restless, his skin was hot as a hearth stone, and he was so congested that he couldn't breathe through his nose. She had tried a few remedies, including smearing Huxley's chest with goose grease ointment and three times making the sign of the cross, like her mother had taught her to do.[9] She mentioned neither the cross nor the Irish origin of this cure to the doctor, of course, but he had approved of the goose grease, saying that it resembled a similar American country practice using candle tallow (Townsend 1847:3–4). She had also given Huxley brandy and administered an enema to drive out any worms that might be causing his illness, a frequent cause of childhood complaints, in her experience. To build up his strength, she had bought and prepared fresh meat, fish, and potatoes, and she had encouraged her boarders to let him have anything from their plates that he desired, since he had shown little interest in food for days (Townsend 1847:1–5). She was pleased that her boarders were good people of her own kind from the old country (Townsend 1847:1) who also adored her little boy. It made managing such a large household a little bit easier. None of her trusted remedies or her boarders' doting had cured Huxley, however, so she feared that his illness was especially dangerous.

Although her boarders were Irish too, most of them were young and had not been as blessed as she to have received so much healing knowledge from her mother and grandmother. In fact, the young adults usually looked to her for help, since she was their elder. She had been working so hard keeping house that she had had few chances to discover where there might be an "herb doctor" (herbalist), *bean feasa* or *bean leighis* (wise woman or healing woman), or "seventh son" (the seventh-born son in a family, who possessed healing power, especially over worms) to approach for stronger cures. She had heard that her Anglo-American neighbors directed a lot of hostility toward the keeners at a recent wake (Ladies of the Mission 1854:203) and imagined that folk healers would keep a low profile.[10] The only way to find out about them would be through friends and acquaintances, since healers would not advertise, even in the Irish newspapers her boarders occasionally told her about. Healers shied away from notoriety, lest they lose their friends and healing gifts by their shameless self-promotion (Buckley 1980:17, 33-34).

Yet, something had to be done, and soon. Huxley couldn't go on much longer this way. In Ireland, she had heard elders say that the fairies loved to take away young children, especially fair little boys like Huxley (NFC 1974[1837]:43). She had little doubt that there were fairies in America but hoped that they weren't as powerful in New York City as they were near their forts on the Emerald Isle.[11] Besides, she still thought that this illness might have a more natural cause. One of her boarders had mentioned that worms had been troubling children in the neighborhood and that local physicians had good medicines to cure them.[12] After the enema failed to remove worms, she summoned Dr. Peter S. Townsend, the physician she had heard was an expert on some kind of deadly fever and who lived down the street (Townsend 1847:1). It's true that he was a native-born New Yorker and professional physician who might prescribe something strange and fearful and who might charge a fortune for it, but he had successfully treated one of her boarders the previous summer. The doctor had diagnosed him with "jaundice" and prescribed that he "go immediately to the seashore" (Townsend 1847:1), a reasonable enough remedy.[13] And, she could afford to pay for good care. She and her husband were doing well, him at his tailoring and her in running the boardinghouse, and they had put some money away. So, she was prepared to listen to the doctor's advice and pay his fee, with the hope that he could cure her boy.

Principles of Irish Popular Ethnomedicine

Although there were some Irish professional physicians who immigrated to New York City bringing ideas about medicine that were similar to their American counterparts (MacNeven 1842a,b; Kraut 1996:163-164), the average Irish immigrant, like Mrs. Huxley, possessed popular Irish conceptions of health and healing. These ideas were part of a pragmatic and eclectic popular ethnomedical system that was spread by word of mouth and practiced throughout the Irish countryside and its towns and cities. Based on my analysis of thousands of popular Irish "cures" (remedies intending to relieve ailments) collected from a variety of folklore and ethnographic records (see Introduction), the following section sketches out the contours of Irish popular ethnomedicine and how it differed from that practiced by 19th-century American physicians, such as Dr. Townsend.

Irish popular ethnomedicine (the medical ideas and practices of "ordinary" Irish people) in the 19th century was syncretic, incorporating ideas from a variety of sources, including European professional medicine, continental European folk traditions, and Roman Catholicism, but it viewed them all through an Irish lens. The mixing of these influences is noticeable in popular Irish explanations for illnesses, as reported to various folklore collectors: bodily imbalance, contamination or invasion (typically by worms or poison), transference of an illness from one being to another, human bewitchment, and intervention by God or fairies.[14] Thus, some of their ideas about illness causation clearly overlapped with those of American physicians, such as bodily imbalance, contamination, worms, and perhaps even divine intervention.[15] Others, including fairy intervention and human bewitchment, probably did not.

Even points of agreement, such as bodily imbalance, differ in the details of how they were understood and treated, however. For example, Irish informants frequently mentioned the dangers of overwork, undernourishment, becoming cold or wet in the rain, and overheating in the sun, but in the approximately 3,500 cures I have reviewed, almost never did informants reference humors, humoral theory, or its principles. Unlike American physicians' first approach of *removing* bodily fluids to help reestablish a humoral balance, Irish people's usual first approach was to *add* things to the body (externally and/or internally) to strengthen and restore the patient to a healthful state. Irish popular methods of counteracting colds and respiratory ailments, for example, included applying ointments made of goose grease, like Mrs. Huxley used, camphorated oil, or chopped garlic to the chest to lessen congestion; warming the body by placing compresses made of warm potatoes or oats on the chest or wrapping the head and feet in a scarf; and feeding warm food, mustard, alcoholic beverages (such as whiskey, brandy, rum, or elderberry wine), homemade cough medicines, and/or hot infusions of plants (including garlic, onions, or dandelions) thought to nourish the body or drive out sickness.[16]

The popular Irish approach to treating illnesses, in general, favored strengthening remedies over depleting ones, and hearty food and drink was an essential element in strengthening. Many Irish in the 19th century had experienced hunger firsthand; seasonal food shortages and even chronic undernourishment were common well before the Great Famine (Miller 1985:281). Even those who did not have personal experience of starvation no doubt understood the debilitating effects of malnourishment. The popular Irish perspective about the importance of food in healing seems to have influenced professional medicine in Ireland. The renowned Irish physician Robert Graves (1796–1853), for example, became famous, in part, because he saved many fever patients in Dublin by going against the widely accepted official medical prescription of bleeding and withholding food to "starve a fever" (Logan 1994:9). Graves's nourishing treatment was so controversial in professional medical circles and so successful that legend has it that Graves jokingly said he wished to have "he fed fevers" inscribed on his tombstone (O'Brien 1983:145). As I will show, Mrs. Huxley's treatment of her grandson was consistent with this Irish restorative approach to healing.

This is not to say that Irish remedies did not include emetics or purgatives—or diuretics, diaphoretics, and narcotics, for that matter. In fact, Irish informants noted many mixtures that could bring upon these actions, but they typically used milder-acting plant, animal, and whiskey-based ingredients, and aimed to expel worms and poisons, rather than to rebalance humors. For example, an Irish recipe to induce vomiting (an emetic) was to drink a strong infusion of chamomile (Purdon 1895a:215). Another to induce purging was to drink boiled nettle roots (NFC 1941[782]:349; Logan 1994:35).[17] In contrast, American professional medicine used antimony and calomel (mercurous chloride) as emetics and purgatives (Townsend 1847:8, 44; NYHMCB 1848–1852).

Irish popular healers also erred on the side of caution. Instead of administering multiple medicinal remedies or doses in quick succession (Dr. Townsend's approach), ordinary Irish people and even Irish folk healing specialists, such as wisewomen, gave single doses of their mixtures or other treatments over the course of several days, and only if necessary. As medical doctor and folklore collector Patrick Logan (1994:1–2) pointed out, time is a great remedy, even if the prescribed medicine is not. And the kind attention of a trusted healer and/or active engagement with a substance regarded as curative can relieve anxiety and speed healing. The next section briefly returns to Mrs. Huxley's boardinghouse and the substances she administered to her grandson to

Back to Mrs. Huxley's Parlor: Interpreting a Frustrating Encounter

These different Irish popular and American professional medical conceptions about the causes of illnesses and how to treat them led to Dr. Townsend's frustration with Mrs. Huxley. It is quite likely she returned his sentiments. As mentioned previously, Dr. Townsend's descriptions of Huxley's symptoms and his prescription of antimony make clear that he aimed to rebalance Huxley's humors, beginning first by depleting. Mrs. Huxley, on the other hand, had treated Huxley with a goose grease ointment, a common Irish remedy to relieve Huxley's congestion (National Folklore Collection—Schools Manuscripts Collection [NFCS] 1938[918]:179; O'Regan 1997:21). She also administered an enema, an Irish remedy for worms (Purdon 1895a:215), and told the doctor outright that she thought her grandson was sick from worms (Townsend 1847:1).[18] Irish from rural backgrounds were likely well-acquainted with intestinal worms. In fact, archaeoparasitologist Karl Reinhard (2000:391) determined from his analysis of night soil in Five Points privies that infection rates of worms decreased with the influx of the Irish, suggesting the Irish possessed effective remedies against the giant intestinal roundworm, *Ascaris lumbricoides*, in particular.

Although Mrs. Huxley and the doctor did not agree about the cause of Huxley's illness, she probably permitted him to administer his antimony emetic and purgative because purging fit with her own perspective as another method to treat worms. Irish informants reported using a decoction of boiled nettle roots, for example, for such purposes (NFC 1941[782]:349; Logan 1994:35). After Dr. Townsend's medicine did its job, Mrs. Huxley probably hoped that her grandson had evacuated the worms and believed that the best thing to do to rebuild his strength was to keep him warm and give him hearty food. Although Dr. Townsend did not appreciate the benefits of potatoes, cod, and meat, these were all highly valued foods in Ireland. Fish, in particular, was recommended for children and pregnant women (Logan 1994:14). Cod liver oil, in fact, was used for centuries by coastal peoples in Europe to strengthen children, and it became the leading professional medical treatment for tuberculosis in the middle of the 19th century and for rickets in the early 20th century (Rajakumar 2003:e134; Grad 2004:107).

When Dr. Townsend visited a few days later, on what became his last visit, Mrs. Huxley asked the doctor for a medicine to treat worms specifically (Townsend 1847:48). Although Dr. Townsend was angry at her for feeding Huxley a rich diet, he begrudgingly gave her a prescription for a worming infusion, composed mostly of senna root. Dr. Townsend believed that it would not really help the child; but it also would not harm him (Townsend 1847:47), likely because senna was gentler than other purgatives in his medical bag, and it might rid Huxley of the hot "animal foods" the doctor so opposed. What Dr. Townsend did not seem to understand during his last heated exchange with Mrs. Huxley was that Mrs. Huxley was not blindly disregarding his advice. Instead, she had her own ideas about the cause of Huxley's illness and how to treat it that were informed by her own cultural background, and these ideas did not match Dr. Townsend's. She believed the cause of her grandson's illness was worms, and she followed the widely held Irish prescription to "feed fevers."

The Irish Popular Medical Toolkit: Ordinary to Extraordinary

The little that Dr. Townsend recorded about the remedies Mrs. Huxley administered to her grandson only scratches the surface of 19th-century Irish popular cures. As an informant told a National Folklore Collection folklorist in County Cork in 1938, the Irish had a system of medicine of their own and were especially skilled and resourceful: "In olden times when doctors were not numerous persons were obliged to rely largely on their own local remedies in cases of illness, and had to procure home manufactured medicine for the cure of certain diseases. In those times the people of Ireland were famous for their cleverness in the preparation of medicine and poultices made from certain herbs mixed with spring water" (NFCS 1938[345]:13).

Irish popular ethnomedicine developed in response to the needs of a mostly rural population that was generally poor in money and limited in access to professional physicians but rich in natural, supernatural, and human resources. They drew upon all of these for healing. Mrs. Huxley's goose grease, codfish, potatoes, and brandy are only a few examples of the myriad ordinary natural substances utilized for extraordinary healing purposes. Others include additional animal parts and products, marine resources, stones, water, other liquors (especially whiskey), and hundreds of plants, including many that American physicians would have categorized as weeds, such as nettle, dandelion, chickweed, and plantain. Anthropologist Conrad Arensberg, who observed Irish folk medicinal practices in the 1930s, noted that "the things of greatest 'power' are not by any means always wondrous, unusual or fearsome things, but the homely articles of use and familiar associations.... These 'tried and true' objects of ordinary life ... bring peace of mind" and "restore emotional equilibrium" (Arensberg 1937:199, 200–201).

The Irish transformed homely ingredients into compresses, ointments, poultices, decoctions, and infusions. Mothers and grandmothers, like Mrs. Huxley, prepared ointments each year to have on hand for treating sprains, strains, burns, colds, and congestion by mixing particular plants with rendered animal fat (NFCS 1938[45]:247; O'Regan 1997:21). Goose grease was a frequently mentioned ointment base, likely because it was typically made from the remains of a Christmas meal, adding spiritual power to this fat with a low melting point that easily absorbs into the skin (O'Regan 1997:21). Women (and some men) also mashed freshly gathered plants into poultices and applied them to the skin to cure cuts, bruises, and skin infections; chickweed and plantain were frequent choices (Egan 1887:11; Purdon 1895b:294; Barbour 1897:388; Verling 2003:63; Allen and Hatfield 2004:91–92, 247–248). As the informant from Cork (mentioned above) noted, they also created infusions by steeping specific herbs in spring water to remedy illnesses ranging from common colds and coughs to more serious ailments, such as jaundice and consumption (NFCS 1938[345]:13). To these infusions, the Irish often added whiskey, which they believed could drive away sickness (see Chapter 2 for more about this). The Irish also made use of many household products, such as cloth and string to cure sprains and turpentine to relieve backaches and toothaches (NFC 1935[265]:597; NFC 1955[1389]:201; Logan 1994:124).

Objects, places, or actions believed to have spiritual power by virtue of a perceived connection with God, saints, or fairies were also important elements in the Irish popular ethnomedical toolkit. These "supernatural" remedies were not necessarily exclusive from "natural" remedies.

Goose grease ointment made from a Christmas goose is an example, as is the plantain plant, associated with St. Patrick; both were believed to possess power, not only because of physical properties but also by virtue of connection with Jesus and a saint, respectively (NFCS 1938[35]:129; Gregory 1920:149). Additional sources of healing included holy water from churches, scapulars, gold rings (once required in Ireland for church weddings), earth from priests' graves, holy well water, iron objects, and special stones (such as rock outcroppings, boulders with man-made impressions, and standing stone monuments or ancient buildings) thought to be the forts of fairies or places where events of religious significance had occurred. The Irish also used actions in healing that they believed to be powerful, including making the sign of the cross, repeating something three or nine times (invoking the power of the Trinity and/or native pre-Christian sources of power), performing a cure on a special day (e.g., feast days of major Irish saints, some of which the Roman Catholic Church had intentionally placed on the same dates as Celtic holidays), completing a pilgrimage, and saying certain prayers. Some cures consisted entirely of a saying and/or ritual motion; these were called "charms." Charms were often passed down in families. For example, the Keogh family possessed a cure for erysipelas, and the McGovern family possessed one for rabies (Barbour 1897:387; O'Connor 1943:278–279; Maloney 1972:68; Logan 1994:12, 70). Other charm cures circulated more widely, such as one for fever that Mrs. Huxley might have known and used.[19]

Such cures attempting to harness supernatural power were typically used in conjunction with herbal or other remedies to cure conditions believed to be caused by supernatural or personalistic forces, often determined by their unresponsiveness to other remedies (McClafferty 1979:1; Linn 2014). Fairies, for example, were said to cause fever, sudden paralysis, difficult childbirth, consumption, and failure to thrive in children (NFC 1935[54]:204; NFC 1937[463]:44-45; NFC 1941[782]:258; Fleming 1953:61; Gregory 1920:169–246). Fairies were enamored with pregnant women and children, especially handsome baby boys, and would kidnap them and replace them with a fairy woman or child, respectively, called a changeling, who wasted away and eventually disappeared (Wilde, L. 1887a:40, 73, 84, 121, 123, 172; NFC 1941[782]:258; Hand 1981:145). To keep fairies away, Irish mothers dressed boys in skirts to fool them about the children's gender (Figure 1.2), sewed bits of iron or iron nails into the hems of children's clothing, or placed iron tools near their beds (NFC 1941[782]:192; NFC 1951[1220]:4, 18; NFC 1974[1837]:42, 59; Dorian 2000:267; Evans 1957:289). When folklore collectors inquired about these practices, informants explained that fairies fled in fear of iron objects, because iron nails once came into contact with Jesus's body during his crucifixion (NFC 1941[782]:248; Fallon 1994:13). This suggests that for many Irish, a metonymic connection with the divine imbued iron with healing power.[20] Such measures, along with invoking the Trinity three times or spitting three times on the ground, prevented children from being harmed by the "evil eye" or being "overlooked" by a jealous onlooker. These are detailed further in Chapter 7.

On this side of the Atlantic Irish immigrants did not have access to the same sites of healing power in the Irish landscape, but historical and oral historical records show that they continued to believe certain conditions were caused by supernatural or personalistic forces and continued to use corresponding cures. The *New York Times* ([*NYT*] 1908:9), for example, reported that an Irish priest named Father Thomas Adams had "used relics of the saints in treating the illnesses of members of his flock."[21] American folklorist Wayland Hand (1981:145), moreover, recorded that masons in California embedded horseshoes and other iron items in buildings to ward off fairies and witches well into the 20th century. It would thus not be surprising if the concerned Mrs. Huxley said a charm or made signs of the cross to give extra potency to the medicine she administered to her sick grandson. Huxley had recently suffered from whooping cough, and she might have worried he had been "overlooked" or was in danger of fairy capture. She might have sewn an iron nail into the hem of his clothing or placed an iron object near him while he was sleeping. She would have had little incentive to mention such tactics to Dr. Townsend, given that many native-born Americans viewed beliefs in fairies and Roman Catholic rituals to be superstitions of ignorant people unlike themselves (Linn 2014). In the next chapter, I will show how other Irish popular medical practices exacerbated the epidemic of anti-Irish prejudice in New York City.

Although scorned by American physicians like Dr. Townsend, and the American public, Irish remedies, both natural and supernatural, would have brought significant comfort to those who believed in them through the placebo effect/meaning response. Some remedies were also likely empirically effective. Even ones that were not, however, operated positively by the same principle as some of Dr. Townsend's prescriptions; they showed the patient that something was being done. Visible action, audible words, and tangible medicines are vital aspects of healing. As medical anthropologists Sjaak van der Geest, Susan Reynolds Whyte, and Anita Hardon (1996:154) explain, "Medicines are tangible, usable in a concrete way: They can be swallowed, smeared on the skin, or inserted into orifices—activities that hold the promise of a physical effect. By applying a 'thing,' we transform the state of dysphoria into something concrete, into something to which the patient and others can address their efforts. . . . Practicing medicine, after all, is the art of making disease concrete." Making ailments concrete is an important part of giving meaning to them which also can include diagnosis and/or the attention of a healer. Together, they can have positive effects upon healing. In fact, recent scientific studies have estimated that the placebo effect/meaning response accounts for 10% to 90% of even modern pharmaceuticals' efficacy (Van der Geest et al. 1996:167). "Meaning can make your immune system work better, and it can make your aspirin work better, too" (Moerman 2002:20). Virtually any kind of treatment that decreases the patient's anxiety can reduce blood pressure and hormones released when under stress to better enable the body to heal itself (Rabin 1999). As many healers, both popular and biomedical, know, time is a great healer. Irish Physician and folklorist Patrick Logan elaborates, most "physical illnesses—over 80% of them—will get better no matter what treatment is given to them." "Even today, the best medicine is reassurance and the ability to reassure a patient does not always go along with a medical degree" (Logan 1994:1).

IRISH HEALERS

Irish women, like Mrs. Huxley, were their family's first line of defense against illnesses and injuries. They devised preventive measures, diagnosed ailments, and created and administered treatments (Jones 2012:39). They learned recipes passed down in their own and neighbor's families for ointments, cough medicines, poultices, and herbal infusions to treat aches and sprains, colds and coughs. As mentioned previously, some families also possessed special charm cures. Other individuals had greater knowledge of herbal cures and/or specialized skills, and people sought them out when their own home remedies failed or when they encountered a particularly serious ailment. People had tremendous faith in these cures.

These healers with more advanced knowledge and skills included midwives, bonesetters, herb doctors, and fairy doctors or wisewomen. They learned their skills through informal apprenticeship, usually with a family member, although it was said that some wisewomen and fairy doctors could communicate with the fairies and learned from them (Gregory 1920:43; Ó Crualaoich 2003:71–76). Even professional physicians recognized the skill of some of these practitioners. For example, according to Logan (1994:90–93), traditional bonesetters knew better techniques and were more skillful in their execution than 19th- and early 20th-century orthopedists. Other individuals were thought to have curative powers as a result of divine gift, circumstance of birth, life experience, or occupation. These included priests (to cure strokes, paralysis, and fever); the seventh consecutively born son or daughter in a family (to cure worms or illness, in general); a "posthumous child," a child born after his/her father's death (to cure headache, thrush, ringworm, sore eyes, or whooping cough); a woman married to a man with the same surname as her maiden surname, or such a couple (to cure whooping cough or lockjaw); a blacksmith (to cure abscesses, bleeding, chilblains, liver complaints, sores, or warts); a person who had licked a lizard or a frog (to cure burns); and a man riding a horse, usually a white horse (to cure whooping cough).[22] Most Irish popular healers were thus neighbors, relatives, or friends with whom the afflicted already had some kind of social connection. They shared the same cultural perspectives and usually similar backgrounds. Patients sought out particular healers because of the healer's previous successes that had built a good reputation. Mrs. Huxley seems to have sent for Dr. Townsend for similar reasons; he lived nearby, had successfully treated one of her boarders, and had a reputation as a yellow fever expert. Unfortunately, she soon discovered that his perspectives about illness and healing were different from hers, and his manner did not appear to inspire her confidence in his prescriptions.

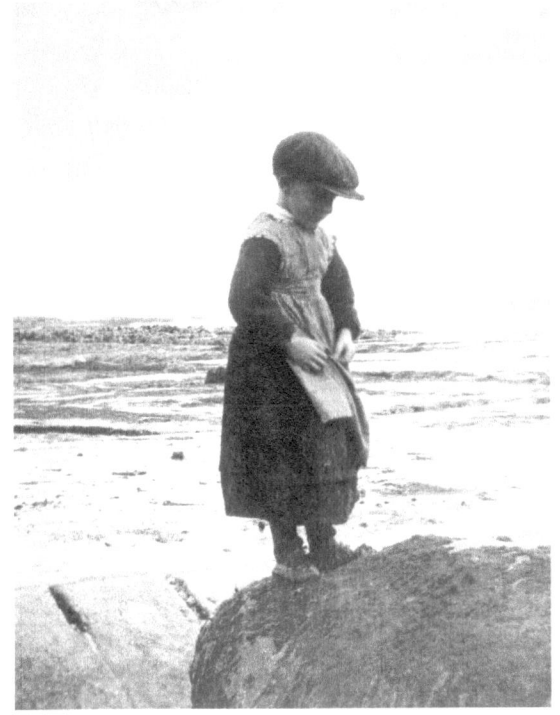

FIGURE 1.2. "Aran boy on a rock, Insihmaan, Co. Galway" (National Folklore Collection 1930). This photograph shows an Irish boy dressed in what appears to be girls' clothing, a traditional strategy to prevent fairy capture. Courtesy of the School of Irish, Celtic Studies, Irish Folklore and Linguistics, University College Dublin and the National Folklore Collection.

Professional physicians like Dr. Townsend marketed themselves in both the U.S. and Ireland as formally educated generalists able to treat a wide variety of ailments. Ordinary Irish people, however, did not revere an academic medical education or ascribe to the same notions of expertise. They were, in fact, highly skeptical and even fearful of professional physicians, whom they generally saw as egocentric outsiders, possessing little practical knowledge, who could cause more harm than good. As Lady Wilde (1887b:110) explained, "The fairies have an aversion to the sight of blood; and the peasants, therefore, have a great objection to being bled, lest the 'good people' would be angry. Besides, they have much more faith in charms and incantations than in any dispensary doctor that ever practised amongst them." Another collector of oral history reported in 1899 that doctors were distrusted because "it is very generally believed among the Irish peasantry in Macroom, County Cork, Ireland, that medicine of any sort is made of dead men, some persons have a horror of taking doctor's medicine because they believe it to be thus concocted. Corpses taken by body-snatchers from the grave are popularly supposed to be used by doctors in manufacturing medicines" (Bergen 1899:159).[23] Additionally, the Irish believed that healing knowledge had been fragmented (Blake 1918:218) and that different people possessed different portions of this knowledge, which they gained from others or through circumstance and/or supernatural inspiration.[24] Many Irish immigrants, likely including Mrs. Huxley, thus viewed physicians' prescriptions not as the correct or only way to treat an ailment, but as one of many approaches that they could reject or modify at will on the basis of their own ideas or those of others.

This perspective of the fragmentation of healing knowledge was part of a much broader rural Irish understanding of society and personhood that generally favored egalitarianism and collectivism over hierarchy and individualism, a perspective that ethnographer Estyn Evans and historian Robert Scally have called "throughother." Throughother describes both the complex rundale system of unmarked Irish agricultural plots in Irish hamlets (or *clachans*), such that a person literally had to walk through another's plot to get to his own, and the communal aspects of Irish life. Within this social world, reciprocity, generosity, and humility were obligations (Evans 1973:60; Scally 1995:13, 235). Scally (1995:235) affirms that "of course individuals in a townland [Irish village] possessed egos, but these were restrained to a remarkable degree by collective taboos against vanity and selfishness." As I will elaborate upon in subsequent chapters, especially Chapter 7, from this Irish perspective, individuals who did not conduct themselves according to these norms faced not only social censure but also supernatural punishment that could interfere with their health.[25] Irish healers interviewed in the 1970s by folklorist Anthony D. Buckley adhered to the expectations of throughother. They stressed that their healing powers were gifts, not their own achievements, and stated that bragging or charging a monetary fee could cause them to lose their healing abilities and their friends. Most accepted token gifts or verbal expressions of thanks for their work. Some also mentioned that their abilities came with negative repercussions for them personally, such as poor personal health, and emphasized that their gift of healing did not put them above others (Buckley 1980:24, 28).

The relationship between Mrs. Huxley and Dr. Townsend was thus quite different than that between a patient (or a patient's family member) and a traditional healer in Ireland. In trying to keep his "stiff upper lip" and in bragging about his antimony prescription, it is likely that Dr. Townsend's demeanor appeared distant and haughty to Mrs. Huxley. Dr. Townsend also charged Mrs. Huxley a hefty fee of $15 (Townsend 1847:51), more than a laboring Irish man would be able to make in two weeks and about as much as a female seamstress could make in two months in New York City (Groneman 1977:36). Dr. Townsend did not fit Mrs. Huxley's expectations of an Irish healer. He did, however, conform quite well to Irish expectations of an American physician, as I will describe further in the next chapter. In summary, from an etic, outsider's perspective, Irish popular cures and healers addressed the symptoms and anxiety of sick and injured individuals, and some remedies would have helped to resolve underlying causes. They effectively attended to *illness*, the subjective "experience of disvalued changes in states of being and in social function," even if they were not always effective against *disease*, the biomedical concept of "abnormalities in the structure and function of bodily organs and systems" (Eisenberg 1977:11).

The Broader Context of Huxley McGuire's Case and Immigrant Life in New York City

Lower Manhattan in 1847

In addition to recording Huxley's illness and treatment, Dr. Townsend's notes document other features of the Huxley family's life that point to the broader context of Irish immigration in New York City. This section will use Dr. Townsend's notes to sketch out this important background about the physical, social, and economic landscape, as well as health risks and treatment options to set the scene for the chapters that follow. Even the most basic details of Huxley's case record, the date and location, are significant. The year was 1847, also known as "Black '47," because it was the worst year of the Great Famine (1845 to 1852). Many historians have chronicled the famine and its ramifications in Ireland (e.g., Miller 1985; Neal 1998; Ó Gráda 2000; Donnelly 2001; Kinealy 2006; Ó Murchadha 2013), so I will not elaborate further here, except to emphasize the suffering and horror that many Irish refugees experienced and carried with them to places of resettlement.

New York City was chief among those places, as noted in the Introduction. Some of Mrs. Huxley's boarders, including her niece, Mary Ann, or perhaps even little Huxley himself, could have been famine refugees. Mrs. Huxley likely emigrated before the famine, given that she had established a boardinghouse by 1847. Her first husband's surname was McGuire, a name associated with Counties Fermanagh and Cavan—the Ulster counties neighboring Connaught's County Leitrim, where the family of Mary MacLean, whose story begins this book, originated.[26] The mechanization of the linen industry caused many makers of linen cloth to emigrate from this region in the 1830s, and they, in turn, sponsored additional immigrants in subsequent decades (Kenny 1998:27–28). It is likely that Mr. and (then) Mrs. McGuire were part of that initial group.[27]

The location of Mrs. Huxley's boardinghouse (on Church Street between Vesey and Barclay Streets) is also significant relative to the landscape of Irish New York. As Dr. Townsend's casebook notes, it was close to the Astor House (no. 46 in Figure 1.1), an employer of Irish immigrants in service, the second most common form of Irish immigrant employment behind unskilled labor (Griggs 2000:35). It was also the nation's most famous hotel, where politicians from the adjacent City Hall (no. 82) frequently dined. In the following decades, the growing Irish population would dominate New York City politics through the Tammany Hall, the Democratic Party political machine, which offered Irish immigrants jobs and assistance in return for votes and loyalty. A few blocks to the north of Mrs. Huxley's house was the city's leading hospital, New York Hospital (no. 70), where thousands of seriously ill and injured Irish immigrants sought care yearly. For spiritual care, her home was conveniently located only a few steps from St. Peter's Church (no. 47), one of several Roman Catholic churches in Lower Manhattan serving the Irish Catholic immigrants who tended to settle in the lower wards.[28] Only a few more steps to the east took her to Broadway, the city's main thoroughfare lined with shops selling all kinds of products, including several pharmacies, and the street where people of all backgrounds came to see and be seen. Crossing Broadway led to the Sixth Ward, home to numerous tailors' shops, secondhand goods stores, groceries, oyster cellars, saloons, and street vendors, as well as the city's jail, "The Tombs," where Irish immigrants were overrepresented among inmates. Along with the First and the Fourth Wards, the Sixth Ward was heavily Irish, and it was home to the Five Points neighborhood. By 1855, over 50% of the population of the Sixth Ward was foreign born; the Irish (especially from counties Cork, Sligo, Kerry, and Tipperary) outnumbered the Germans, the next largest immigrant group, by about three to one (Groneman Pernicone 1973:34–36; Baics 2016:217; Anbinder et al. 2019a:1610). Lower Manhattan was also populated by many native-born Americans, Black and White, and immigrants from England, Scotland, Italy, and Poland.[29] Thus, while Mrs. Huxley was surrounded by Irish neighbors, she did not live in an exclusively Irish enclave, but in a diverse and cosmopolitan city. She probably chose to keep an intimate Irish social circle, but her daily interactions on the street, in shops, and in her boardinghouse would have put her in contact with non-Irish neighbors, including Dr. Townsend. This physical, if not social, proximity between Irish and native-born Americans likely contributed to anti-Irish sentiment but also ultimately aided the incorporation of the Irish as well, as I will elaborate upon in the chapters that follow.

Economic and Social Relations

New York City's economy grew dramatically during the 19th century, and demand for labor and housing was high. Mrs. Huxley's taking in of boarders was a viable economic strategy adopted by women of many backgrounds in Lower Manhattan (McGowan 2000; Stansell 1986). By renting space and preparing meals, women could earn money and still care for children too young for work or school. Keeping boarders was more profitable than other respectable home-employment options, such as sewing, rug making, or laundry. Some boardinghouse proprietors amassed substantial savings.[30] In the 1850s, the average boarder paid $1.50 a week. Thus, even one boarder generated funds equal to the meager wages of lower-ranking seamstresses, although some of the fee covered the cost of providing meals (Groneman Pernicone 1973:152). This occupation, not always visible in documents such as censuses, was especially appealing to widows or women whose husbands were absent or unable to work. Even in two-income homes, monetary contributions from wives and children were often necessary, however, because the typical wages of male laborers of about $1 per day could not support a family (Groneman Pernicone 1973:153; Stansell 1986:117). To make ends meet, women often needed to take in multiple boarders; this was grueling work. Dr. Townsend (1847:1, 42) described Mrs. Huxley's residence as a "large boarding house," and noted she kept several boarders.

One of the people who lived in Mrs. Huxley's residence, in addition to her grandson, was her niece Mary Ann (Townsend 1847:42). It was common for Irish immigrants in New York to take in newly arrived or struggling relatives or neighbors from their home villages and to help care for children whose parents had died or were unable to support them.[31] Many Irish immigrants, especially those from rural areas or from towns in Kerry and Cork, also settled near one another in the same city neighborhoods and were more economically successful than those who did not.[32] Earlier arrivals often assisted the immigration of family and friends and provided vital intelligence about city life and employment; the latter is visible in the dominance of people from particular regions in particular jobs. Examples include immigrants from Donegal clustering in peddling and Morocco leather dressing; from Tyrone in the charcoal trade; from Castlegregory, Kerry, in the gas works; and from the Lansdowne estate in Kerry in construction (Groneman Pernicone 1973:70; Anbinder et al. 2019:1597, 1612; McMahon 2021:223–226).[33] Obligations of kinship, community, and reciprocity, as well as affection, that had characterized life in Ireland, especially in rural areas, continued to be very important in New York City.

While the employment niches described above often had little to no relation to immigrants' previous occupations in Ireland, those who emigrated with a profession or trade usually attempted to find related work in New York City. It is possible that Mrs. Huxley's first husband, Mr. McGuire, and perhaps Mrs. Huxley herself, had been involved in linen production, given his surname common to southern Ulster, pre-famine immigration, and her second husband's occupation as a merchant tailor (a person who engaged in the buying and tailoring of cloth) (OED 2001b). These connections raise the possibility that Mr. Huxley had been a former (and possibly English, given his surname) business associate of Mr. McGuire (Townsend 1847:7). Mr. and Mrs. Huxley might have been brought together through mutual grief and/or perhaps Mr. Huxley viewed caring for his friend's widow as a personal obligation. Such an arrangement might explain Dr. Townsend's (1847:7) observation of a large age difference between the Huxleys: "Madame's husband is... quite young for her and a very decent father to appearances." In Ireland, it was more common for men to marry later than women, and beginning in the 1830s, financial insecurity led many men and women to delay or never marry. Increased possibility of marriage and choice of spouses attracted immigrants to the U.S. before and after the famine (Miller 1985:57, 219, 408). The records of the Transfiguration Church in the Sixth Ward suggest that many famine-era immigrants chose spouses from their own home counties, which describes nearly 50% of the marriages at the church between 1853 and 1860 (Griggs 2000:48).

For many in Ireland and New York, marriage was an important economic arrangement for spouses and their families. Mrs. Huxley's marriages along with her boardinghouse might have contributed to her better financial position relative to many other Irish women in Lower Manhattan. Dr. Townsend noted that she slept in a feather bed (with Mary Ann and Huxley), provided meat and fish daily to her family and boarders, and was able to pay his hefty $15 bill. Mr. Huxley's occupation as a merchant tailor, if he was successful, would have put him in a higher income bracket than most of the Irish men who began arriving in the 1840s, the majority of whom found work in manual labor or service. In 1850, for example, nearly 80% of Irish men in the Sixth Ward worked as laborers (Groneman Pernicone 1973:115). If the Huxleys had not been able to pay the doctor's bill, they could have turned to friends and family or a local pub or saloon owner. These entrepreneurs often gave short-term loans and/or were connected to one or more of several Irish immigrant aid organizations and the Democratic Party (Rosenzweig 1983). Borrowing from others was a common practice among Irish immigrants, as it was in Ireland (and in many other parts of the world), to survive short-term scarcity. While elite lenders often expected repayment in favors or votes, lenders of more equal rank could expect their generosity to be returned in roughly equal measure and to have the right to call on the borrower for future assistance. Male laborers, who were often their family's major breadwinners, were subject to frequent unemployment, seasonal layoffs, and lost income from illness and injury (Roney 1931; Shumsky 1976; Stott 1990). These informal networks helped many families to get by and to navigate some of the many risks they encountered in the city.

Health Threats and Treatment Options in New York City

Dr. Townsend did not offer any details about how little Huxley came to live with his grandmother, but he did note that the boy was well taken care of. The fact that Huxley was ill and the possibility that he was orphaned points to the serious health threats Irish immigrants encountered while emigrating and once living in New York City. The following chapters will provide more details about these conditions. Here I will sketch out an overview, led by the details of Huxley's case. Lower Manhattan in the late 1840s and early 1850s was not a healthy place. Mortality rates were high. Between 1845 and 1854, the death rate in the city reached an all-time peak of 40 deaths per 1,000 (Blackmar 1995:57). Contemporaries pointed to epidemic disease, such as cholera and typhus fever, and often pointed their fingers at the Irish (see Chapter 2), but the majority of excess mortality citywide was generated by endemic illnesses, including tuberculosis (see Chapter 6) and dysentery, accidents, maternal death in childbirth, and infant death (Condran 1995; Haines 2001). Immigrants fleeing famine and death in Ireland arrived to a city in the midst of an ongoing public health disaster. They suffered disproportionately, and young children were at greatest risk.

Health threats were exacerbated by the city's inability to keep up services and housing for a population skyrocketing from domestic migration and international immigration; the population grew from 124,000 in 1820 to 516,000 in 1850 (Stott 1990:11). Wealthier neighborhoods and less densely populated areas on the northern fringes of the city, which reached to about 14th Street in the 1830s and to 42nd Street by the mid-1850s, were healthier. Some Irish immigrants settled on the fringes or in the villages even further to the north of the island, such as Bloomingdale, Yorkville, and Seneca Village, but Lower Manhattan, where the Irish were most concentrated, was overcrowded and lacked good sanitation and regulation of housing and industry. Much of the Sixth Ward had been created by infilling the Collect Pond and surrounding marshy areas, after the pond had become polluted with industrial, animal, and human waste. Problems with dampness and drainage persisted for decades.

Refuse and horse manure littered most streets to several inches in depth and raw sewage seeped into tenement yards, basement apartments, and wells (Keeney 1865; Thoms 1865; Maguire 1868; Milne 2000). Even when laws were passed requiring tenement owners to increase apartment ventilation or connect privies to sewers, few made changes in poorer neighborhoods, such as the Five Points, where most landlords did not reside in their buildings (Milne 2000:355). In mid-19th-century New York City, "access to health depended primarily on the personal ability to be able to pay for a healthy environment" (Blackmar 1995:43). Most Irish immigrants could not afford a healthier neighborhood, and too many paid the ultimate price.

The environment surrounding Mrs. Huxley's residence in the Third Ward was better drained and thus somewhat healthier, yet details from Huxley's case record reveal he was unable to escape all of Lower Manhattan's health risks.[34] In addition to Huxley's fever and bronchitis, Mrs. Huxley told the doctor that her grandson had recently recovered from a case of whooping cough (pertussis), an infection causing a wheezing cough and difficulty breathing that can be life threatening for children. Dr. Townsend instructed Mrs. Huxley to boil her grandson's milk, suggesting the doctor knew that much of the milk sold in the city was dangerous. In response to complaints since the 1840s, *Frank Leslie's Illustrated Newspaper* (1858a) published an exposé in 1858, showing that many local producers sold milk from sickened cows fed on distillery waste that they adulterated with plaster and other substances to make it appear more wholesome. It was estimated that this "swill milk" caused thousands of infant deaths each year (McNeur 2014:153). Although it was not known at the time, it is likely that many of these cows were infected with bovine tuberculosis (*Mycobacterium bovis*), one of several related types of bacteria that can cause tuberculosis in humans by ingesting infected milk or meat or inhaling air exhaled by infected animals or humans. Tuberculosis reached epidemic proportions among the Irish in New York around the middle of the century and was a leading cause of morbidity and mortality (see Chapter 6).

Thus, even inside the Huxleys' residence, little Huxley was not safe, because of germs carried by boarders and the potential of drinking tainted milk or eating spoiled food. The term "summer complaint" was coined in the 1840s to describe an acute condition of diarrhea that could be fatal to children, caused by food contamination and spoilage common during warm summer months before reliable refrigeration (OED 2017). Ireland has a more temperate climate, and newly arrived Irish immigrants were unaccustomed to dealing with the extreme temperatures they encountered in New York City. This posed problems beyond food. Laboring men complained of being forced by bosses to work at dangerously fast paces, and they were frequently admitted to New York Hospital with sunstroke (NYHAR 1846–1853). Newspapers reported deaths from falling off fire escapes and roofs, where people slept to avoid the heat of overcrowded tenements in the summer, and deaths from freezing in the winter.

The winter, thus, also had its challenges, aggravated by seasonal layoffs in many industries employing Irish immigrant men. Families sometimes had to choose between spending money on food or fuel. Irish immigrant laborer and later labor leader Frank Roney expressed in his diary his worry that his wife and son's health would be compromised because they could not afford enough fuel (Shumsky 1976). Even those who could keep their houses warm faced other dangers. During one of Dr. Townsend's visits in December, Mrs. Huxley pointed out what she feared was blood coming from Huxley's nose. The doctor determined it to be soot from the coal fire used for cooking and heating the house (Townsend 1847:42). Particulates from coal fires, gas lamps, and other pollution only worsened respiratory problems, including bronchitis and pulmonary tuberculosis. Serious burns from these fires and gas lamps also were common, most often injuring women and children (NHMCB 1847–1853, 1865).

The medical options to treat illness and injury in 19th-century New York City were multiple although, as noted previously, the state of professional medicine was such that few treatments effected cures, and some were downright harmful. Mrs. Huxley had access to a number of different kinds of healers. They included professional, trained and licensed physicians; physicians trained in alternative medicine, such as homeopathy; untrained and unlicensed so-called physicians; licensed and unlicensed pharmacists; midwives; faith healers (including priests); folk healers (such as wise women); and friends and relatives with knowledge of home remedies or charm cures. Consistent with the popular Irish view that medical knowledge had been fragmented, available evidence suggests Irish immigrants often sought out multiple healers and self-medicated. Mrs. Huxley, for example, continued to administer her own treatments to Huxley alongside Dr. Townsend's, despite his objections. Self-medication was typical, and options included popular home remedies originating in Ireland, pharmaceuticals purchased from a druggist/drugstore, and patent or proprietary medicines, which were enormously popular and heavily marketed at the time (see Chapters 3, 5, and 7).

Requesting a house call from a professional physician was the most expensive of these treatment options. Mrs. Huxley's willingness to summon Dr. Townsend suggests she was concerned about her grandson and felt she had exhausted other options. A benefit of a house call was that it allowed Mrs. Huxley to have more control over her grandson's treatment than in either an outpatient dispensary or an inpatient hospital setting, the places where people could access professional physicians for lesser costs. As I will describe in subsequent chapters, most New Yorkers, including Irish immigrants, feared American hospitals for good reason and used them only in the most desperate of circumstances. New York Hospital and the New York Dispensary, both well-regarded institutions, were within a few blocks of Mrs. Huxley's boardinghouse and within easy walking distance from the Five Points and the Sixth Ward. The city's public hospitals, Bellevue and Ward's Island, were farther away and had poorer reputations. As of 1849, Mrs. Huxley would have had an additional hospital to consider. To address the staggering needs of Irish famine refugees, the Sisters of Charity, a Roman Catholic order of nuns, established St. Vincent's Hospital during that year at 102 East 13th Street between 3rd and 4th Avenue (Walsh 1965:9). As I will show, St. Vincent's, and the sisters who provided nursing there, more often met Irish immigrants' expectations of care. Over time, St. Vincent's and other hospitals established by and for immigrants changed healthcare in the U.S.

Despite the efforts of the Sisters of Charity, physicians, including Dr. Townsend, Irish grandmothers, such as Mrs. Huxley, and many other healers, illness and injury were unavoidable elements of Irish immigrant life in New York City from the 1840s through the 1860s. Dangers included unsanitary and overcrowded living conditions, grueling and dangerous labor, industrial and household pollution, extreme temperatures, anti-Irish prejudice, and more. All these hazards, when combined with economic instability and emotional and/or physical trauma from immigration, proved to be a toxic potion. Irish mortality rates were the highest in the city. Children, such as Huxley, suffered especially. Women and men, too, faced premature death, illness, and disability. This was the context of Irish immigrant life in Lower Manhattan in the middle of the 19th century and the backdrop of the strained interaction between Dr. Townsend and Mrs. Huxley.

Conclusion

This chapter used the medical case record of a young boy to detail the differing medical perspectives of Irish immigrants and native-born American physicians and to describe the broader health-related context of Irish life in mid-19th-century New York City. Details of the case show that while Dr. Townsend and Mrs. Huxley agreed upon little Huxley's symptoms—extreme congestion and fever—their understandings of the causes of and proper treatment for these symptoms diverged. Mrs. Huxley viewed the ultimate cause as worms and opted for mild treatments to drive them out and strengthen her grandson. Dr. Townsend saw humoral imbalance as the cause, aggravated by an overly indulgent diet, and advocated harsh chemical depletion and little food. That Dr. Townsend was so perturbed by potatoes, in particular, is revealing and again points to the broader context of Irish immigration.

Consternation about potatoes most obviously evokes the Great Famine, which was happening at the very moment the doctor attended to Huxley and which was brought on by a pathogen that devastated the potato crop, the main source of food for much of Ireland's population. As historian Cormac Ó Gráda (2000:17) notes, the "Irish were Europe's 'potato people' *par excellence*." This association was well known by the 18th century, when some English cartoonists even depicted Irish people as potatoes. In Ireland, potato consumption crosscut divisions of class and religion, and the Irish maintained their preference for potatoes even after emigration. Among other European groups, potatoes were not nearly so popular, in large part because they associated potatoes with poverty and considered them to be a dirty and crude food unfit for people with delicate or genteel constitutions, as most middle-class Europeans and Americans preferred to think of themselves (Ó Gráda 2000:14–18). The association that the English, and then Americans, made between the Irish and potatoes only reinforced the perceived crudity of both. When faced with the flood of Irish famine refugees, many Americans found the Irish, like the potatoes upon which they so depended, to be difficult to digest.

Dr. Townsend's concern over Huxley eating potatoes was ostensibly related to Huxley's fever but spoke to these broader American concerns about incorporating Irish immigrants, and perhaps even more importantly, their children, into American society. Many Americans feared that carrying on practices such as eating potatoes, drinking whiskey, waking the dead, and adhering to Catholicism would reproduce Irish culture in the U.S. and prohibit assimilation. If the lines between nature and nurture were permeable, as some well-intentioned Americans hoped, their greatest chances of Americanizing the Irish lay in "properly" cultivating their children. Huxley's unrelenting fever thus might have been concerning to Dr. Townsend, not only because he feared a poor health outcome, but also because it suggested the boy possessed an overheated sanguine humoral temperament, inherited from his Irish parents and fostered by his grandmother's care. The next chapter fleshes out these American ideas about Irish temperaments and how they informed prejudicial stereotypes, which intensified in response to a particular fever that afflicted many famine refugees.

CHAPTER 2

"Irish Fever"

Typhus Fever and an Epidemic of Anti-Irish Prejudice

WHILE DR. TOWNSEND and Mrs. Huxley disagreed about her grandson's fever inside her New York City boardinghouse (see Chapter 1), outside, hundreds of immigrants arrived daily, most from Ireland and the German States, hoping to escape the famine, economic inequality, and political instability affecting these regions during the late 1840s. The poor conditions in their home countries and during their long journeys took a toll on their health. Many arrived suffering from a particular serious illness, epidemic typhus fever.[1] In a rare firsthand account of a steerage passenger, William Smith, a Manchester native and "power-loom weaver," recorded how he became ill with the disease while aboard the ship *India* between Liverpool and New York in the winter of 1847–1848.[2] He described the characteristic symptoms, including high fever, weakness, headache, myalgia, reddish rash, and delirium. Smith attributed the outbreak that took the lives of twenty-six of his fellow passengers at sea and put him and another 122 into the Staten Island Quarantine Hospital to filthy and crowded shipboard conditions, poor ventilation, lack of a physician, and inadequate provisions, all not unusual on immigrant ships of this period. After surviving poor treatment in the hospital, he sought lodging but was refused. One family said his "looks were enough to frighten anyone, and if their neighbors saw, they would say that [he] had just broke loose from the grave." The following day Smith observed people move away and stare at him in a railway car. A stranger warned him not to tell anyone that he had had typhus: "I might say that I was ill with dysentery, (which was true), but by no means admit that I had ever had the ship-fever" (Smith 1850:8, 15, 29). Why was admitting to having active dysentery acceptable, but admitting to having recovered from typhus unacceptable? Why would typhus leave a lasting stigma?

Smith was not alone in observing that typhus fever proliferated in crowded and unsanitary places. Although the cause of the disease was not known until the late 19th century, for centuries typhus had been called names that reflected the places where it was observed, such as [military] camp fever, gaol fever, hospital fever, and ship fever. Yet in 1847, during the height of the Great Famine in Ireland, it acquired a new name. Public officials in Liverpool, concerned by outbreaks among Irish famine refugees huddled along the docks and in crowded boardinghouses, dubbed it the "Irish fever" (Hardy 1988:405; Scally 1995:206; Gallman 2000:87; Darwen et al. 2020). This name was significant because, unlike previous names, it correlated the disease not with a place but with *a people*. This fear that Irish themselves, and not necessarily the ships in which they immigrated or the places where they sought refuge, were sources of typhus quickly crossed the Atlantic to the U.S.

A variety of sources suggest that Irish immigrants experienced considerable suffering from typhus fever, the leading cause of deaths aboard immigrant ships originating in Europe during the famine years (McMahon 2021:148). Major typhus outbreaks in New York City corresponded with peak years of Irish immigration, 1848, 1851, 1864, and 1865; thousands of Irish were treated with the disease in the city's hospitals; and eyewitness accounts from healthcare officials, firsthand experiences in immigrant letters, and mortality data from Ireland, Canada, and New York attest that typhus was a major threat to health in Ireland and the places the Irish sought refuge (NYHAR 1849–1854; Smith 1850; Commissioners of Emigration 1861:12; McArthur 1956; MacShane 1958; Maguire 1868; O'Connell 1980; Condran 1995; Crawford 1999). Yet, historians, including Raymond Cohn (1984:296–297; 1987:390), Cormac Ó Gráda (2000:106–107), and Cian McMahon (2021:147–160) have shown that during the famine years overall, greater mortality on immigrant ships was not statistically correlated with any one national group. Typhus fever also infected English, German, and other passengers on the same and other ships, many originating in England, but it was not called the "English fever" or the "German fever" or even the "immigrant fever."

This chapter explores how Americans initially reacted to Irish immigrants in the late 1840s and early 1850s and why many saw a meaningful and stigmatizing connection between typhus fever and the Irish, focusing on New York City. It suggests that humoral theory guided their interpretations in important ways, an idea that has not been investigated previously. Humoral theory offered authoritative medical support for preexisting Irish stereotypes and anti-Irish prejudice; fit within British, American, and Irish nationalist discourses about an age-old struggle between Celts and Saxons; and responded to American nativist concerns, including how to categorize and absorb poor Whites in a context in which Americans increasingly looked to race "science" to try to find natural, physical roots of racial, ethnic, and class difference. Typhus fever, and its particular symptoms, offered visible evidence to Americans that there was something essentially different and dangerous about the Irish that was manifest in their physiology, in their sanguine temperaments. "Irish fever" fed a "second epidemic" of prejudice (Farmer 1993) that increased the challenges the Irish faced in New York City and prompted harmful misdiagnoses in the very hospitals where they sought care.

From Ship Fever to Irish Fever: Public Health and Quarantine in 19th-Century New York City

In the mid-1840s news of deadly epidemic fever spotted among Irish immigrants in Liverpool and Quebec reached New York City and became a leading concern among the residents of eastern cities, an "object of everyday conversation and not a little dread" (Knobel 2001:3). These cities, and New York especially, were already struggling with high morbidity and mortality. Between 1810 and 1845, New York City's death rate had nearly doubled and, according to a statistician reporting to the state assembly, was "greater than in any city and at any period where life was valuable enough to be numbered" (Blackmar 1995:42). In the previous few decades there had been outbreaks of yellow fever, malaria, smallpox, and cholera (Condran 1995). This did not stem the flow of newcomers from other parts of the U.S. and the world from crowding into the city. The population swelled from 124,000 in 1820 to 313,000 in 1840, and then soared to 516,000 in 1850, largely from Irish immigration (Stott 1990:11; Blackmar 1995:42). Crowded and run-down housing and poor sanitary conditions in many neighborhoods, combined with the limited medical knowledge and tools of the day, made controlling disease nearly impossible, even before the arrival of the fever. The average New Yorker blamed both the city and newcomers for outbreaks of disease.

Memories of the terrifying 1832 cholera epidemic, the very same that afflicted Mary MacLean and her family, still haunted New Yorkers in the 1840s, and those of more advanced age might have remembered the yellow fever epidemic of 1795 as well. Like yellow fever, cholera had been brought to North America by ship. An Irish family was said to have had the first identified cases of cholera in New York City. Infection rates were highest in the Five Points neighborhood, and according to the Board of Health, the "low Irish suffered the most, being exceedingly dirty in their habits, much addicted to intemperance and crowded together in the worst portions of the city." Cholera quickly spread and spared neither the wealthy nor the native born, however, taking the lives of more than 3,500 New Yorkers that year (Rosenberg 1987a:25–26, 33, 62). Epidemic disease and even cholera contributed far less to overall mortality than endemic disease and accidents, but as demographer Gretchen Condran (1995:33) explains, epidemic diseases "elicited such widespread fear and response that their psychological and political impact is only partially measured by the resulting death rate." Thus, as famine refugees began to arrive in unprecedented numbers only a little more than a decade later, New Yorkers were already concerned about public health, and they were primed to view ships as conveyors of deadly epidemics and immigrants, particularly impoverished Irish newcomers, as sources of disease.

As in the case of the 1832 cholera epidemic, New Yorkers had advance warning of outbreaks of typhus fever at other ports. Newspaper reports and correspondence from England and Canada painted dire pictures. Several ships arrived in Quebec from Cork and Liverpool in late 1846 and early 1847 with unusually appalling numbers of typhus infections and deaths; 15% to 19% of passengers died at sea or in hospitals on land. The *Ceylon*, originating in Liverpool, sailed into New York Harbor with shocking levels of disease a few months later. Dr. John Griscom—quarantine inspector, New York Hospital physician, and public health reformer—described how in the steerage, he encountered scores of "emaciated half-nude figures, many with the petechial rupture [of typhus fever] disfiguring their faces . . . present[ing] a picture of which neither pen nor pencil can convey a full idea." These ships were atypical even in 1847, as others had only a few cases of fever or none at all, but they made a strong impression upon New Yorkers (The Select Committee of the Senate of the United States 1854:54; McMahon 2021:155).

Contributing to the alarm was the fact that few American physicians had previously seen outbreaks of the disease.[3] From time to time there had been cases aboard previous immigrant ships, but typhus was considered foreign to the Americas. Historians of medicine suspect there had been outbreaks among British soldiers during the Revolutionary War and among English and Irish immigrants in Philadelphia in the 1830s, but for reasons yet unknown, they were limited and short-lived (Humphreys 2006:271–278). Familiarity with typhus did not lessen fear, however, because even in Europe, where the disease had long been known, physicians did not understand its cause or how to cure it. Competing theories included miasma, "noxious vapour rising from putrescent organic matter" (OED 2001a); peculiar atmospheric conditions; and *de novo* generation "from any number of predisposing factors."[4] Physicians identified filthy and unventilated conditions as dangerous but could not explain why certain individuals and not others became infected. Old notions about predisposing temperaments, and even divine punishment, filled this gap (Murchison 1862:265; Hamlin 1992:48).

Today, scientists understand epidemic typhus fever to be caused by *Rickettsia prowazekii* bacteria and spread by body lice. Lice eat blood of an infected person and excrete the bacteria in their feces. When an infected louse moves to a new human host, its bites cause the individual to scratch their skin, enabling the bacteria to enter their body. Lice can move from person to person by direct contact or by shared clothing or bedding. Inhaling the feces of infected lice on clothing and bedding can also spread typhus, and this method of transmission is a particular danger to healthcare providers. Typhus thrives in unsanitary and cold environments where malnourished or otherwise ill people are crowded together and the cold encourages wearing of clothing and huddling together (Goldman and Bennett 2000:1769; Humphreys 2006:271). It is thus not surprising that cases of typhus on famine-era immigrant ships peaked during cold months (McMahon 2021). This etiology was not proven until 1909, however. Adding to the confusion, until at least the 1860s, physicians had trouble distinguishing epidemic typhus fever from fevers with some similar symptoms, including marine typhus, typhoid, relapsing fever, and pellagra (J. P. 1872; Crawford 1981, 1999; Hardy 1988; Condran 1995).[5] As I will show, many New Yorkers, including physicians, considered Irishness to be a predisposing factor of typhus fever and the presence of Irish immigrants to distinguish typhus from other fevers.

Another aspect of epidemic typhus that differentiated it from other fevers and raised alarm was its comparatively high lethality. Today, death rates among infected people range from 10% to 60% in the absence of antibiotic treatment, the cure for the disease which was not available in the 19th century. Adults, especially the elderly, are more likely to die from typhus than children. Historians of medicine estimate that death rates in 19th-century Europe, where the disease was more prevalent, ranged from 20% to 45%, with a lower upper end of the range because of acquired immunity from previous exposure. Typhus fever survivors can experience a recurrence, now called Brill-Zinsser disease, years or even decades later, which can make them a source of a new outbreak, if they become infected with lice (Goldman and Bennett 2000; Humphreys 2006:271–272). The lower end of 19th-century typhus mortality is estimated to be higher than in the present, in part, because physicians' treatments were often more harmful than helpful, as will be described later in the chapter. Some physicians openly acknowledged that there was little they could do for typhus patients. "Typhus fever cannot be arrested by any drug or medical means," declared Dr. William McLeod of the prestigious Royal College of Physicians, Edinburgh in 1847, for example (*Scientific American* 1847:43).[6] Most agreed it was contagious, however, and their recommendations to isolate the sick and wash, burn, or, later, disinfect their clothing and living spaces had some success (Hardy 1988:408). Thus, in the 1840s, public health officials concentrated primarily upon two measures to try to avert an outbreak on U.S. soil, limiting the number of immigrants allowed on ships and intensifying an old, but tried-and-true, method to contain disease: quarantining sick foreigners.

The federal government did little to regulate immigration in the mid-19th century, but it responded in 1847 with a new passenger law. The new regulation expanded the amount of space required per passenger, with the goal of reducing crowding and increasing air circulation and sanitation that had been lacking on many British emigrant ships (like the one upon which William Smith sailed), which had higher rates of illness among passengers than American or German ships.[7] To meet the demands of an unprecedented number of emigrants in the late 1840s, especially 1847, some British ships had been pressed into service that were woefully inadequate for transporting people across the ocean. Lax enforcement, overwhelmed inspectors, and a laissez-faire approach to business in Britain enabled them to set sail. The new U.S. passenger law, followed in subsequent years by additional U.S. and U.K. regulations, improved conditions. It also reduced the total number of passengers a ship could carry and thus the number of arrivals at American ports. Irish immigrants' own increasing preference for superior American ships, especially packet ships that departed Liverpool on regular schedules, also helped to decrease overall rates of shipboard deaths. By 1849, American emigrant ships outnumbered British ships arriving in the port of New York by two to one (McMahon 2021:5–11). American ships were not immune to typhus, however, and their more expensive fares meant that poorer emigrants continued to travel on poorer ships. Shipboard outbreaks thus continued.

Individual states controlled immigration during much of the 19th century (Hirota 2017). New York, Boston, and other eastern port cities ramped up enforcement of laws requiring ships carrying immigrants to moor in harbors until quarantine officers could examine passengers. From 1800 through the mid-1840s, most passengers who failed inspection in New York City, including William Smith, were sent to the Marine Hospital on Staten Island, also known as the "Quarantine Hospital." Their care was funded by a tax on incoming immigrant ships and no other aid was provided to immigrants when they passed inspection or were released from the hospital. This situation was a threat to public health and was also dangerous for newcomers, who were vulnerable to a variety of scams perpetrated by swindlers, as well as latent illness. In response to the wave of famine-era immigration and fears of typhus on American soil, concerned citizens—including John Hughes, the Irish-born Catholic Bishop of New York; Andrew Carrigan, a wealthy Irish-born businessman and later president of the New York Irish Emigrant Society; and prominent politicians—lobbied the New York State Legislature to create a commission to manage newcomers. The Board of the Commissioners of Emigration was established in 1847 to provide for the "relief and protection" of immigrants up to five years after their arrival. They supplied emergency medical care, temporary shelter and food "in cases of apparent, absolute necessity," and advice and job placement. The Commissioners took charge of the Marine Hospital and established the State Emigrant Refuge on Ward's Island that same year (Commissioners of Emigration 1861:iv, 115; Hirota 2017:66).

These two hospitals were designed to hold only a few hundred patients each, and they were quickly overcrowded and overwhelmed, largely by typhus fever patients. Between May and December of 1847 alone, 5,740 immigrants were diagnosed with typhus fever and treated at the Marine Hospital, comprising nearly 83% of admitted patients and representing about 4.5% of the total immigrants who arrived at the port during that time, according to Commissioners' (1861:290) records.[8] New York, Bellevue, and later St. Vincent's Hospital (established in 1849) were marshalled to accept overflow and recently arrived sick or injured immigrants already in the city who could not be transported to a quarantine hospital.[9] Challenges continued into the 1850s. During the harsh winter of 1851–1852, there was another spike in typhus fever cases; the Marine Hospital was so overcrowded that physicians were unable to classify newly admitted patients. Its official capacity was 556 beds, but for months it housed more than 1000 patients, some of them in unheated and unventilated adjacent warehouses that one physician described as "sepulchers for the dry bones of the living" (Duffy 1968:493, 496).[10] The need was so great that the Commissioners of Emigration created three shelters within the city center, one on Centre Street, another on Canal Street, and a third in an abandoned church on Duane Street.

Despite good intentions, the Commissioners' measures were underwhelming in the face of so many sick immigrants in the late 1840s and early 1850s, and they met a variety of complaints. Survivors of the quarantine hospitals complained of poor treatment (see Chapter 3). Newspaper editors and members of the public complained that quarantine measures were ineffective: ship-board inspections were lax, especially for wealthier passengers, and put the resident population at risk (Kraut 1996:157; *Citizen* 1854a:225).[11] Of several explanations for how recent immigrants could pass quarantine inspections and fall ill shortly afterward, one is the incubation period of typhus, which is now understood to be one to two weeks. Many such individuals became patients at Bellevue or New York Hospital, but some suffered without formal medical attention in run-down boardinghouses, tenement apartments, private "hospitals" set up by ship brokers, or even in public on the street (Maguire 1868:185–186). "The condition and habits . . . as well as their state of health . . . prove[d] a subject of annoyance or alarm to the neighborhood" (Commissioners of Emigration 1861:115).[12] In response to some of these complaints, Castle Garden at the southern tip of Manhattan was made an official landing depot and location for immigrant assistance in 1855. That did not prevent local Staten Island residents from burning down the Marine Hospital (after evacuating the patients) in 1858 to express their fear of immigrants bringing foreign diseases that could wreak havoc in the U.S. (Figure 2.1).

Each of these imperfect New York City institutions treated immigrants from many nations for typhus fever in the late 1840s and early 1850s. Among them were German and English immigrants, who often traveled

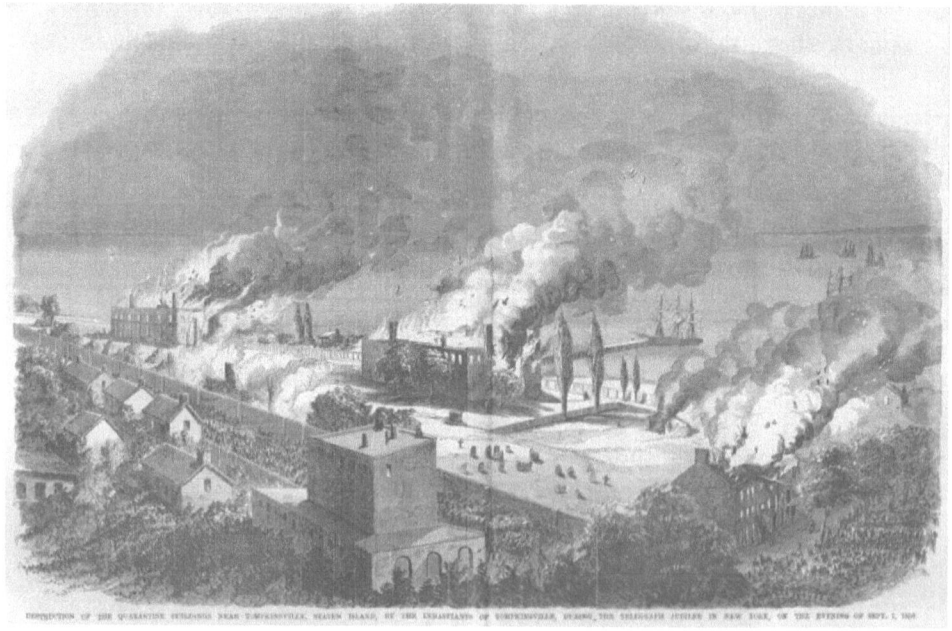

FIGURE 2.1. "Destruction of the Quarantine Buildings near Tompkinsville, Staten Island, by the Inhabitants of Tompkinsville, During the Telegraph Jubilee in New York, on the Evening of Sept. 1, 1858," *Frank Leslie's Illustrated Newspaper* (1858b).

on the same ships as the Irish, but the Irish consistently outnumbered other groups sent to hospitals. This greater numerical presence certainly contributed to the perceived connection between the Irish and typhus fever, but other important factors emerge with a closer examination of preexisting anti-Irish prejudices and Americans' visceral reactions to immigrants' physical appearances.

Anti-Irish Prejudice in the U.S. and American Practical and Ideological Concerns

Anti-foreign sentiment has existed in the U.S. in one form or another since the nation's founding. Max Berger's (1946:174–175) study of over 230 19th-century British travelers' accounts found a "dislike for all foreigners" and a particular mistrust of British visitors was commonplace, but by the late 1830s, a disdain for Irish immigrants emerged. Then the "Famine Emigration fanned this sentiment to a white heat." Other historians have also noted an increase and hardening of anti-Irish prejudice coinciding with the arrival of famine-era immigrants. Their explanations have focused largely on the practical economic, social, political challenges many Americans believed this group posed, as well as religious conflict (Knobel 1986, 2001; Kenny 2006; Hirota 2017). In addition to these concerns, I propose that the shocking appearances of some famine-era Irish immigrants drew out deep ideological concerns about American identity and citizenship.

In the 1830s, the demographic composition of Irish immigrants shifted such that less prosperous and Catholic individuals became predominant. Historians have suggested that American nativists, who were largely Protestants of real or imagined Anglo descent, feared that this group's Catholicism, cultural practices such as drinking alcohol, and frequent need of assistance upon arrival indicated they would become perpetually dependent upon public resources. This could lead to a permanent underclass, bringing unwanted European class stratification to the U.S. Reports from American and other travelers to Ireland reinforced such views. They portrayed the Irish populace as poverty-stricken and the depths of Irish poverty to be lower than anywhere else. Also influencing this Irish pauper narrative were British stereotypes of the Irish as irrational, ignorant, lacking desire for self-improvement, prone to

66 "Irish Fever"

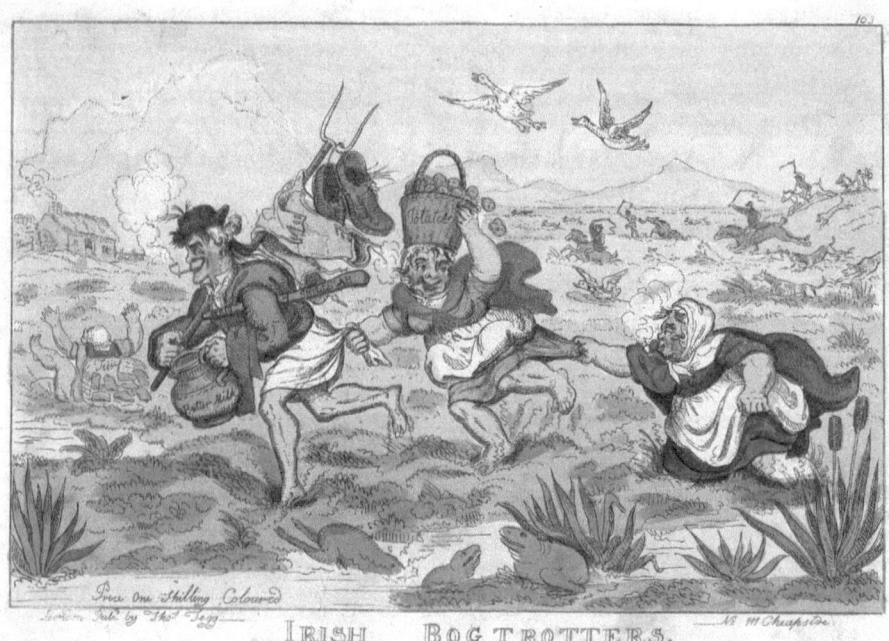

FIGURE 2.2. Hand-colored etching attributed to William Elmes and published by Thomas Tegg in *The Caricature Magazine or Hudibrastic Mirror* in London in 1812. It depicts Irish people as ruddy-complexioned, clumsy, barefoot, immodest (exposing their legs), pipe-smoking, pugnacious (note the shillelagh), and generally uncivilized people who live close to the earth. Courtesy of the Digital Commonwealth, Massachusetts Collections Online, Boston Public Library.

violence, and generally culturally inferior and uncivilized (Figure 2.2). These prejudices had been refined in the crucible of the British colonialist struggle to dominate Ireland, as I will explain in the next section. Such views facilitated the British government's tepid response to the potato blight in the 1840s, including Parliament's Poor Law Extension Act in 1847 that placed the burden of famine relief upon the Irish themselves, resulting in additional suffering and emigration. Poverty was already synonymous with the Irish on both sides of the Atlantic (Berger 1946; Knobel 1986; de Nie 2004; Hirota 2017). On top of that, as historian Kevin Kenny (2006:367) describes, the Irish came to "symbolize immigration and its attendant problems."

American nativists called Irish immigrants "leeches" who would drain public funds (Hirota 2017:1). American workers, whose status had been lowered in the early-to-mid-19th-century shift from artisanal to industrial production, also worried about job competition from Irish immigrants willing to work for lower wages. This was an issue that drew many craftsmen to the nativist Native American Party, or the "Know-Nothings," which achieved sweeping victories in the 1854 elections and aimed to restrict immigration and naturalization. "It was much easier [for nativists] to find villains [in the Irish] than to grapple with understanding large, impersonal forces of economic and social change" (Knobel 2001:8–9 quoted in Kenny 2001:28). The party's support for the abolition of slavery in the South (New York State had emancipated enslaved residents in 1827) was also favored by many working men in New York, despite considerable proslavery sentiment among wealthy New Yorkers whose fortunes were tied to Southern and Caribbean plantations.[13] The unwillingness of the Catholic hierarchy and some prominent Irish nationalists in New York to condemn slavery, and most Irish immigrants' willingness to support the proslavery Democratic Party, also fomented the ire of some nativists. Relatedly, many feared the Catholic Irish were not rational thinkers loyal to the U.S. and instead were easily manipulated by priests and politicians and members of the Pope's supposed secret army (Knobel 2001; Kenny 2001, 2006; Hirota 2017).

The appearances of newly arrived famine-era immigrants and Americans' reactions to them were also important factors in the acceleration of anti-Irish prejudice that deserve greater attention. Irish immigrants who could afford to travel as cabin passengers and outfit themselves in fashionable and clean clothes probably caused Americans little alarm, but a sizable proportion of steerage passengers made a very different impression. Despite attempts to tidy the ship and self upon arrival, many lacked proper clothing by New York City standards and were in poor condition from the myriad trials of their journeys.[14] Those who fared the worst were typically among the thousands of tenants whose emigration had been assisted by landlords, and who were impoverished, malnourished, sick, very old, or very young even at the beginning of their journeys (McMahon 2021:157–158, 196, 226). The appearances of the poorest of the famine Irish immigrants, especially, left lasting impressions on many observers. Just as epidemics had a larger psychological effect than their actual death rates, Hirota (2017:37) notes that "assisted emigration . . . had a much bigger psychological impact on Americans than its size may have warranted."[15]

The vivid language many native-born Americans used to describe them, including comparisons to animals, insects, and ghosts, forms of life that were not human, attests to strength of feeling and suggests their exceptional wretchedness hit deep nerves. For example, writer Nathaniel Hawthorne wrote of his revulsion toward Irish families awaiting ships in Liverpool: "You behold them, disgusting, and all moving about, as when you raise a plank or log that has long lain on the ground, and find many vivacious bugs and insects beneath it" (Scally 1995:208). An anonymous author penned a letter to the Boston City Council that similarly demeaned Irish immigrants in Liverpool, alluding their behavior was similar to that of apes; he/she saw them "picking the vermin from under their arm pits . . . they are too lazy to wash themselves" and opined that they should be given scrubbing brushes instead of bread (Hirota 2017:59). Many nativists, including this author, blamed the Irish for their own misery and categorized them as "unworthy poor." Other 19th-century writers and artists compared the Irish to other animals, particularly pigs and rats, both imagined as dirty scavengers. The ape metaphor was especially long-lasting in pictorial depictions.[16] It was reinfused by Charles Darwin's publication *On the Origin of Species* (1859) and the well-known political cartoons of John Tenniel in London's *Punch* and of Thomas Nast in New York's *Harper's Weekly* in the 1860s and 1870s, especially during episodes of Fenian violence in Britain and Ireland and riots and violent collective action in New York (Gray 1993; Curtis 1997; de Nie 2004:17, Stallybrass and White 1986:132–133; Garner 2015).[17]

Such dehumanizing comments during the famine era conveyed concerns about poverty and recycled timeworn tropes of the Other as dirty animals in a context in which a new level of personal cleanliness had become critical to American notions of citizenship, civility, and personhood. As historian Kathleen Brown (2009) details, by the early 19th-century, Americans, and especially the middle class, had come to embrace bodily cleanliness—not just clean clothes, which had long been important—as a critical aspect of their identity. They interpreted cleanliness as a sign and embodiment of not only health but also morality, rationality, and civility. This resulted from many factors, including Protestant religious movements, new ideas about the benefits of immersive bathing for personal and public health, domestic reform, and the technology (e.g., municipal water systems) and largely female domestic labor power (including African American and immigrant servants) that enabled more people to meet higher standards. Middle-class White women seized leading roles in this endeavor, redefining ideal femininity as exemplarily clean and moral and rejecting long-held Western notions that the female body was naturally filthier than the male and the feminine gender more naturally susceptible to irrationality and sin than the masculine (Jordanova 1980; Wall 1994; Fitts 1999; Brown 2009). For many Americans, personal cleanliness distinguished people from beasts and Americans and the salubrious American natural environment and democratic government from "dirty" foreigners and the filth and inequality of European cities and aristocracies.

It is thus perhaps not surprising that even Americans who felt compassion for the shockingly poor condition of some Irish immigrants still instinctively recoiled. A "prominent and much respected" citizen of New York said, for example, "he could never forget the appearance of a miserable old Irish woman who . . . was begging one Sunday morning in Broadway. Her hair was almost white, her look that of starvation, and the clothing . . . as scanty as the barest decency might permit. This half-naked, starving, shivering creature was one of a ship-load of human beings who had been 'packed off to America' by an absentee nobleman. . . . She was but a type of the thousands . . . consigned to the fever-ship and the fever-shed, or flung, naked and destitute, on the streets of New York, objects of pity or terror to its citizens." Despite feeling sorry for the woman, the citizen confessed he did nothing to help (Maguire 1868:186). Her appearance terrified him too. What if she passed her "Irish fever" on to him, rendering him squalid and unable to care for himself or his family?

The ability to take care of and support oneself was a fundamental element of American identity and of Northern "free labor ideology" (Foner 1995:ix–xxxix; Matthews 2015; Hirota 2017:52). As a number of scholars have shown, White Americans saw it as essential to White—and especially masculine—identity and to U.S. citizenship, which was limited to White men until the passage of the 14th Amendment after the Civil War in 1868. Cases of dependency among White women and children or among African Americans of all ages and genders were economic issues for Northern cities, but comprehensible. Americans of this time recognized the difficulty of women to support themselves on their own, given their job options, and many also imagined dependency on men to be the "natural place" of women. Most White Americans expected that Blacks would be prone to poverty and in need of assistance from Whites, either because enslavement had inflicted trauma, limited education, and cultivated dependency, as many White abolitionists believed, or because of supposed fixed, essential differences between Blacks and Whites that had been used to justify slavery and white supremacy from the 17th century onward.

Race "science"—and its attempts to identify and quantify biological differences between fabricated, but socially and culturally significant, racial categories of Black and White—gained momentum and popularity in the decades leading up to the Civil War. Leading American race scientists, such as Samuel Morton and Josiah Nott, aimed to prove that "Caucasians" and "Negroes" were different, unchangeable species with separate origins and the former were naturally superior. For them and other race scientists, heritable biological difference—supposedly reflected in differences in skin color, cranial volume, facial profiles, etc.—was the substrate of other differences.[18] Nott even argued that such differences made "Negroes" naturally suited to enslavement. To "prove" the idea of separate species they also searched for "degeneration" in mixed offspring. The supposed propensity of people of "pure" or mixed African descent toward disease, low intelligence, dependency, and unsanitary habits were key parts of the race science discourse (Jacobson 1998:34–35; Erickson 109–110).[19] Poor Whites—especially poor White men—had long posed a conceptual challenge to the racial ideology and racial boundaries that structured American society, however, because they did not fit into either the category of White/self-sufficient or Black/dependent (Reilly 2019:40–43). The tremendous number and misery of Irish famine refugees, combined with the growth of race science, raised the visibility and stakes of this conceptual problem and provoked strong reactions against the Irish. It is important to be clear, however, that Americans and the American legal system have always considered the Irish to be White; they were never as a group subjected to the extreme forms of racism—including enslavement and denial of human rights—systematically inflicted upon Black Americans and Native Americans (Jacobson 1998:38, 52–53; Arnesen 2001; Fields 2001; Kenny 2001, 2009:70–72; Dawdy 2005:157–158; McMahon 2015a; 2015b).

Unlike many African Americans and other non-Europeans who Americans could often categorize upon quick glance—and split-second categorization of strangers was increasingly important to social life in urban areas—a healthy and well-outfitted Irish person could pass as a White, Anglo American. To White Americans, sickly, dependent Irish immigrants presented shocking specters of what they, themselves, could be if similarly infected with disease and poverty and what their families could become if infiltrated by such Irish people. Foreign and superstitious Irish customs, such as wakes, seemed even more threatening when performed by people who shared white skin and Northern European origin. Anthropologists have shown how the combination of mimesis and alterity also prompted profound confusion and disturbance among European and European American colonizers in their encounters with Indigenous peoples in many parts of the world. In those cases, colonizers were usually stunned by the sight of unfamiliar and "uncivilized" people engaged in activities that appeared so familiar (Taussig 1993). In this case, White Americans were distressed by White, and therefore supposedly civilized people, existing in degraded states and engaging in "primitive" behavior and how to explain it. Most American nativists focused on Catholicism, poverty, and British domination of Ireland to account for this situation; for them the problem was one of culture and local environment (or *nurture*) that might be reversible with exposure to American society and culture, including conversion to Protestantism, temperance, thrift, and work and bodily discipline (Berger 1946:175–178; Knobel 2001:7, 10). But, as Knobel (2001) and Hirota (2017:122) point out, by mid-century the idea that Irish paupers could be reformed was largely rejected, and the arrival of the famine-era Irish was a significant factor in that shift. In the 1840s climate that fostered race science, many came to view the problem of

Irish poverty as one of Irish *nature* and looked beyond skin color for its source (Knobel 2001:10). Typhus fever, I propose, revealed that source. Americans interpreted the fever as vivid evidence of essential Irish difference and as the key to explaining it.

Humoral Theory and the Roots of Irish Stereotypes

Typhus fever was deadly and contagious, physicians were powerless against it, and New York City's quarantine measures were inadequate, but typhus did not wreak the havoc of the 1832 (or 1849) cholera epidemic. There were no similar outbreaks of typhus among the resident population in the late 1840s and early 1850s, although some American health-care workers who treated immigrants succumbed to the disease. Some reasoned the "exciting" causes that promoted typhus did not exist on American shores, while others asserted that Americans lacked predisposition (Humphreys 2006:279). In this tumultuous period when medicine was also undergoing major transition, Americans looked—consciously and unconsciously—to the timeworn, familiar theory of humoralism to understand why typhus seemed to afflict the Irish differently than Americans (Table 2.1). This section will investigate how, facilitated by 16th-century British revisions of the phlegmatic and sanguine temperaments, this holistic theory appeared to Americans to offer both an explanation for the pattern of typhus infection and authoritative support for important elements of American identity and Irish stereotypes.[20]

As noted in Chapter 1, humoralism was still influential in the 19th century among both the public and physicians. According to the theory, humoral balance was necessary for good health, and a variety of internal and external factors, such as climate, age, diet, activity, and even state of mind, could disrupt balance. Regular exposure to the same stimuli produced habitual imbalances, or temperaments, that not only predisposed an individual to particular illnesses but also shaped character and appearance. Thus, for example, an individual with a phlegmatic temperament would be prone to respiratory ailments, cool and rational in character, and appear pallid and plump, while an individual with a sanguine temperament would be prone to fevers (such as typhus), warm and passionate, and ruddy-complexioned and muscular.

TABLE 2.1. Humoral Temperaments and Their Associations.

Temperament	Humor	Element	Season	Quality	Color	Organ	Character
Sanguine	Blood	Air	Spring	Hot & wet	Red	Heart	Optimistic, passionate (pleasure-seeking, unreliable)
Choleric (Bilious)	Yellow bile	Fire	Summer	Hot & dry	Yellow	Liver	Easily angered, aggressive
Melancholic (Nervous)	Black bile	Earth	Autumn	Cold & dry	Black	Spleen	Despondent, creative
Phlegmatic (Lymphatic)	Phlegm	Water	Winter	Cold & wet	White	Mind	Calm, unemotional (rational, courageous)

Note: This table outlines associations between humors, elements, seasons, qualities, colors, organs, and character as generally understood from Classical period Greece through the 19th century. Details of humoral theory varied across time and place. Nineteenth-century terms and ideas are in parentheses below those of the Classical period.

Sources: Thomas (1830); Puckrein (1981); Stelmack and Stalikas (1992).

Humoral theory was not just used to diagnose individuals. Importantly, it was also used to explain observed and imagined differences between human groups. Hippocrates and Galen hypothesized "the strength of the sun in the Southern Hemisphere made humans black; its weakness in the Northern Hemisphere left humans white" and that "the closer one moved toward the North Pole," the more one would find people who were "white of colour, blockish, uncivil, fierce, and warlike.... In the Southern Hemisphere, travelers encountered people who were black, wise, and civil, but weak and cowardly" (Puckrein 1981:1755). In response to cold climates, the bodies of "Northerners" tended toward hot humors and thus sanguine and choleric temperaments, while "southerners" responded to warm climates by developing more cold humors and thus phlegmatic and melancholic temperaments. Some believed these characteristics became hereditary over a number of generations. Humoralism's holistic approach to explaining the mutually influential relationships between the interior and the exterior and between the mind, body, and environment in both individuals and groups made it attractive and long-lived well beyond medical circles. It was embedded within Western popular consciousness for centuries and underpinned how many Europeans and Americans understood themselves and others; "the theory lent to social thought a vocabulary that became a source of metaphor, if it did not actually dictate social values" (Haller 1981a:3).

The English began to adjust classic humoral ideas to fit their own self-definitional desires in the 16th century. Classical formulations of the temperaments proposed that the Greeks—who resided in the warm Mediterranean and possessed great learning, culture, and the first so-called democracy—were phlegmatic in temperament, while the "barbarian" Germans and Celts of the colder regions of northern Europe were sanguinous (Isaac 2006:72). Historian Gary Puckrein (1981:1756) describes how the English embraced the idea that they were "white of color, showed great boldness in war . . . and strong and sincere'" as a consequence of living "near the North Pole," yet they were also "generally inclined to phlegm." They altered the classic formulation that the weakness of the sun in the northern latitudes had a negative effect on brain development, causing those who lived there to be "of little wit and incapable of governing themselves" by arguing that education had equally strong effects on national temperament. The English poet and scholar John Milton contended, for example, "the sun, which we want, ripens wit as well as fruits; and as wine and oil are imported to us from abroad, so must ripe understanding and many civil virtues be imported into our minds from foreign writings and examples of best ages."[21] In short, the English claimed a phlegmatic temperament and expanded its characteristics to include what they saw as the best qualities from the North and the South, the physical prowess of barbarians and the learning and civility of ancient Greeks.

British nationalism and contemporaneous efforts to colonize Ireland were significant in this reformulation. Jean Feerick (2002:103–104, 107) describes how Edmund Spenser, author of the *Faerie Queene* (1590 and 1596), portrayed the Irish as "explosive," "enslaved to the body's passions," and "propelled by a forceful heat," in contrast to Englishmen, whose chief virtue was temperance. Spenser made the sanguine nature of his Irish characters especially clear by their names and physical descriptions: Pyrochles (from the Greek "fire disturbed"), who has reddish locks, and his henchman Atin (from the Gaelic *athainne* [embers] or *aithinne* [firebrand]), who rides a "bloudy red" steed and carries a shield displaying a "flaming fire in the midst of a bloudy field." Meanwhile, in his geographical and historical survey of Great Britain and Ireland, *Britannia* (1586 [Latin], 1610 [English]), William Camden described the Irish as "having both a hotter and moister nature than other nations." In classical formulations, a sanguine temperament was understood to produce positive character traits, such as optimism, generosity, amorousness, quick-wittedness, and courage. In their depictions of the sanguine Irish, the British exaggerated these traits to the point that they became negative: unrealistic optimism, irresponsible generosity, animalistic sensuality, inability to concentrate, and propensity to anger and violence.[22] In these characterizations, the British marshalled a trusted scientific theory to defend their own violent colonial actions and to argue that the Irish were unfit to govern themselves. Many English hoped that colonization and conversion to Protestantism could civilize the Irish, that exposure to an environment rich in English culture would shift their humoral balance toward the phlegmatic (Feerick 2002). Unyielding Irish opposition combined with the adoption of Irish language and culture by older English settlers, however, suggested that Ireland's environment produced a character that was obdurate, at least while on Irish soil.

During this same period, Camden and his contemporaries also helped to popularize the myth of the Anglo-Saxon origins of England, initially developed, according to historian Reginald Horsman (1976:387–391), to validate the English Church's break from Rome as a return to a "purer" Anglo-Saxon church. The myth cast the English as a freedom-loving, democratic Anglo-Saxon people, who had inherited a unique reverence for individual freedoms from their Germanic/Teutonic ancestors, in contrast to inferior, savage Celtic people who did not share the same love of freedom and whose descendants populated Ireland. These descriptions of Anglo-Saxons and Celts mapped onto and were inseparable from the contemporaneous British reformulations of the phlegmatic and sanguine temperaments, and with their stereotypes of the Irish. I suggest that the fusion of the Anglo-Saxon myth with humoral theory increased the myth's power and longevity as a tool of nationalist discourse and its success in permeating public imagination. English nationalists used this synthesis to interpret their achievements as the results not only of historical victories and cultural superiority but also of embodied (temperament + character) differences that were inseparable from that history and culture. This discourse traveled to North America with English colonists, and they adapted it to their circumstances. American nationalists, including Thomas Jefferson, were intensely interested in Anglo-Saxon origins, which could address the conundrum of how to divorce themselves from British domination during and after the Revolutionary War without severing claim to the elements of Anglo culture and ancestry that were essential to American identity. Irish nationalists, meanwhile, created countermyths about the greatness of Celtic peoples and positioned their own fight for freedom as part of an eternal struggle between Celts and Anglo-Saxons, as historian Cian McMahon (2015a) has detailed (see also Jacobson 1998:48–52).

Over time, British, American, and Irish nationalists all placed greater emphasis on the supposed natural origins of the superiority of their respective so-called "races." As members of each group dispersed away from their native soil, the British/"Anglo-Saxons" via colonization and the Irish/ "Celts" via colonization and diaspora, they described the traits of their respective people as inborn and passed down via blood, de-emphasizing the importance of environment and education. Their views drew upon, and probably also to some degree influenced, the work of race scientists and ethnologists in the U.S. and Europe. In the 1840s and early 1850s, while Samuel Morton and Josiah Nott were looking for physical proof of determinative innate differences between "Negroes" and "Caucasians" in the U.S., for example, they also considered differences between "Caucasian" peoples. Morton's skull experiments, which had vast and lasting impacts on American anthropology, ranked Anglo-Saxons at the top and Celts at the bottom (Mitchell 2018). Meanwhile, the influential anatomist and ethnologist John Knox (1850:7) was busy in England publicizing his theory that "race is everything": physiological differences were the source of cultural differences. Knox argued there was no such thing as a Caucasian race, but instead numerous European races. He, too, ranked Anglo-Saxons—which he saw as a subset, along with the Germans, of the Scandinavian race—highest and Celts the lowest. Knox described the Scandinavian race as the "only one which truly comprehends the meaning of the word liberty," and the Celtic race as one of "furious fanaticism; a love of war and disorder; a hatred for order and patient industry; no accumulative habits; [they are] restless, treacherous, uncertain: look at Ireland" (Knox 1850:26 cited in Horsman 1976:406–407).[23]

Knox's ideas were popular among many audiences; he published books and in medical and science journals, gave public lectures, and corresponded with influential Americans including Ralph Waldo Emerson, for example. According to McMahon (2015a:29), Knox's ideas heavily influenced Thomas Campbell Foster (1845), a correspondent of the *London Times*, who reported on the famine in Ireland in a regular and widely read column. Foster described the dreadful situation and attributed it to "the characteristics of the [Celtic] race." Such nationalist-racial ideas incorporated enduring ideas about British identity and Irish difference expressed in earlier British reformulations of humoral theory. Knox, Foster, and others readily applied them to their concerns about Irish poverty in the 1840s and 1850s in arguing that the Irish would remain a poor class of people because of their innate character. The Irish, of course, disagreed with these negative assessments of their character, but they did not question the core premise that they were a people different from the English and their descendants in the U.S. and that those differences were ultimately rooted in blood (McMahon 2015a:3).

Ideas about gender were also marshalled in support of racial nationalism and provided a rich set of metaphors. In a famous 1854 essay, English poet and cultural critic Matthew Arnold wrote, for example, "If it be permitted us to assign sex to nations as to individuals, we should have to say without hesitance that the Celtic race . . . is essentially a feminine race," while Anglo-Saxons were a masculine race. He elaborated that Celts were "sensuous, impetuous, and 'ineffectual in material civilization and politics'" (de Nie 2004:24). Such comparisons can be understood as simply referencing preexisting gender hierarchy to elevate one group over another, but the supposed naturalness of that hierarchy and how it related to humoral theory was part of the analogy. Scholars had long proposed that humors were ultimately responsible for the differences in anatomy and character between men and women. Historian Gale Kern Paster (1998) describes how heat and dryness was thought to be critical in the formation of male anatomy and masculine character traits, including sounder minds and stronger bodies, whereas the lack of heat and wetness produced females and their "imperfect" anatomy and character traits, including weaker minds and bodies that made them naturally dependent. Within this framework, "hot" behavior among women, such as expression of anger, was seen as a symptom of pathology (Paster 1998:423).[24] Portraying men as effeminate or infantile and women as masculine were tropes used in the U.S. and England in the 19th century to denigrate "non-White" Blacks and Asians as well as the Irish (see Figure 2.4).[25] Deeply embedded ideas about humoral theory and supposed naturalness of gender norms made these tropes all the more powerful. Deviations from such norms were seen as not simply unusual but pathological and thus supported lower ranking in the racial hierarchy.

Stereotypes of Irish immigrants in both the U.S. and England around the time of the famine were rooted in a long history of interactions between the British and the Irish. Much, although not all, of this history was antagonistic, prompting both groups to frequently stress their differences, real or imagined, instead of their many similarities. More vicious portrayals of the Irish as exceedingly violent or inhuman corresponded with periods of heightened altercation (Curtis 1997; Kenny 2006). Each group used the other as a foil in creating and maintaining their own national identities, a project still in process in the 1840s and 1850s. The traits that they imagined in themselves and in the "Other" were inspired by and, in turn, supported contemporaneous ideas in history, literature, and in the growing field of race science. Interwoven into all of them was humoral theory. Humoral theory was a foundational element of Western worldviews that was frequently resorted to—consciously and unconsciously—to explain relationships between categories that were perceived to be binary: sick/well, interior/exterior, physiology/character, us/them, male/female, culture/nature, etc., and in this case, Irish-Celtic/English-Anglo-Saxon. Humoral theory's own binary structure—hot/cold and wet/dry—remained fixed and authoritative, but the qualities assigned to the four resulting permutations of temperaments and characters proved to be somewhat malleable and conveniently applicable to social and political endeavors. There has been discussion among historians about whether most American, British, and Irish people widely believed that Anglo-Saxon and Celtic races truly persisted into the 19th century or if they interpreted such ideas as purely rhetorical. Certainly, many were well aware that there had been a great deal of mixing of these "races," and many used the term race loosely to describe "a people" or what might be defined today as an ethnic or cultural group, rather than how race scientists used the term to indicate a group with fixed, hereditary characteristics that correspond to differences in body, mind, and behavior (Kenny 2006; McMahon 2015a). While it is beyond the scope of this book to try to answer that question, I suggest that the prevalence of typhus fever among the wave of Irish immigrants to Britain, Canada, and the U.S. in the late 1840s and early 1850s prompted many Americans to consider the possible reality of meaningful innate physiological differences between themselves and the Irish, and they, too, fell back upon humoral theory for clarification and support.

Fever, Rash, and Delirium: Typhus Fever and Irish Sanguinity

When thousands of Irish immigrants arrived in New York City in visibly dreadful condition, many suffering from an unfamiliar and deadly fever, physicians and immigration officials—and the American public—paid close attention to the fever's symptoms and who it afflicted. The prevailing view was that the disease arose from filth or miasma, individuals with predispositions were most likely to fall ill, and people with sanguine temperaments were predisposed to fevers. Such a temperament could be possessed by any person at a given time, depending on the previously mentioned factors influencing humoral balance, and children were thought to tend toward sanguine temperaments (Thomas 1830:13).[26] Additionally, as described, the British had long portrayed the Irish as a group who possessed sanguine temperaments all the time; this idea had traversed the Atlantic well before the famine-era immigrants arrived. From this cultural perspective, it would not have been surprising that such immigrants would be susceptible to fever. Typhus was not a run-of-the mill fever, however, and the famine-era Irish were not the usual group of newcomers. This section proposes that typhus among this group of immigrants pushed Americans to ponder whether physiological difference was the foundation of differences in character and practices between the Irish and themselves, and whether such a foundation was changeable in the American environment. Three prominent symptoms of typhus—high fever, rash, and delirium—were especially important in their considerations.

Fever, an increase in body temperature in response to an illness, was the foremost symptom of epidemic typhus fever, included in most, if not all, of its 19th-century alternate names. This symptom underscored that those most likely to suffer from the disease possessed temperaments that made their bodies especially susceptible to overheating, and their minds to over-excitement, passion, or frenzy (Haller 1981a:18). One medical guide of the era, for example, described that among the sanguine, "the diseases most readily induced are those of excitement. Inflammations of every degree, fevers of every type.... As the diseases of the melancholy are chronic, those of the sanguine are acute. Inflammation once begun rapidly proceeds, fever once kindled burns with an exterminating flame" (Thomas 1830:16, 19). One of the ways typhus fever differed from other fevers was literally by degree; in cases observed today, very high temperatures of 105 degrees Fahrenheit are not uncommon. Such high temperatures would have left little doubt about the temperament of those afflicted with the illness and raised alarm about the degree of their humoral imbalance. The correlation between the Irish and this particular fever thus reinforced the idea that Irish blood consistently ran too "hot" and could easily erupt into pathological conditions of body, mind, and behavior, including mania and alcoholism, two conditions evoked by another symptom of typhus: delirium.

Delirium has been frequently observed in typhus fever patients in the past and present. It is the symptom for which typhus was named, from the Greek for smoke, because of the disease's frequent neurological side effects, understood in the 19th-century as resulting from cerebral inflammation (Murchison 1862:263). Physicians today also view inflammation as a cause but explain it as an immune response to the bacterial infection. Manifestations of delirium include disorientation, hallucination, hyperactivity, drowsiness, emotional changes, decreases in memory, and changes in speech. Such symptoms were not unlike those manifested by people suffering from mental illness or by heavily inebriated individuals or habitual heavy drinkers suffering from withdrawal (*delirium tremens*). It was not just neurological symptoms that these conditions were thought to share, but also their origins in a sanguine temperament. Scottish physician Robert MacNish argued in an 1835 study, for example, that "the sanguine temperament seems to feel most intensely the excitement of the bottle." A health reformer in 1840s

Liverpool subsequently remarked: "Spirits produce a greater effect on the Irish than on others. It makes them in fact insane when under its influence and they are so violent as to be regardless of the consequences of their acts" (Scally 1995:209).

The issue here was not alcohol itself. There were some temperance leaders who felt alcohol was a dangerous substance and advocated abstinence for everyone, but that was a minority opinion. For the vast majority of physicians, alcoholic beverages were important substances in patient care. For convalescing patients, they prescribed beer and wine, which they believed to be nourishing, and they used hard liquors to "revive" nonresponsive patients and to "warm" individuals who had been overexposed to cold (NYHMCB 1847–1853 and New York Hospital Surgical Casebooks [NYHSCB] 1848, 1851–1853). Thus, at issue was the mixture of alcohol, especially warmer and more stimulating hard liquors, on people with already overheated sanguine temperaments. The delirium of typhus fever provided yet more support for the idea that the Irish were especially prone to excited mental states, including mental illness not necessarily caused by overindulgence of alcohol.

Mania was then understood as an overly excited and irrational state, akin to long-term delirium, to which people with sanguine temperaments were especially susceptible. It was a diagnosis that likely included mental illnesses categorized today as bipolar disorder and schizophrenia (Haller 1981a:18). The connection between the Irish, sanguinity, and mania helps to explain why so many Irish individuals were sent to insane asylums in the 19th and 20th centuries in England, Ireland, and the U.S. Other scholars have studied these problematic rates and exposed them as the product of anti-Irish prejudice, a means to subdue potential political agitators, or even a result of child-rearing practices, but to my knowledge none have considered how humoralism might have informed physicians' disproportional diagnoses (Malcolm 1999; Scheper-Hughes 2001). This connection suggests a significant reciprocal relationship between medical models and widespread stereotypes and underscores that neither medical science nor individual physicians were unaffected by popular prejudice, a topic I will explore further in the next section.

The prominent rash observed among most typhus fever sufferers was additional visible evidence of sanguine temperament. The rash usually begins on the trunk and is light red in color and then spreads to other parts of the body, but usually not the face, and deepens to a darker red or "mulberry" color (Goldman and Bennett 2000:1770; Murchison 1862:127–130). As the disease progresses, the rash can become petechial, from broken capillaries under the skin. Such eruptions of blood, through the logic of humoral theory, suggested that the hot and wet interiors of the many Irish afflicted with typhus could not be contained in their interiors nor restrained in their character. British and American caricatures of the Irish often depicted them as ruddy-complexioned and redheaded, even though both groups recognized that fair skin and dark hair were at least as common.[27] These stereotypical reddish features clearly signaled sanguine temperament and character. Ruddy complexions also conveyed the rural and manual laboring origins of most Irish immigrants of this period. Working outdoors produces darker and redder complexions from sun, wind, and physical exertion. By the circular logic of humoralism, this kind of work both best suited and cultivated sanguine temperaments (see Chapter 4). In their study of New York Hospital typhus case records from 1847, Geltson and Jones (1977:815) found that physicians believed typhus was "more prevalent among people living closer to organic emanations arising from the earth." In the 19th-century American imagination, there were few groups who lived closer to the earth than the Irish, many of whom dwelled in semi-subterranean homes with earthen floors and thatch roofs and dug their primary food source out of the ground (Figure 2.2).

The classic symptoms of typhus fever were highly visible and severe. When read through the lens of humoral theory, they suggested that famine-era Irish immigrants were sanguine in temperament and character to a greater degree, and thus physiologically different to a greater degree, than Americans had previously imagined. Such intense and constant sanguinity put emphasis on the more hostile aspects of Irish stereotypes and stoked American fears of not only epidemic disease but also mania, alcoholism, and violence that could erupt from such hot interiors. By this humoral logic, all Irish immigrants harbored fever within themselves. Case records from New York Hospital suggest that physicians embraced this idea, leading to misdiagnoses that exaggerated typhus infection rates among the Irish, which, in turn, further solidified stereotypes.

Misdiagnosing Typhus at New York Hospital: Irishness as a "Usual Symptom of Typhus Fever"

New York Hospital opened in 1791 at 319 Broadway, between Duane and Reade Streets, as the first dedicated hospital in New York City (Figures 2.3 and 1.1, no. 70). Prior to its establishment, there had only been a small infirmary in the city's almshouse, then located in what is now City Hall Park. From its beginnings, New York Hospital's board made great efforts to distinguish the institution as a center for excellent medical care, unlike almshouses, which were seen as places where only the most unfortunate sought food, shelter, and a place to die. By the 1840s, New York Hospital was preeminent in the nation. It attracted the best physicians and surgeons, educated students from the prestigious affiliated College of Physicians and Surgeons, utilized the most advanced techniques, and provided "state-of-the-art" facilities, including spacious and well-ventilated wards, gas lighting installed in 1838, steam heat in 1844, and toilets connected to sewers in 1845 (Duffy 1968: 481–482; Larrabee 1971:213). New York Hospital enjoyed a far better reputation than the city's second hospital, Bellevue, inconveniently located about two miles uptown between 26th and 28th Streets and 1st Avenue and the East River. Bellevue had been established initially as a hospital for yellow fever victims in 1795 and became the city's new almshouse in 1811.[28] Despite the quality of New York Hospital, a close examination of the hospital's records suggests that physicians there misdiagnosed a significant number of Irish patients with typhus fever, when they likely suffered from an ordinary fever. These misdiagnoses exacerbated Irish immigrants' already difficult adjustments to New York both by subjecting them to unnecessary, and even life-threatening, harsh medical treatments and by providing additional medical "evidence" for ideas about Irish difference.

From New York Hospital's founding, it treated both private paying patients and nonpaying sick or wounded patients on a charitable basis.[29] Admitting the latter enabled the hospital to secure vital state funding in addition to what it raised from private donors (Roosa 1900). As mentioned previously, New York Hospital, like Bellevue, also had an agreement with the Commissioners of Emigration to care for recent

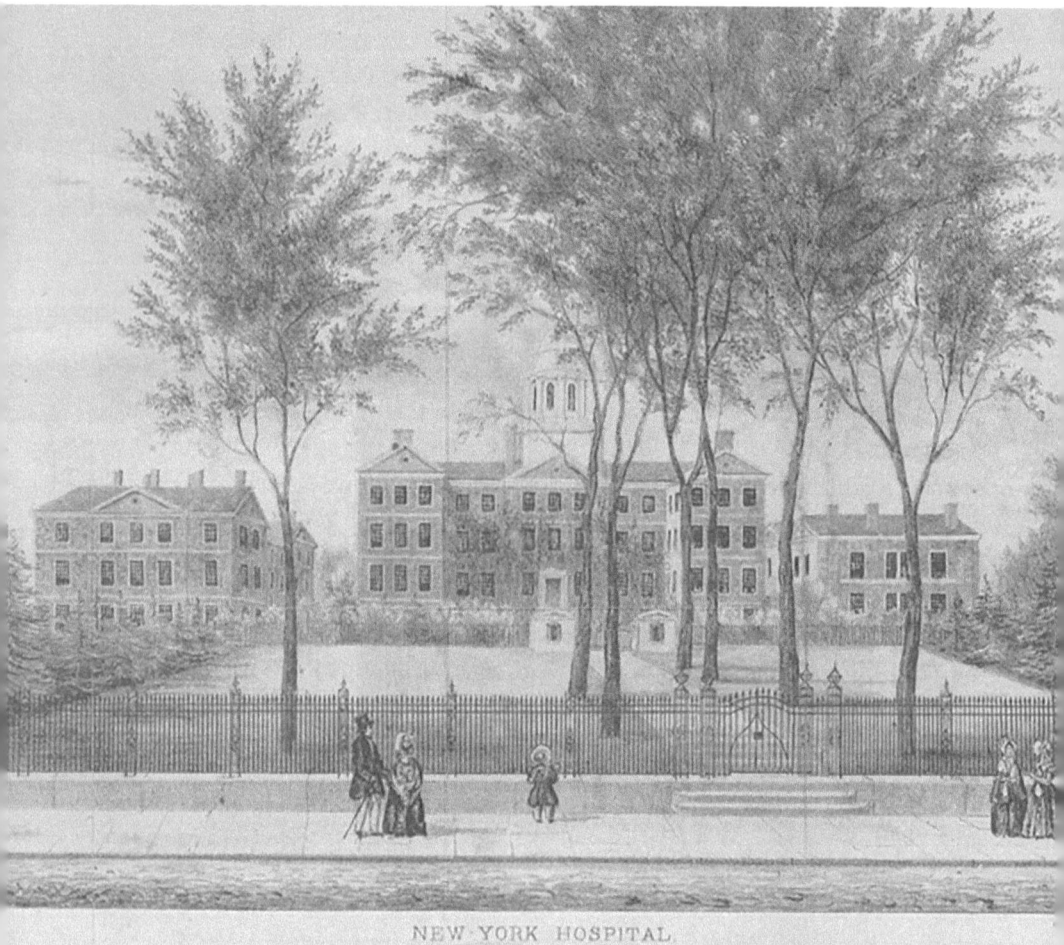

FIGURE 2.3. Print of New York Hospital viewed from Broadway circa 1845 by the artist George Hayward and lithographer Thomas Wood. At the center is the Main Building, erected in 1775 and opened in 1791. The South Building, left, was erected in 1808 as the "insane asylum" and later used as the Marine Department to care for sailors. The North Building, right, was erected in 1841 to accommodate more patients, and wounded soldiers were cared for there during the Civil War (Larrabee 1971:203). Courtesy of the New York Public Library.

immigrants when the quarantine hospitals on Staten or Ward's Island were full, or when emergency prevented safe transport to them. Such individuals amounted to a very small percentage of the total number of patients treated at New York Hospital from 1847 to 1852 (0 to 2%), with the exception of the challenging winter of 1851, when the Commissioners sent 589 sick immigrants, accounting for 25% of the total number of patients that year (NYHAR 1848–1853; Commissioners of Emigration 1861:67, 74). The much larger number of Irish immigrants who were treated at the hospital during the whole famine period reflects the limited reach of the Commission and the fact that many Irish fell ill in the city after passing inspection, as Americans feared.

Irish-born patients outnumbered any other single group admitted to New York Hospital from 1844 to 1860, averaging 43% of patients yearly over those nearly two decades when they made up an average of less than 28% of the general population (Rosenwaike 1972:41). During the famine years, the proportion of Irish treated at the hospital was even larger. Between 1847 and 1852, 49% of patients treated at New York Hospital had been born in Ireland, whereas 9% had been born in the German States (the next largest immigrant group), 27% had been born in the U.S., and 15% had been born in other nations (NYHAR 1845–1861).[30] Typhus fever was a leading diagnosis of Irish-born patients. From 1841, when typhus first appeared in annual reports as a diagnosis, until 1852, when the reports no longer keep track of illness by place of birth, Irish immigrants accounted for an average of 70% of typhus patients, with yearly percentages ranging from 44% to 95%. In contrast, German and U.S.-born patients accounted for an average of 10% of typhus patients during each of these years, with yearly percentages ranging from 1% to 25% and 2% to 21%, respectively (NYHAR 1842–1853). From a present-day perspective, the terrible conditions of Irish emigration combined with poor health or malnourishment even at the outset of journeys might explain why the Irish seemed to suffer more from typhus. However, a close examination of both individual case records and statistics from the hospital's annual reports reveals curious inconsistencies in typhus fever diagnoses, treatment, and mortality rates that suggest the number of infected Irish were inflated.

New York Hospital was staffed by house physicians and nurses who worked full time and by private physicians who visited daily for consultation and to perform difficult procedures. "House physicians" kept records about each patient's case that typically included diagnosis, number of days spent in the hospital, outcome of the case, and patient's place of birth used for yearly quantitative analysis in annual reports. Additionally, they recorded into bound ledgers details of individual cases that they, or a visiting private physician, deemed to be particularly interesting or representative, and useful for teaching or research. Most case records contain the date, diagnosis, attending physician, patient name, age, gender, country of birth, occupation, history of the complaint gathered from patient or those who brought him/her to the hospital, treatments and medicines prescribed, patient reactions and progression of the ailment, and how the case resolved. There are more than 100 cases of Irish immigrants diagnosed with typhus recorded in the 1847 medical casebook alone, outnumbering all other ailments in that year's casebook, and revealing that the physicians found typhus, and typhus patients, to be interesting. New York Hospital treated close to 1,000 patients for typhus that year, 80% of them Irish.[31] Case notes of immigrant typhus patients include additional information about the ships they arrived upon—ship name, numbers of total and sick passengers aboard, and number of days or weeks since landing—suggesting physicians were interested in how ships might have been involved in the fever. Nevertheless, curious patterns in recorded symptoms and case outcomes also suggest that these same physicians considered a patient's Irish ethnicity to be a relevant factor when assigning a typhus diagnosis. It appears they considered shipboard conditions to be "exciting causes" of typhus and Irishness to be a "predisposing cause."

In many of the case records of Irish immigrants diagnosed with typhus, physicians noted only the symptoms of *simple fever*—such as pain in the head and/or body, hot skin, thirst, weakness, and chill—not the classic diagnostic symptoms of epidemic typhus fever: fever, rash, and altered mental state. Physicians' infrequent mention of a rash is suspicious, because, according to contemporary studies, 90% to 95% of people who suffer from epidemic typhus develop the rash (Goldman and Bennett 2000:1767–1770). British physician Charles Murchison (1862:130) reported that rash was observed in 90% of patients treated at the London Fever Hospital in the 1840s and 1850s, suggesting that typhus fever has not changed radically since the 19th century. At New York

Hospital, however, physicians noted an "eruption," pink- or red-colored rash, or petechiae, in only 23% of patients they diagnosed with typhus fever and recorded in the 1847 casebook. In another approximately 33% of cases, physicians simply wrote "taken with the usual symptoms of typhus" (NYHAR 1848; Geltson and Jones 1977:817). Even if New York Hospital physicians considered rash to be one of the "usual symptoms," that would still mean that approximately 44% of patients diagnosed with typhus fever did not exhibit a rash, compared with between 5% and 10% observed elsewhere. This is a substantial difference. Absence of this characteristic symptom of typhus in otherwise thorough case notes (with no accompanying statement that the case was unusual because of lack of a rash) suggests that physicians misdiagnosed a significant number of Irish patients or leaned heavily toward a diagnosis of typhus fever whenever they were unsure and if the patient was Irish.

Comparison of the case histories of Irish-born patients with those of German and American-born patients also shows that physicians rarely diagnosed German or U.S.-born patients with typhus fever, even if they presented with the same symptoms as Irish-born patients they diagnosed with the disease. Instead, physicians usually determined German- and U.S.-born patients to be suffering from either simple "fever" or "remittent fever," a term used in the 19th century to describe a fever that fluctuated by several degrees daily, and was of an unknown origin (NYHMCB 1847–1848:C7, C39, C43, C58, C424, C717; 1851–1852:C326, C381; 1865:92; Schroeder-Lein 2008:107). Between 1845 and 1852, German immigrants were almost twice as likely to be diagnosed with simple fever than Irish immigrants, and U.S.-born patients were about one and a half times more likely to be diagnosed with remittent fever than Irish immigrants (NYHAR 1846–1853).[32] Both of these ailments had lower associated death rates and neither carried the same stigma as typhus fever.

Mortality rates of typhus patients at New York Hospital during the famine years were unusually low, also suggesting frequent misdiagnoses (Table 2.2). During the years of the largest outbreaks (1847–1849 and 1851) when the total number of typhus patients and the proportion of them who were Irish were the largest, the mortality rate hovered around 16% and was as low as 13% in 1847 (NYHAR 1848–1850 and 1852). These rates are considerably lower than the 20% to 45% typhus mortality rate in the 19th century estimated by scholars, based on rates at other hospitals (Hardy 1988:406). At the London Fever Hospital between 1848 and 1862 the average rate was 21%. In Edinburgh between 1846 and 1848 it was 25% and in Glasgow 21%. Among French troops in the Crimean War between 1853 to 1856 it was 50% (Murchison 1862:50–51). While New York Hospital had lower patient death rates overall than Bellevue Hospital during this time period due to better conditions and care, that does not fully explain such low typhus mortality rates compared with European peer institutions. The unusually low typhus mortality rates at New York Hospital thus also suggest that some of the Irish patients who were diagnosed with typhus had a different and less life-threatening illness that skewed the "typhus" mortality rate. The Marine Hospital on Staten Island also recorded an unusually low mortality rate of 17% among 3,040 patients treated for typhus, all of them immigrants, suggesting prejudiced misdiagnoses were not limited to New York Hospital (Humphreys 2006:278).[33]

Mortality rates for simple fever at New York Hospital also show unusual patterns suggesting misdiagnoses. Mortality rates for simple fever at New York Hospital ranged from between 1.5% and 2.5% during non-epidemic years in the 1840s and 1850s. In contrast, during the typhus epidemic years of 1847 and 1848, simple fever mortality rose to 8% and 7%, respectively (NYHAR 1846–1853). Since patients born in the U.S. or German principalities were more likely to be diagnosed with simple fever than typhus fever, this spike in simple fever mortality implies that physicians misdiagnosed some U.S. and German-born patients with simple fever when they might have been infected with the deadlier typhus fever. Physicians missed this diagnosis because these patients lacked what they appear to have considered a characteristic symptom: Irishness.

Misdiagnosis of Irish immigrants with typhus during epidemic years might be partially attributable to overcautious physicians aiming to retain patients in the hospital to contain the outbreaks and/or anxious physicians who worried typhus was everywhere. The fact that Irish immigrants alone appear to have been the targets of this type of misdiagnosis is critical, however. Like the American public, the top American physicians at one of the country's best hospitals seemed to have understood typhus to be primarily an Irish disease, reflecting their shared views about the sanguine Irish temperament and character.

TABLE 2.2. Percentage of Deaths of Typhus Fever Patients at New York Hospital (1845–1852).

Year	1845	1846	1847*	1848*	1849*	1850	1851*	1852
% of Typhus Patients Who Died	22	33	13	18	16	26	14	16
% of Typhus Patients Who Were Irish	77	77	80	55	84	81	95	48
Total Number Of Typhus Patients	96	99	1034	436	224	169	596	99

*The table ends at 1852 because after that year, the hospital's annual reports no longer tabulate patient illnesses by nation of origin. An asterisk indicates year of a major typhus outbreak. Sources: Data from NYHAR (1845–1852).

The vast majority of case records written by physicians at New York Hospital do not contain disparaging remarks about Irish patients or other indications of conscious prejudice. Instead, most read as earnest attempts to attend to suffering patients. There are, nevertheless, a few remarks that suggest physicians shared some of the negative views of Irish immigrants that circulated outside the hospital, including an understanding that the Irish were sanguine in temperament. One physician, for example, seemed surprised by a young Irish woman's appearance. He noted, "Patient has a rather handsome countenance . . . hazel eyes, and fair skin" (NYHMCB 1848:C1632). It was not common for physicians to record the attractiveness of patients in case records, therefore, this statement suggests a noteworthy deviation from the physician's expectation of a "typical" brutish and ruddy-complexioned Irish woman. Another physician, frustrated by being denied an autopsy, scribbled in the case record of a deceased Irish patient, "Irish ignorance defeats the ends of science. No autopsy is granted" (NYHMCB 1865:C232).[34] This remark suggests the physician believed that ignorance was a characteristic of all Irish people, an erroneous and prejudiced generalization that was also part of Irish stereotypes. Several physicians also commented that Irish patients had been "drinking freely" before admission, referencing the supposed connections between alcohol, Irishness, and fever (NYHMCB 1847–1848:C100; 1865:249).

Physicians' assumptions about Irish temperament and habits, even if some were well-meaning, endangered individual patients on a microscale and relations between Irish immigrants and Americans on a macroscale. On the individual level, the "medicines" physicians prescribed for typhus fever were harsher and more dangerous than their prescriptions for simple or remittent fever, and likely complicated their cases. They purged typhus patients with castor oil; induced volcanic vomiting and purging with calomel (mercurous chloride) or Dover's Powder (a mixture of ipecacuanha, powdered opium, and potassium sulfate); sweated them with spirits of Mindererus (ammonium acetate); withheld food; and, more rarely, bled them using the cupping technique (NYHMCB 1847–1848; Geltson and Jones 1977:819).[35] Such therapies were not effective against the disease or most others, a point the physician and writer Oliver Wendell Holmes remarked upon in an 1860 speech at Harvard Medical School: "If the whole materia medica, as now used, could be sunk to the bottom of the sea, it would be so much the better for mankind—and all the worse for the fishes" (Gibian 2001:171). In addition to mercury poisoning, such typhus fever remedies also could have caused dangerous dehydration and drops in blood pressure; clinical research on epidemic typhus during WWII found that dehydration increased the severity and duration of the disease and could cause cardiac arrest or kidney failure (Coates 1963; Larrabee 1971:119). New York Hospital physicians' prescriptions conformed to the medical logic of the day, however; the more severe the disease, the more severe the action required.

Assumptions about Irish patients possessing sanguine temperaments might have also subjected them to even more aggressive treatment. Dr. F. Thomas (1830:22) noted in an award-winning essay about temperaments, for example, that for sanguine individuals "treatment must be adopted early, and vigilantly pursued. Depletion must be liberally employed when necessary, mental excitement and physical stimuli religiously avoided when injurious. . . . Evacuants are the best class of medicines for the sanguine." Patients diagnosed with simple fever, who were more often American or German born, received far gentler treatment at New York Hospital. For them, physicians usually prescribed a regimen of cold water, brandy, gruel, and rest. Patients misdiagnosed with typhus fever, therefore, were subjected to unnecessary harmful treatments that complicated their cases and probably resulted in longer hospital stays and even some deaths.[36] They also cost the hospital more; the Commissioners of Emigration (1861:55) noted that in 1848 New York

Hospital spent more than twice as much on typhus fever patients than the $3 per week they spent on most other patients.

On a macroscale, misdiagnoses elevated the rates at which Irish immigrants were thought to have been afflicted with this new and frightening epidemic fever, thus making even stronger the perceived connection between this disease, the Irish, and the sanguine temperament. Stronger connections generated more bias among physicians that propelled more misdiagnoses. News of so many Irish immigrants afflicted with typhus spread by mouth and official reports fed negative Irish stereotypes outside the hospital. Although this was a period in which the American public challenged the authority of the professional medical establishment, it still had considerable influence, especially when it supported preexisting public opinion. Infection rates had the weight of "science" behind them. "Science is one of the most convincing tools to persuade others" because in modern societies it appears to be the most objective means of justification (Latour 1999:259). These seemingly high rates of typhus infection combined with anecdotal stories of sick Irish immigrants and such visible symptoms created a compelling case for Irish sanguinity and all the negative stereotypes about Irish character that were intertwined with it. Public opinion and medical science were mutually influential and aligned to malign the reputation of Irish immigrants in New York City.

Conclusion

The full-blown American stereotype of an Irish immigrant woman, often glossed as "Bridget," the female counterpart of "Pat," is arguably most vividly rendered in a cartoon created by Frederick Burr Opper for the American humor magazine *Puck* in 1883 (Figure 2.4). Opper's cartoon unfavorably contrasts an Irish domestic servant on the right with her White American mistress on the left. The servant is large and muscular, redheaded and ruddy-complexioned, with a prognathous face (meant to resemble an ape), gigantic feet, and dressed in a gaudy orange shamrock frock that indecently exposes her thick calves and bulging forearms. She resembles the depiction of Irish women in "Irish Bogtrotters," the British etching from about 70 years earlier (see Figure 2.2) in her clumsiness, inappropriate dress, large facial features, and complexion. In that etching,

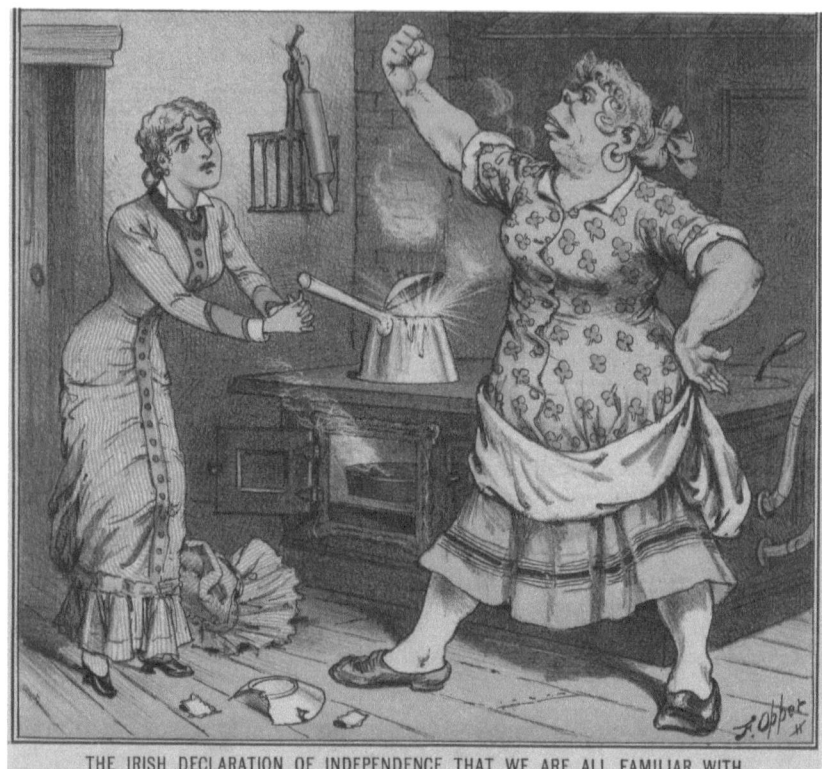

FIGURE 2.4. Cartoon by Frederick Burr Opper from the cover of the May 19, 1883, edition of the American humor magazine *Puck*. Courtesy of the Library of Congress.

the British artist depicted Irish women, and their male companion, as naturally suited to the boggy Irish landscape, not unlike the happy frogs in the foreground. The man carries a shillelagh and thus the potential for violence, but the group is portrayed more as backward and comical than dangerous. Opper's cartoon, in contrast, depicts the Irish woman as ill-suited to her new, urban American environment and a pain, if not a threat, to her employer. Her body is too large and awkward for the kitchen; she lacks the grace and intelligence required to put together a meal without breaking or burning something; and she is angry. The written caption of the cartoon, "The Irish Declaration of Independence That We Are All Familiar with," makes clear that the artist expected his middle- and upper-class American readers to understand and find relatable this negative caricature of a working-class Irish woman, the kind of woman many employed in their homes. The contrast with the mistress, representing the American feminine ideal—pale, dainty, modest, and fashionable in her cool-colored dress—not only amplifies the servant's faults, it also clearly draws on humoral theory to make visible the deep, natural differences between them and the broader implications of the disruption that can be caused by inviting (or allowing) the sanguine Irish into one's home (or country).[37] Like the boiling-over pot on the stove and the smoking pie in the oven, the hot Irish temperament was a source of impending danger and ruin. There was no reasoning with it, and it could shatter domestic (and national) tranquility like a dish on a kitchen floor. This image of the Irish immigrant woman was one not entirely inherited from the British. It was also shaped by the initial encounter between Irish immigrants and native-born Americans in the late 1840s.

This chapter has focused on the importance of epidemic typhus fever in this encounter in New York City, from the perspectives of White native-born Americans. Historians have shown that prior to the arrival of this unprecedentedly large wave of immigrants, Americans had formed negative stereotypes of the Irish, viewing them as likely to become paupers and thus a people unsuitable for U.S. citizenship, a seminal aspect of which was self-sufficiency. Many Americans believed the combined influences of Roman Catholicism and British colonialism had cultivated poor habits among the Irish, thus centering their faults on the cultural practices and political conditions that shaped Irish character. Anti-Irish prejudice intensified with the massive increase in immigration from Ireland during the famine that brought more unskilled, previously rural-dwelling, poorer, Catholic Irish to American shores. Consequences of this increased prejudice included a surge in nativism and changes to state immigration policies that permitted rejecting (from New York) or even deporting (from Massachusetts) immigrants inspectors deemed likely to become public charges. Such policies later shaped federal immigration policies (Hirota 2017).

This chapter suggests that Americans' reactions to typhus fever among famine-era Irish immigrants played an important role in not only increasing prejudice but also in the shift that historians have described toward greater emphasis on more dangerous aspects of Irish character and toward justification of such stereotypes in inherited physiological difference. The visibly terrible conditions of many famine-era Irish immigrants upon arrival attracted attention and prompted visceral reactions among Americans. Some struggled to recognize the equal humanity of these newcomers, comparing them to animals and insects, while others were sympathetic but terrified of another deadly and unfamiliar disease and what to do with so many who would need help. In New York, city officials, physicians, and the public fell back on updated versions of old strategies and ideas to meet their new needs: quarantine, humoral theory and British stereotypes of the sanguine Irish, and rhetoric about descent from ancient Celts and Anglo-Saxons reinvigorated by nationalism and race science. From these perspectives, the easily discernible symptoms of typhus fever—high fever, red rash, and delirium—were evidence that the Irish were intrinsically different from the British and their American cultural descendants. Typhus fever vividly revealed naturally overheated Irish interiors, explaining a "predisposition" not only to poverty and being misled by priests and politicians but also to mania, alcoholism, and violence.

It is, of course, difficult to assess how widespread such views of essential Irish difference actually were among Americans at this time and the impacts of such views on Irish immigrants in the U.S. when they did not lead to government policies, aside from the important immigration policies mentioned above. As many scholars have pointed out, anti-Irish prejudice never produced the extreme racial legal discrimination imposed upon other groups of people Americans categorized as non-White, particularly African Americans and Native Americans. The Irish were never legally considered eligible for enslavement, never permitted to be tortured with impunity, never not allowed to testify in court on their own behalf, never considered permanently ineligible for citizenship, etc. While not at all comparable to such discrimination, this chapter has proposed that the idea of essential Irish difference did infect the minds of the most well educated American physicians at one of the nation's leading hospitals. This prejudice had real effects in misdiagnoses and harsher treatments that increased the suffering of individual patients and in hospital reports that inflated the incidence of typhus fever among the Irish and thus supplied authoritative evidence of supposed intrinsic, pathological difference.

The distinction between the ideas that the source of Irish difference was inside their bodies versus in their culture and practices mattered, although not as much as skin color, in an American context where ideas about supposed physiological differences between "Black" and "White" races had been used to defend permanent enslavement and other atrocities. Ideas about culture, class, and physiological difference were always intertwined, and which caused which was debated, but in the 1840s and 1850s, as the popularity of race science increased, more people in the U.S. and Britain viewed the body as a relatively fixed substrate, formed through biological inheritance, and the ultimate source of other differences. In the case of Irish immigrants, always categorized as White, such a distinction put into question the American nationalist myth about how the unique American environment and culture—including Protestantism, democratic government, and an ethos of self-reliance—had produced an exceptional nation, able to successfully integrate and foster prosperity among (White) people from many places and of many backgrounds. The famine Irish tested this myth. At the time, it was unclear whether exposure to the American "climate" could cool their sanguine temperaments and make them suitably American in character. Typhus fever combined with the continuance of Irish practices, such as imbibing alcohol and participating in wakes (see Chapter 3), suggested to New Yorkers that Irish temperaments were hotter and more hardwired than imagined. Chapter 4 considers the implications of such ideas in the kinds of work Irish immigrants were able to find in New York City and how many Americans believed they were naturally suited to manual labor. The next chapter will shift perspectives and explore aspects of how Irish immigrants themselves experienced arrival and settlement in New York City, focusing again on typhus fever and drawing on a combination of documentary, folkloric, and archaeological resources.

CHAPTER 3

Irish Immigrant Perspectives of and Remedies for Typhus Fever

SIX WEEKS into his harrowing crossing between Liverpool and New York City in 1847, Manchester native William Smith, introduced in Chapter 2, fell ill from the dreaded "ship fever." In his subsequent publication, Smith (1850:23) wrote: "I was so dizzy that I could not walk without danger of falling. I was suffering from a violent pain in my head, my brains felt as if they were on fire, my tongue clove to the roof of my mouth and my lips were parched with excessive thirst. Cheerfully I would have given all the world . . . for one draught of water." He also described the delusions the disease caused among the passengers. Smith imagined his family (then still in Manchester) standing sadly before him; one Irish passenger fancied himself a Catholic priest and blessed all on board; another believed he had become a wealthy New Yorker; and a third tried to stab his wife because he imagined she threatened him.[1] Each of these hallucinations arguably reveals the desires and anxieties—about their souls, bodies, families, and fortunes— that immigrants carried with them to America.

This chapter investigates Irish immigrants' perspectives and experiences of typhus fever, in contrast to the previous chapter that examined the views of native-born Americans. This chapter does not provide a direct response to American nativism and Irish stereotypes, but instead focuses on the difficult conditions Irish immigrants faced and their attempts to manage them. It draws from historical and folklore records as well as archaeological remains from the Five Points site to uncover how Irish immigrants understood typhus fever and responded to it in New York City. These records suggest that in their new urban environment, Irish immigrants initially sought out familiar healing practices for fever, and drinking alcoholic beverages was a leading remedy. This practice that many Americans believed was dangerous for the sanguine Irish, related to their propensity for typhus fever and central to negative stereotypes, was a vital healing strategy in many Irish immigrants' views. This interpretation draws attention to Irish immigrants' agency, especially to women's roles in healing and in a possible "hidden industry" to support themselves and their communities.

Through the Lens of Typhus: Experiences of Emigrant Ships and New York City Hospitals

William Smith was English, but he came from Manchester, England, a city heavily populated with Irish immigrants laboring in the textile industry in which he also labored. As a steerage passenger, he shared tight quarters (Figure 3.1) and shipboard experiences with poor Irish passengers. Upon arrival in New York City, he was quarantined like so many Irish immigrants. This section sketches out the general contours of many Irish immigrants' immigration experiences as they relate to typhus fever as gathered from firsthand accounts of Smith and others as well as secondary sources.

Smith described his experiences aboard the *India* to include: airlessness, fetid odors, intense heat, and constant near darkness in the steerage; violent storms that destroyed passengers' possessions and caused miscarriages; injuries from ship equipment and falls; shortages of food and water; absence of a physician or adequate medicines; witnessing deaths of other passengers; chronic seasickness; acute diarrhea; and finally typhus fever. In the end, Smith's ship arrived in New York in better shape than some, which he attributed to the efforts of a skillful and compassionate captain, who himself succumbed to typhus fever.

While not every Irish immigrant had horrible shipboard experiences, and some even claimed their health improved while at sea and others made important alliances (McMahon 2021:1, 131–145), many immigrant letters and journals describe events similar to those Smith detailed, or other horrors.[2] These include abuse by the crew or other passengers, childbirth in terrible conditions, fires, leaks, running aground, and collisions with other ships or icebergs.[3] All of this was on top of traumas encountered before embarkation, including: malnourishment, sickness,

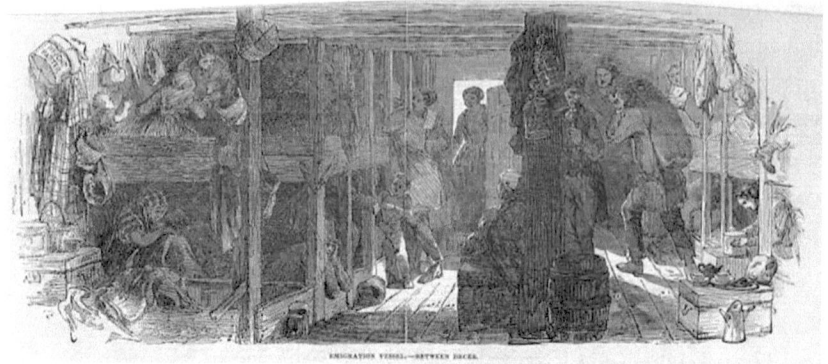

FIGURE 3.1. Drawing of the interior of an emigrant ship printed in the *Illustrated London News* (1851:387). Courtesy of the New York Public Library Digital Collections.

eviction, separation from family and community, and for some, a stay in a workhouse and/or arduous and distressing journeys to the Irish coast, encountering corpses along the roadsides.[4] Some ships departed Irish ports for North America, but the majority arriving in New York departed from Liverpool. To reach those ships required crossing the notoriously rough Irish sea, and put emigrants at risk in Liverpool, if their ships did not set sail immediately.[5] Liverpool was among the most unhealthy and dangerous cities in England, reportedly so filthy that "sailors claimed they could smell Liverpool on the horizon" and so crime ridden that gangs of criminals robbed and assaulted people in daylight (Scally 1995:187).[6] An English health official dubbed Liverpool in 1847 "the cemetery of Ireland" (Neal 1998:142). The workhouses and boardinghouses that harbored Irish emigrants in Liverpool as well as the ships that brought them across the Atlantic provided perfect conditions for contracting (or experiencing a recrudescence) and spreading typhus: cramped, dirty, and filled with people who were already depleted.[7] All of these experiences took heavy tolls on passengers' health before they reached New York City.

When Dr. John Griscom entered the steerage of the ship *Ceylon* in 1847 upon its arrival in New York (see Chapter 2), he found scores of sick and emaciated passengers "just rising from their berths from the first time since Liverpool having been suffered to lie there all the voyage wallowing in their own filth" (Select Committee of the Senate of the United States 1854:54). While this ship was a particularly egregious example, nearly all immigrant ships during this period lost at least some passengers to illness or injury; 1% to 2.5% mortality was "normal," according to historian Cian McMahon (2021:148–49, 151), and typhus fever was a leading cause of death, along with cholera and dysentery. Immigrants remarked how watching loved ones or even strangers perish at sea was traumatic, and many were particularly distressed about the treatment of the deceased, "buried" at sea in a watery grave far from home with little or no funeral rites (McMahon 2021:151, 165–167, 170–176). Such emotionally debilitating experiences also increased their susceptibility to disease; scientific research has shown that stress depresses immune function (Dressler 1996:265). Many probably continued to suffer from what would be diagnosed today as post-traumatic stress disorder, complicating their adjustment to life in New York. Some were sent directly to New York City's quarantine hospitals and subjected to further trials there.

William Smith described the abuses he encountered in the Staten Island Marine Hospital, including the poor heating system that made some freeze and others swelter, scant bedding on iron beds that cut and bruised his emaciated frame, poor quality and quantity of food, the doctors' apathy, and the nurses' cruelty. The nurses were "the most hardhearted and cruel set of men there ever was. . . . I saw no kind feelings, no generous actions shown to us . . . every opportunity was taken by these miscreants to display their little brief authority" (Smith 1850:25; 27–28). Smith was not alone. Others complained of mistreatment there and on Ward's Island (Hirota 2017:92). At such quarantine hospitals, historian of medicine Morris Vogel (1985:291) wrote, "the welfare of the patient was often secondary to the well-being of the society that required his isolation." The cruelty Smith suffered was magnified by how it shattered his expectations. "Little did I think that in this glorious land of freedom I should meet with such a reception," he wrote (Smith 1850:28). Like many Irish immigrants, Smith distrusted hospitals at home, but was optimistic about all aspects of life in America. The U.S. had a reputation as a land of opportunity that rewarded hard work, an idea reinforced by remittances and some rosy immigrant letters, containing what Miller (1993:269) describes as "highly selective use of information."[8] Between Smith's cruel treatment at this hospital and the unfriendly receptions he received from some Americans once in the city (recall his being rejected from lodging and feared by streetcar passengers), he felt dismayed and rejected. Smith resolved to seek help at hospitals thereafter only if absolutely necessary.

For Smith, and many Irish immigrants of the famine era, typhus fever was integral to their experience of immigration. Whether or not they suffered from the disease themselves, they viewed others who did and/or were suspected of harboring the disease. As described in the previous chapter, typhus fever influenced how Americans received them. Such receptions made at least some feel alienated, a sentiment exacerbated by prior hopes of acceptance and prosperity, as well as by profound trauma and suffering during their travels that could not be fully appreciated even by the most sympathetic of Americans. For many, the appropriate response was to seek out familiar people and medicines for healing.

Popular Irish Views of Hospitals and Physicians

Hospitals and professional physicians would not have been familiar to most Irish immigrants, unless they had lived in or near Irish cities: Dublin, Belfast, Galway, and Cork.[9] Professional medicine in Dublin was on par with London and included several hospitals.[10] Dublin medical schools turned out many graduates relative to the general population, but most left Ireland for better job opportunities elsewhere (Malcolm and Jones 1999:4). In rural areas, from where the majority of famine-era immigrants to New York had come, professional medical services were limited and inadequate. Choices there included poorly equipped infirmaries and dispensaries offering free care and staffed by overextended doctors, notorious workhouse/poorhouse hospitals, or expensive and rare private physicians.[11] Cormac Ó Gráda (1994:187) optimistically estimates that in Connaught there was one doctor per 10,000 inhabitants, compared with 1.8 doctors in Munster, 2.1 in Ulster, and 2.9 in Leinster in 1851, only slightly higher ratios than in 1841.[12] Private physicians charged from 7 shillings to 1 pound for a home visit in 1855 when the average wage of a laborer was 8 pence a day (Fleetwood 1983:134). Given these options, it is not surprising that most rural Irish had infrequent access to professional medicine and chose to avoid it.

Written and oral histories suggest people in rural areas distrusted physicians for several reasons including: lack of frequent contact, unaffordable fees, religious differences, physicians' harsh treatments (purges and bleedings), fears of being subjected to experimentation, and "unshakable faith . . . in traditional remedies" (Connell 1975:188).[13] Distrust of physicians was so great that a popular rumor in Ireland during the 1832 cholera epidemic was that physicians had created the disease and poisoned patients to exact a profit; the discoloration of those who died was interpreted as proof of mistreatment. In Dublin, people "rescued" patients being taken to hospitals, assaulting carriers and throwing carriages into the River Liffey (Robins 1995:74–75). A satirical article published later in the century in *Harper's Weekly* (1879:806) highlights the rural Irish's lasting lack of confidence in professional physicians. Supposedly written by an Irish dispensary doctor, the article illustrates how nearby villagers refused to follow his directions and showed him little respect. They tested his prescription on the family cat, adjusted doses, exchanged the medicines amongst themselves, and told the doctor his advice had hastened the deaths of their neighbors.

Given most rural Irish people's negative views of physicians and hospitals, the fact that so many Irish immigrants *were* treated in New York City hospitals attests to the gravity of their illnesses (and injuries) and their desperation. Contrary to the opinion of nativists, who framed Irish immigrants as dependent and desirous to accept charity, the vast majority tried to avoid the hospital. Analysis of New York Hospital medical case records from the late 1840s and early 1850s shows that the majority of Irish immigrant patients had been sick for many days, if not weeks, before arriving at the hospital; others had been forced there by authorities. Irish typhus fever patients, for example, waited an average of a week of feeling ill before seeking hospital care (NYHMCB 1847–1852), likely only after they had exhausted familiar remedies or could no longer care for themselves. It is probable, though the case records do not supply adequate information to definitively assert this, that immigrants unable to connect with family or friends in the city sought care in the hospital earlier than those who had a network of people to take care of them. The Irish were not alone in considering the hospital as a place of last resort. Native-born Americans reportedly "would not allow even a hired member of his or her 'family' to be cared for by strangers" in such institutions. Fears of rampant infection and experimentation on patients, alive and dead, were high on the list of concerns (Duffy 1968:484, 496; Vogel 1979:106; Rosenberg 1987b:16). If they had any choice in the matter, most New Yorkers of all backgrounds preferred home care. Irish immigrants who fell ill after passing quarantine likely tried to cure themselves of typhus first with trusted home remedies, and then with help from others in their community, before going to the hospital.

Historical studies show that many Irish immigrants had friends and family in New York who could help them, even upon first arrival. Some traveled with family, others met those who had immigrated before them, many of whom sent remittances back to Ireland to assist the immigration of others. Chain migration and landowner-assisted emigration fostered the concentration of family and former neighbors into particular neighborhoods (see Chapter 1) (Anbinder et al. 2019a). Previous connections helped many newcomers to quickly find community in New York City. Evidence of such ties might be seen in instances in which families took in children of relatives or friends who could not care for them. Mrs. Huxley's adoption of her grandson is one example (Chapter 1). Another is the adoption of an 8-year-old girl by John and Catherine Ward of 474 Pearl Street (NYSC 1855). Even more distant connections could aid a newcomer in finding help in New York; reference to a mutual acquaintance or origin in a common county or parish in Ireland, for example, could be enough. "Runners" for boardinghouses found such shared knowledge was often enough to persuade the newly arrived to follow them, often not to the benefit of the newcomer. Personal job referrals were critical to Irish immigrants in finding jobs, resulting in the clustering of individuals from particular regions or townlands in particular occupations (Anbinder et al. 2019a:1597, 1612). Obligations of reciprocity and mutual aid so important for survival in rural Ireland (see Chapter 1), and in agricultural communities worldwide, were also vital for the Irish in New York City, providing "bulwarks against disaster" in this and other urban areas too (Arensberg 1937:69, 84).[14]

When disaster struck in the form of illness in New York City, such obligations informed immigrants' expectations of help that they could receive from (and later return to) their neighbors. Archaeological remains, discussed later in the chapter, also support the idea that familiar people and substances formed the first line of defense for the residents of 472 and 474 Pearl Street. Distrust of hospitals and physicians and trust in home remedies and neighbors help to explain the observed delays between when Irish immigrants fell ill from typhus and when they resorted to hospital care.

Popular Irish Understandings of and Cures for Typhus Fever

If hospitals and physicians were unfamiliar, what were the familiar Irish approaches to treating serious fevers in the 19th century? The rich archives of the [Irish] National Folklore Collection (NFC) and other folklore sources can be used to piece together how fevers were popularly understood and treated. These records rarely distinguish between different fevers, suggesting that popular approaches to most fevers were the same. Working from these records, I propose that like their American contemporaries, most Irish people explained typhus fever to be a result of "exciting" and "predisposing" causes. Their perspectives differed, however, in the factors they placed within these two categories. Instead of miasma as the exciting cause of typhus, most Irish people attributed it to a poison from a variety of possible sources, such as bad air or food, witchcraft or fairy malevolence. Similarly, the Irish shared the idea that an already imbalanced body could predispose an individual to sickness, but they rarely mentioned humors or temperament, or hereditary predisposition. Instead, they focused upon near-term conditions, such as overwork, exposure to cold or wetness, and inadequate diet, as harmful and leading to greater susceptibility to illness (see Chapter 1). Additionally, in Ireland, people considered fevers to be transferable from person to person and from people to animals (Logan 1994). The most commonly mentioned method of transfer was through a shared drink (Ó Súilleabháin 1970:312). Some reported that fever could be removed from a house by filling it with sheep, the logic presumably being that the disease would be taken up by the sheep (NFC 1941[782]:360).[15]

Irish physicians and laypeople understood fevers to be dangerous and to frequently afflict the poor, especially during periods of famine. Nineteenth-century physician William Wilde studied Irish censuses of 1841 and 1851 and found fevers to be the leading cause of death, accounting for nearly 20% of all deaths nationwide (Farmar 2004:94).

Four major typhus fever epidemics in Ireland corresponded to periods of famine, 1816–1819, 1826–1827, 1836–1837, 1846–1849, as did localized epidemics in 1879–1880 and 1898. "In the popular mind fever and famine were related" (Crawford 1999:121). Popular Irish cures for fever noted by folklore collectors were relatively few compared with those for other ailments, and a greater number of fever cures appear to draw upon supernatural healing power. This suggests that the Irish recognized that some fevers were part of larger calamities and not easily cured. Remedies they did employ focused on both perceived causes and symptoms.

From the perspective of the sufferer, the most pronounced early symptoms of typhus are those that are not clearly visible to others: headache and fever chills. In Ireland and the U.S., Irish people reported that fevers, as well as colds and tuberculosis, began with a cold sensation. They tried to remedy this by warming themselves by a heat source, with more clothes, or with alcoholic beverages, including whiskey, wine, and brandy.[16] Most Irish people understood alcoholic beverages to be warming, strengthening, and able to drive out poisons, making them both good preventive medicine and effective remedies for exciting and predisposing causes of fever. The most commonly mentioned remedy for fever was drinking whiskey or *poitín* (homemade whiskey) (Wilde, L. 1890:42; NFC 1941[782]:196–198; Ó Súilleabháin 1970:312). Whiskey had long been revered in Ireland as a powerful substance; the Gaelic word for whiskey, *uisce beatha*, translates to "water of life." Lady Wilde (1890:42), a late 19th-century collector of folklore, for example, was told by an Irishman that "for ordinary disease there is nothing as good as the native poteen, for it is peculiarly adapted to the climate, and, as the people say, it keeps away the ague and rheumatism, and the chill that strikes the heart; and if the gaugers [liquor tax officers] would only let the private stills alone, not a bit of sickness would there be in the whole country." Whiskey was also the popular remedy of choice for unfamiliar and fearsome illnesses. During the 1832 cholera epidemic in Ireland, for example, many people were observed wandering "blind drunk." A man in Cork went so far as to plunge his cholera-stricken wife daily into a hogshead of distillery wash and made her drink large quantities of brandy and castor oil (Robins 1995:102). Whiskey remained a popular remedy into the 20th century. During the influenza epidemics of 1884 and 1918, *poitín* mixed with honey was a widely used cure (Logan

1994:27). Elderberry flower wine was also regarded as a "cure–all . . . if it failed to clear up the trouble in question, then it could only be that something serious was afoot" (Allen and Hatfield 2004:272).[17]

A number of herbal remedies to treat fever included: a drink made of brewed clover blossoms and sloe leaves or infusions of boneset (*Eupatorium perfoliatum*), centaury (*Centaurium erythraea* or possibly *pulchellum*), common sorrel (*Rumex acetosa*), tansy (*Tanacetum vulgare*), wall lettuce (*Mucelis muralis*), watercress (*Rorippa nasturtium-aquaticum*), or yarrow (*Achillea millefolium*) (Purdon 1895b:295; NFC ca. 1929[35]:247; NFCS 1938[35]:249; Allen and Hatfield 2004:118, 194–195, 272, 287, 296, 302). Alcohol was often an ingredient, said to complement herbal remedies by extracting and preserving their medicinal properties (Logan 1994:38). These herbal remedies addressed perceived symptoms and causes of fever. For example, according to ethnobotanists David E. Allen and Gabrielle Hatfield (2004:302), people in the British Isles believed that yarrow opened the pores and promoted sweating that would bring down body temperature. Other plants, such as sorrel and tansy, induced purging, which the Irish believed would drive fever-causing poisons out of the body. Tansy was also used to remove intestinal worms (Allen and Hatfield 2004:96, 295).

Other remedies could have been used to treat other fever symptoms. There were a number of popular headache cures, including, again, drinking whiskey or *poitín*, eating cabbage, drinking strong tea or an infusion of mint, smoking tobacco, washing the head with an infusion of chamomile or cold water, massaging the head with goose grease, rubbing the temples with crowfoot leaves, applying mustard or pitch to the head to create blisters, applying vinegar to paper and placing it on the head, and tying moss or a cloth around the head.[18] In County Kerry, the cloth used to wrap a corpse was said to be especially effective for curing a headache (NFC 1941[782]:247).

Several fever cures reported to collectors appeared to address perceived supernatural causes and/or were intended to draw upon supernatural healing power (see Chapter 1). A charm cure for fever reported with slight variations in counties Donegal, Cavan, Roscommon, Mayo, Westmeath, and Cork was "when Our Lord saw the cross he was to be crucified upon he shivered and said, 'whoever shall say these words—this prayer—either in word or mind shall never fear a fever or an ache'"

(NFCS 1937[981]:146; NFCS 1938[353]:499; NFCS 1938[1028]:447). Making a vow to abstain from eating meat or from shaving was understood to engage the divine and oblige reciprocation with healing. Physician and folklorist Patrick Logan (1994:8) wrote that many Irish had great faith in these vows well into the 20th century; he once heard a man who "when told his sister had typhoid fever, declared this was impossible because nobody in their family ever ate meat on the second day of Christmas."

Other fever remedies sought to access supernatural power in special places in the Irish landscape, such as holy wells, large stones, grave sites, and the ocean. Numerous wells throughout the country were known for their power to cure or protect from any number of illnesses. St. Brigid's Well near Ballyheigue in County Kerry was famous particularly for curing fever (Logan 1994:8). An informant in County Wexford relayed that there is a coffin stone in Bannow Bay that could cure a person suffering from backache or headache by lying in it (NFC 1935[54]:78). An informant in County Clare advised that dipping one's head in the water on any stone in a graveyard would cure a headache (NFCS 1937[598]:104). Michael Kennedy, a farmer from County Kerry, noted, "If a person has fever it can be cured by carrying him to the sea shore when the tide is in[;] lay him down on the sand and leave him there until the tide is going out and the fever will leave and go away with the tide" (NFC 1941[782]:360).

Most of these fever remedies appear to have been well known throughout the country because they were frequently mentioned and were easy enough to have been administered by family members, neighbors, or the patient. There are other cures that required specialized healers, however. The seventh-born son in a family, for example, was said to be able to cure "illness" with his touch, while a child born after their father's death could cure a headache (Blake 1918:222; NFC 1930[80]:20; NFCS 1937[598]:433; NFCS 1938[345]:15; Logan 1994:47, 53). Some Catholic priests and local saints were believed to channel divine healing power, and the soil from the graves of others was said to be curative (NFCS 1938[345]:8; NFC 1938[514]:30–37; NFC 1974[1838]:274–278). Informants in Northern Ireland noted that in the more recent past, emigrants carried with them a bit of "St. Mogue's Clay" for protection (Glassie 1982:174). "Wisewomen," as I will describe later in this chapter, were sought out for serious illnesses, often after ordinary remedies had failed. The next section applies these insights about 19th-century Irish popular approaches to fevers to interpret archaeological remains from the Five Points site in Lower Manhattan.

Treating Typhus Fever in the Tenements: Archaeological Remains of Popular Irish Remedies at the Five Points, New York

The Five Points, briefly described in the Introduction, was a mixed-use, multiethnic, working-class neighborhood within the city's Sixth Ward where many Irish immigrants settled, especially during their first five to ten years in the U.S. Middle-class native-born New Yorkers regarded it as a slum, a dangerous place to live because of inadequate sanitation and drainage, overcrowding, deteriorating housing, and higher rates of illness and crime (Figure 3.2). Rents were low, however, and the presence of Irish immigrants drew others from their home regions who preferred to live near friends and, like William Smith, often felt unwelcomed by native-born Americans.

A large-scale archaeological excavation in 1993 within the boundaries of the former neighborhood unearthed material traces left behind by residents that challenge the one-dimensional slum narratives in written records. Underneath the present-day city lots, archaeologists excavated features such as privies, cisterns, and drainage ditches that had been in the backyards of tenement buildings. These features contained thousands of artifacts, as well as faunal and floral remains (Yamin 2000 [1–6]).[19] Careful digging, with attention to how remains were deposited and the surrounding soil matrix, combined with analysis of the artifacts and their manufacturing dates and historical evidence of backyard renovations, enabled archaeologists to surmise approximately when the residents discarded the artifacts.

Archaeologists used census records and city directories to determine who had lived in buildings connected to each feature when the artifacts were deposited. They found that the tenements located at 472 and 474 Pearl Street were inhabited almost exclusively by Irish immigrants between 1850 and 1870 (USBC 1850, 1860, and 1870; NYSC 1855). Associated with these buildings were a few artifact-filled features, shown in Figure 3.3. Feature J+Z was a stone-lined cesspool and drainage complex at 472

108 *Irish Immigrant Perspectives of and Remedies for Typhus Fever*

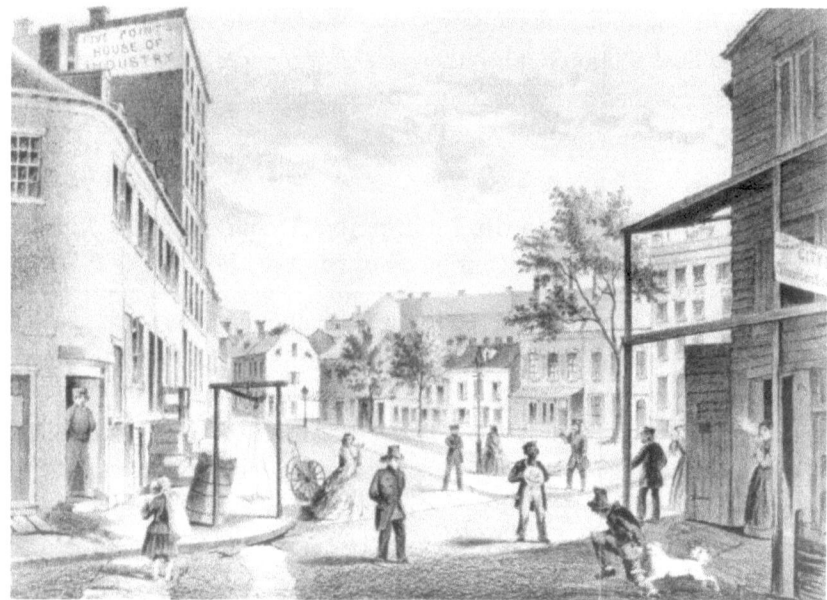

FIGURE 3.2. Illustration titled "The Five Points in 1859. View taken from the corner of Worth & Little Water St.," published in the *Manual of the Corporation of the City of New York for 1860* (Valentine 1860). Courtesy of the Library of Congress.

Pearl (on Lot 6) with two layers, one deposited after 1850 but before the early 1860s and another deposited around 1870. Feature O was a stone-lined privy at 474 Pearl (on Lot 7) with one layer deposited after 1860 (Brighton 2008:143). I will follow archaeological convention and refer to the layers by their *terminus post quem* (TPQ) dates, the earliest dates that the layers could have been deposited—1850, 1860, and 1870, respectively (Miller et al. 2000).[20] These deposits thus contain traces of Irish residents' activities between the late 1840s and the early 1870s that would otherwise be inaccessible. This section analyzes material remains that relate to typhus fever and early adjustment to life in New York City.

Census records show that many of the people who resided in these two buildings had immigrated during the famine period (Brighton 2008:139–140). It is possible that some suffered from typhus fever.[21] Remains unearthed in these contexts included several ingredients used in popular cures in Ireland for fever or headache: liquor (bottles),

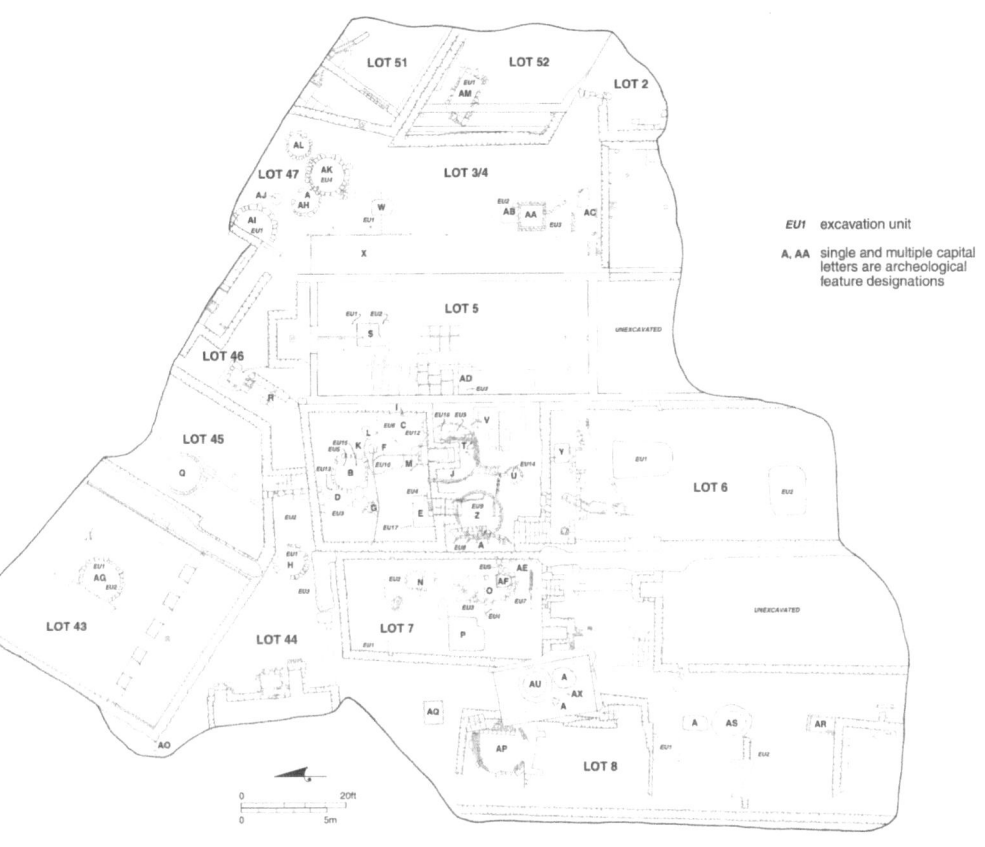

FIGURE 3.3. Plan showing features identified by archaeologists at the Five Points site. Features J + Z and O, associated with the Irish tenements at 472 and 474 Pearl Street, are within Lots 6 and 7 (Yamin 2000[1]:7).

110　*Irish Immigrant Perspectives of and Remedies for Typhus Fever*

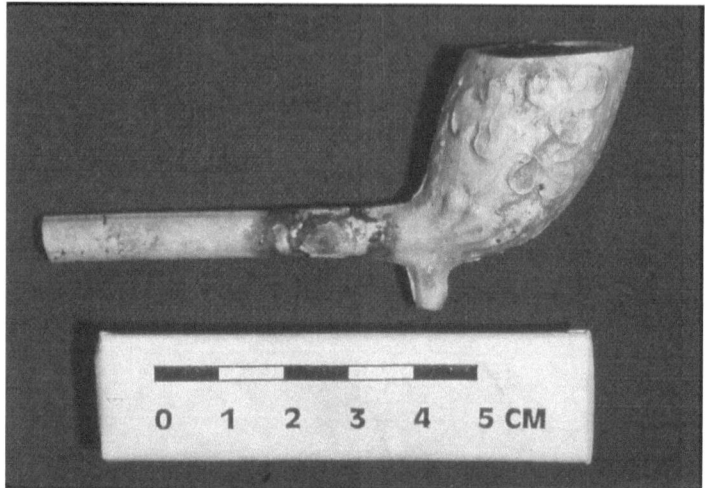

FIGURE 3.4. Photograph of a clay tobacco pipe unearthed in Feature J at the Five Points (Reckner 2000:102). This example was decorated with shamrocks. In County Donegal, it was said that smoking a pipe would cure a headache (Dorian 2000:274). Image courtesy of Rebecca Yamin and the New York City Archaeological Repository: The Nan A. Rothschild Research Center.

mustard (bottles), tobacco pipes (Figure 3.4), cloth, sorrel (*Rumex species*), mint (*Mentha* species—in the 1850 layer of Feature J only), elderberry (*Sambucus canadensis*), and goose bones, possibly left from the process of making goose grease (Milne and Crabtree 2000; Ponz 2000; Raymer et al. 2000).[22] The presence of these ingredients does not mean that Irish residents necessarily used them to cure fevers, because they had other possible uses. Their presence, nevertheless, confirms that residents had access and chose to acquire them, and large numbers of medicine bottles that were contained in the same deposits suggest residents engaged in healing at home.[23]

Medicine bottles stand out to archaeologists as clear evidence of healing practices that resonate with present-day practices. They are usually relatively easily identifiable because of their distinctive shapes; some are embossed with names of pharmacies or brands. Medicine bottles found in the 1850 layer of Feature J+Z at 472 Pearl Street composed almost 35% of the glass vessel assemblage (Figure 3.5). In the 1870 layer from the

Irish Immigrant Perspectives of and Remedies for Typhus Fever 111

same feature, medicine bottles composed 26% of the glass vessels. Next door at 474 Pearl Street, the percentage of medicine bottles in Feature O was even more striking, accounting for 40% of the glass vessels. The proportion of soda water bottles, another medicinal substance discussed in Chapter 7, was high in comparison to other sites in New York City. Soda water bottles accounted for 3% and 14% of the glass vessels at 472 Pearl Street, in the 1850 and 1870 layers, respectively, and 7% of the glass vessels at 474 Pearl in the 1860 layer.[24] The glass artifact assemblage thus clearly indicates the Irish residents of these buildings were actively engaged in healing at home. This pattern increases the likelihood that residents also used the remains mentioned above as medicines and suggests taking a closer look at the alcoholic beverage bottles in the assemblages, given the important role that liquor, and whiskey especially, played in popular cures in Ireland.

Alcoholic beverage bottles made up a smaller portion of the artifacts excavated from the 472 and 474 Pearl Street deposits, amounting

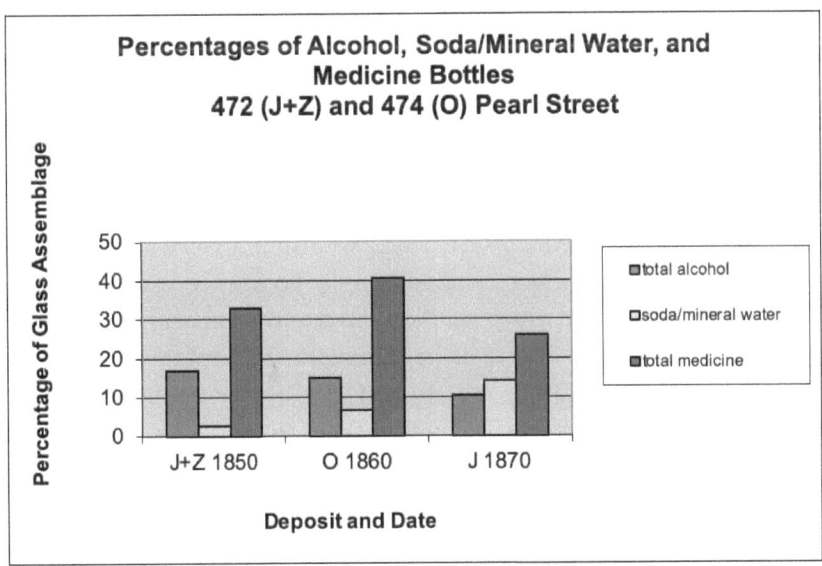

FIGURE 3.5. Graph showing the percentages of alcohol, soda/mineral water, and medicine bottles composing the glass bottle assemblage in features associated with Irish immigrants at 472 and 474 Pearl Street. Compiled by author from Bonasera 2000a, Ponz 2000, Yamin 2000[1 and 4], and Brighton 2005.

to between 11% and 17% of the glass assemblages (Figure 3.5). Wine bottles were most represented, composing between 3% and 14% of the glass bottles in each deposit. A small number of cylindrical liquor-style bottles, a type often used for whiskey, were also found, accounting for between 2% and 4% of the glass bottles. Such bottles are significant because none were found in features associated with German or Polish residents, where archaeologists found glass wine and case bottles (frequently used for gin) and ceramic beer bottles, suggesting they preferred other beverages (Yamin 2000[1]:Appendix A). Whiskey appears to have been a uniquely Irish preference on this Five Points block. A typical interpretation might propose these bottles support the stereotype that the Irish were avid—sometimes too avid—recreational whiskey drinkers, while a typical interpretation of wine bottles might suggest adoption of middle-class values. The remainder of this chapter considers how residents might have additionally, or instead, used the contents of these bottles in healing activities, given that other artifacts in these assemblages indicate residents' concerns with healing, the long tradition of using whiskey and wine as medicines in Ireland, and the health threats to famine-era immigrants.

It is worth noting that some of the *medicine* bottles found in the Irish-related deposits at the Five Points could have contained substances residents used to treat typhus fever. Determining exactly which ailments a consumer acquired a bottled medicine to treat is very difficult. Paper labels on prescription bottles rarely survive. Patent/proprietary medicines (identifiable by embossments on bottles) were often advertised as able to cure a wide range of problems.[25] Additionally, consumers with different cultural worldviews had different ideas about why a particular medicine might be desirable and how to use it (Linn 2022). Chapters 5 and 7 will focus on medicine bottles in the 472 and 474 Pearl Street deposits and suggest that residents more likely used them to manage work-related injuries and tuberculosis—long-term problems—than acute typhus fever. Irish immigrants typically suffered from the former ailments over a longer period of time, during which they became more acquainted with professional medicine and patent medicine brands, whereas most who fell ill with typhus fever had been in the city only a short time. These newcomers likely sought tried-and-true fever cures: alcoholic beverages or mixtures provided by Irish healers. For this reason, and because

Americans interpreted Irish consumption of alcoholic beverages as a contributing factor to typhus fever, alcoholic beverage bottles are more relevant to this chapter.

Irish Immigrants and Alcohol: Social Medicines in the Pub Versus in the Home

Archaeologists have typically followed the leads of historians and interpreted alcoholic beverage bottles found in working-class contexts as traces of recreation, male sociality, resistance, alliance building, and/or maintenance of working-class identities (Rorabaugh 1979; Rosenzweig 1983; Levin 1985; Bond 1989; Mrozowski et al. 1989; Reckner and Brighton 1999; Casella 2000). Overindulgence in alcohol was a prominent aspect of Irish stereotypes, but reformers in the 19th century were concerned about alcohol consumption among the poor and working class more broadly as a source of poverty, worker inefficiency, domestic abuse, and crime; liquor drinking was thought to be a gateway to prostitution for women (Rosenzweig 1983; Stansell 1986:80–81; Bond 1989:138; Fitts 2000b; Stivers 2000). A number of studies have shown that while some Irish immigrants did abuse alcohol, as did some native-born Americans and members of other immigrant groups, involvement in the liquor trade and consumption of alcoholic beverages in drinking establishments was important socially, politically, and economically for Irish immigrants.

Many Irish immigrants found economic success in some aspect of the alcoholic beverage trade. In his classic study of Boston's immigrants, for example, Oscar Handlin (1941:124–125) found that even as early as the late 1840s the majority of liquor dealers in the city were Irish. In New York City, Max Berger (1946:177) estimated that between 1840 and 1860 one-third to one-half of the liquor trade was Irish-controlled. In the Sixth Ward, most of the Irish men who owned land ran saloons or liquor stores (Groneman Pernicone 1973:111). Several saloon owners and liquor dealers became aldermen (Pitts 2000:65). Contemporary American observers portrayed the many Irish-owned liquor establishments in the Five Points—such as Richard Barry's saloon (Figure 3.6) at 488 Pearl Street, just a few doors down from 472 and 474 Pearl Street—as places where Democratic politicians extorted immigrant votes and where Irishmen

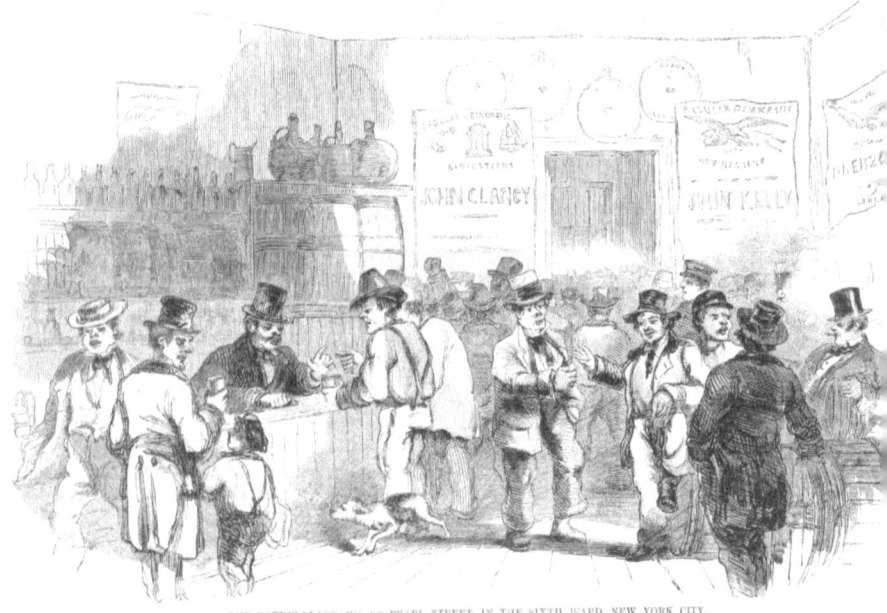

FIGURE 3.6. Illustration Titled "The Voting-Place, No. 488 Pearl Street, in the Sixth Ward, New York City," described in *Harper's Weekly* (1858:724) as a polling place where Democrats extorted Irish working-class votes. Courtesy of the Library of Congress.

wasted their wages on drinks that inflamed their already irrational constitutional tendencies. Barry himself was an assistant alderman from 1860 to 1861 (Pitts 2000:65). But, from an Irish immigrant's point of view, drinking at a neighborhood saloon was an investment in community and an opportunity to build social capital. Irish-owned pubs and groceries were important places of refuge, guidance, economic credit, and social and political interaction for Irish immigrants, and places to relieve homesickness, as other studies have shown (Rosenzweig 1983; Malcolm 1998; Stivers 2000; Diner 2001). Treating friends to drinks and exchanging help and advice in pubs was critical for survival in Ireland and remained so in New York City and other places Irish immigrants settled.

In the 19th century, like today, different drinks had different associations relative to economic status, social acceptability, and nationality, which also depended on who was making the associations. Native-born Americans generally associated wine with wealth and gentility, ales with relatively respectable working men, and rum with poverty and debauchery, for example. Lager beer, introduced by German immigrants, not surprisingly was associated with them and their family-oriented beer gardens. Whiskey was linked to the Irish, who had produced it in their homeland (Rorabaugh 1979; Stivers 2000). In Ireland, whiskey, and especially *poitín*, was an important component of many community-oriented rituals, such as births, weddings, and wakes. Whiskey was a substance that traditionally brought people together in good times and bad, for shared celebrations and sorrows. Additionally, because *poitín* was prohibited by the occupying British government, producing and consuming it was also an act of political resistance and a show of solidarity with the Irish nationalist cause (Malcolm 1998). These associations made public consumption of alcohol, and whiskey especially, an important kind of social medicine, active in constructing Irish community in New York City. Such strong connections to Ireland might have also increased whiskey's potency in the minds of those who used it for healing. With so many grocers, bartenders, and saloon owners in the Five Points, whiskey would not have been difficult to find, even for the newest of newcomers (Figure 3.7). The many motivations and opportunities to drink in public, as well as potential home-production (discussed below), help to explain why relatively small proportion of whiskey bottles, and alcoholic beverage bottles overall, were found in the deposits at 472 and 474 Pearl Street.[26] The residents do not seem to have engaged in frequent solitary or large-scale social drinking at home.

It is also important to consider how alcoholic beverages were used in homes in Ireland. There they were usually reserved for medicinal purposes (described above and in Chapter 1), to host guests, or for special occasions, such as brokering marriages or celebrating wakes. Folklorist Braid Mahon (1991) notes that each Irish household traditionally kept a bottle of whiskey they called the "priest's bottle" to be prepared for unexpected visits. Providing and accepting hospitality was and remains a core value of rural Irish society. As one of folklorist Henry Glassie's (1982:141) informants in 20th-century rural Ulster explained, "If you don't want tea, you must ask not to be asked, because if the tea ceremony begins . . . the host will push you until you take something and

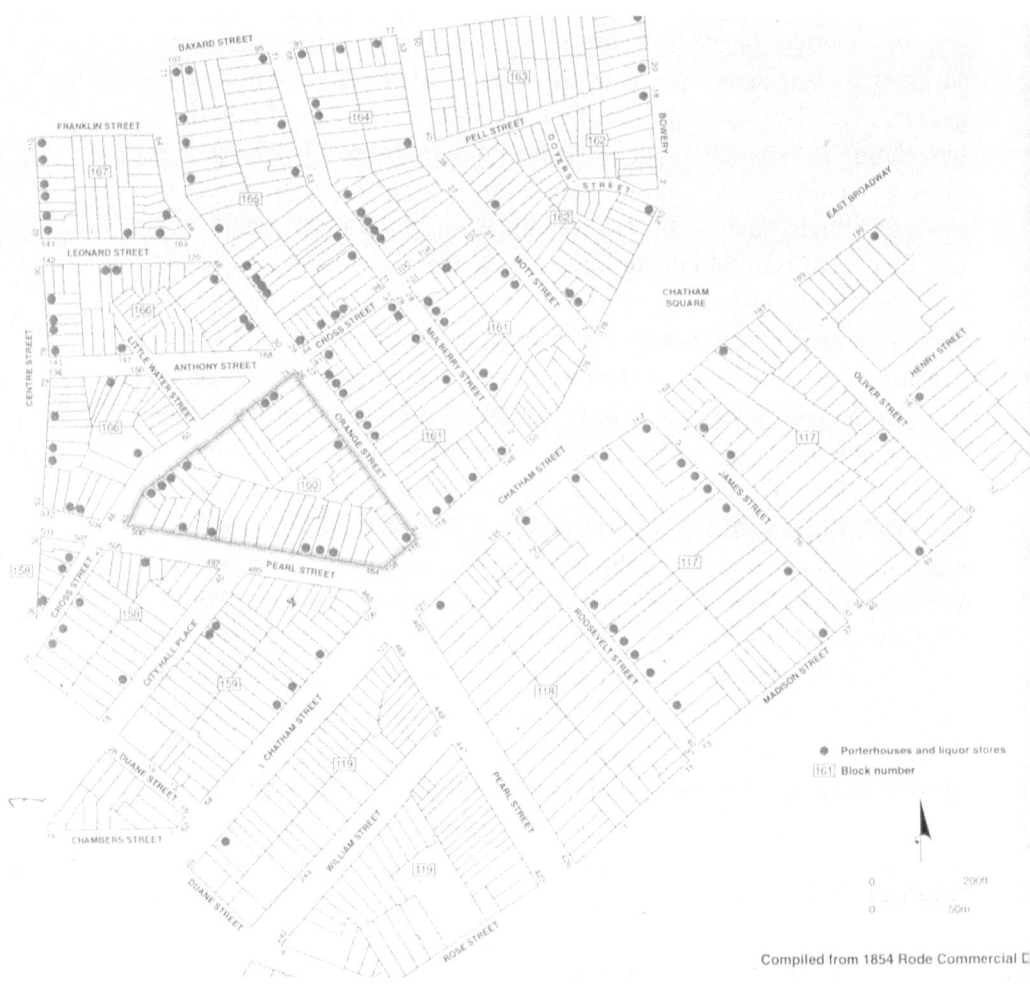

FIGURE 3.7. Locations of porterhouses and liquor stores near Five Points [Block 160 highlighted] at mid-century, compiled from Rode's *New York City Directory, for 1853–1854* (Reckner and Brighton 2000:455). Image courtesy of Rebecca Yamin and the New York City Archaeological Repository: The Nan A. Rothschild Research Center.

offers will become exceedingly embarrassing. Refuse tea and you will be made to drink the house's last bottle of stout." Hosting demonstrated generosity, and it enabled the host to call on the visitor later for a favor in return. Thus, alcoholic beverages were usually used at home to restore health, facilitate socially correct behavior, and generate social ties of personal obligation that could be utilized in times of need. It is no wonder that immigrants recommended to others departing after them to bring a pint or two of whiskey on the ship for medicinal use or to share with the ship's cook or sailors, or that others emphasized how well they were welcomed by old friends upon arrival in New York with "potatoes, meat, butter, bread, and tea for dinner and you may be sure we had a drink after" (McMahon 2021:62, 99, 223).

Whiskey, Wine, and Women

Of the alcoholic beverage bottles in the 472 Pearl Street deposits, wine bottles were the most numerous type: 28 in the 1850 layer and 9 in the 1870 layer. These numbers represent approximately 14% and 5% of the glass bottles in each layer, respectively (Figure 3.8). At 474, there were 3 in the 1860 deposit, representing 4% of the glass bottle assemblage.[27] Such quantities are somewhat surprising, because of the high relative cost of wine. Wine was approximately four times as expensive as whiskey during this period and would have been a significant expenditure for a working person (Williams 1985:134). This suggests that wine, wine bottles, or both, were valuable to the residents who acquired them. Consideration of Irish perspectives and predicaments in New York suggests three overlapping interpretations that draw attention to Irish immigrant women: wine as a genteel beverage for guests, a physician-approved medicine compatible with Irish medical ideas, and wine bottles as receptacles for homemade medicines, including whiskey.

Archaeologists excavating a 19th-century working-class neighborhood of Oakland, California, found a direct correlation not only between better employment and wine bottles but also between Irish female-headed households and wine bottles (Owen 2004:G1). This latter pattern can also be seen in the Five Points. Between 1850 and 1860, at 472 Pearl Street—the tenement associated with the 1850 layer of Feature J+Z where the most wine bottles were found—census records show that 31% of the 35

118 *Irish Immigrant Perspectives of and Remedies for Typhus Fever*

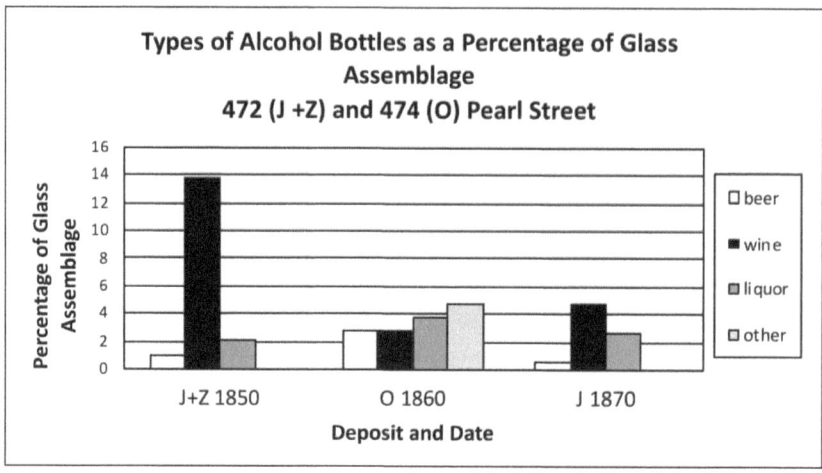

FIGURE 3.8. Graph showing beer, wine, liquor, and "other alcohol" bottles found in association with the Irish tenements at 472 and 474 Pearl Street as a percentage of the total glass bottle assemblage. Compiled by the author from Yamin 2000[1]:Appendix A.

individual Irish households were headed by women (USBC 1850, 1860; NYSC 1855). In the 1870 layer of the same feature, which contained the next highest number of wine bottles, 19% of 16 households were headed by women (USBC 1870). In the deposit with the least number of wine bottles—Feature O, associated with 474 Pearl Street circa 1860—19% of 21 households were female-headed (Brighton 2009:173-176). Irish women were frequently heads of households in both Oakland and the Five Points, because of high mortality rates and high rates of absence among Irish laboring males working away from home (see Chapter 4) (Groneman Pernicone 1973; Praetzellis and Praetzellis 2004).[28] Single working-class women, especially those with children, would most likely not have been able to afford to purchase wine for recreational purposes alone and likely had more weighty uses in mind.

Given that women were central to the emerging middle-class ideology of domesticity (Wall 1994; Brown 2009), it is reasonable to suggest that Irish female heads of house might have used wine to "participate in the genteel rituals of the day," an aspiration that archaeologist Stephen Brighton (2000:30) contends is reflected in Five Points residents' ceramics choices, such as tea wares. Offering wine to guests or using it to remedy illness would have been interpreted positively by middle-class American onlookers. As Pierre Bourdieu (1984) vividly demonstrated with regard to 20th-century Parisians, individuals project class status through use and display of commodities, including food and clothes, as well as through manners. Valued items and actions show "good taste" that can act as cultural capital. Lack of "good taste" can be a bar to social advancement. While there are certainly differences between 19th-century New York City and 20th-century Paris, the principle still applies, and in acquiring wine, Irish women on Pearl Street would have shown good taste. Consuming wine or offering it to others might have helped these women to achieve greater status, particularly among middle-class visitors, such as priests, reformers, or physicians. Irish immigrants in New York City who aspired to middle-class status might have replaced the traditional bottle of whiskey kept for visiting priests, the "priest's bottle," with a bottle of wine that would have been considered "classier" in Ireland as well as in New York (Mahon 1991).

Christine Stansell (1986) and Richard Stott (1990:272) have suggested that working-class women were keener than men to embrace middle-class values because there was little space for them in hyper-masculinized working-class culture. Embracing the ideals of domesticity gave women greater social power. Women were also interested in passing on middle-class tastes to their children, so that their children could achieve greater prosperity and power. Children's tea sets found in Irish features at the Five Points appear to be material evidence of inculcating "good taste" into the next generation (Brighton 2000:27). Historical records also shows that many Irish immigrants encouraged their children to receive more formal education than they themselves had had, and usually chose Catholic schools (Fitzgerald 2006). Upwardly mobile Irish did not imitate the American middle class exactly, but instead adopted elements that also fit within their own values. The use of wine for hospitality and healing might have been one of those elements.

As noted previously, although they shied away from the more "stimulating" hard liquors, physicians in New York regularly prescribed wine to strengthen patients recuperating from illnesses, and even the most radical temperance reformers in New York City did not object to partaking of wine for medicinal purposes (Stivers 2000:32). Physicians in Ireland and England diverged from their New York counterparts in recommending wine specifically for typhus fever. The authors of a report in the *Dublin Quarterly Journal of Medical Science* (*DQJMS*) in 1849 stated that "every practitioner of any experience in fever knows in how many instances he feels wine or brandy to be the *unicum remedium* for his patient" (*DQJMS* 1849:325). English physician and fever expert Charles Murchison (1862:42) also noted, "A few years ago, the name typhus seemed to call for the liberal use of stimulants, and immense quantities of wine were accordingly given." Wine was a remedy that was compatible with Irish professional and popular medical ideas. It is thus possible that some of the wine contained in the bottles uncovered at 472 Pearl Street was used to treat typhus fever, in particular, possibly at the advice of one of a few Irish-trained physicians or pharmacists in New York City.

There are culturally specific reasons why Irish immigrants might have chosen wine as a healing beverage for an illness as serious as typhus fever. Red wine has profound religious significance in Roman Catholicism. During the mass, the priest consecrates red wine, and it is transubstantiated into the blood of Jesus. In Irish folk medicine, red-colored objects were frequently employed for healing because of the color's powerful association with Christ's blood, as were other objects associated with the Church, such as scapulars, holy water, wedding rings, and soil from the graves of priests (Barbour 1897:390; NFC 1930[80]:11; NFCS 1938[345]:8; Logan 1994:58; Linn 2010, 2014). Therefore, although partaking of wine to cure fever might have been approved by physicians for scientific reasons, Irish immigrants might have considered wine to be curative for spiritual reasons. The same observable action could have been underpinned by different reasoning, or by a combination of both perspectives.

Another possible explanation for the abundance of wine bottles in the refuse of Irish tenements in the Five Points is that some of the bottles do not represent wine consumption at all. Instead, the bottles could be evidence of alternative home industries of *poitín* and cure making that the Irish, and likely women especially, used to make ends meet and to care for their friends and family. The thick glass of wine (and soda) bottles makes them ideal for reuse (Figure 3.9). Jane Busch (1987:71, 78) noted that in the 19th and 20th centuries, thick soda water bottles were so often refilled with homemade liquor and sauces that it caused shortages of bottles for soda manufacturers; immigrants were more likely to reuse bottles than native-born Americans, because they were accustomed to doing so in their countries of origin where glass was less available. Historical and archaeological sources indicate glass was scarce in rural areas of Ireland in the 19th century (Dorian 2000; Hull 2004; Brighton 2009).

In Ireland, women played important roles in both *poitín* making and distribution. They sold it from unlicensed pubs that they conducted out of their own houses, called *shebeens* (Malcolm 1998:51). Hugh Dorian (2000:279), in his memoir of 19th-century Donegal, writes that these women filled dark glass bottles with illegal whiskey and hid them around the house, especially in the thatched roof. Nearly all the wine bottles found in the 472 and 474 Pearl Street deposits were made of dark green glass, the most common color of wine bottles during the period (Lindsey 2021a). "The keeping of a *shebeen* was a 'recognized resource of widows' and they had 'privileged status' in the liquor trade" (Rosenzweig 1983:43 citing Connell 1968:18). Rosenzweig (1983:43) found in his study of drinking establishments in Worcester, Massachusetts, that Irish immigrants, even those involved in the temperance movement, "continued to insist upon this form of communal charity, despite the failure of American laws to recognize it."

Similarly, in New York City, selling homemade whiskey or traditional cures could have provided single mothers who needed to stay at home with their children or older widowed women (or men) with income, goods, or favors more significant than those gained from other occupations. Other occupations included part-time needlework or other piecework, rag collecting, peddling, taking in boarders, washing laundry and other service work, and prostitution. It is conceivable that some Irish residents of the Five Points, including women, produced *poitín* in a tenement yard. Such an enterprise was possible because relatively simple and small equipment was required. It would have included a small copper pot, in which the mash (typically made of barley or potatoes) was heated and from whence the liquor derived its name (the diminutive word for the Irish word for pot, *pota*); copper tubing, through which the alcohol vapor ran; and a barrel in which the tubing was placed, immersed in cool water, to condense the vapor. The "run" of liquor that emerged from the end of the tubing was collected in bottles of glass or

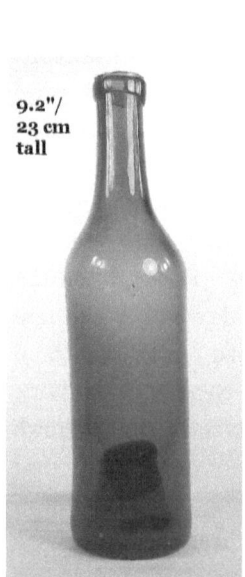
9.2"/ 23 cm tall

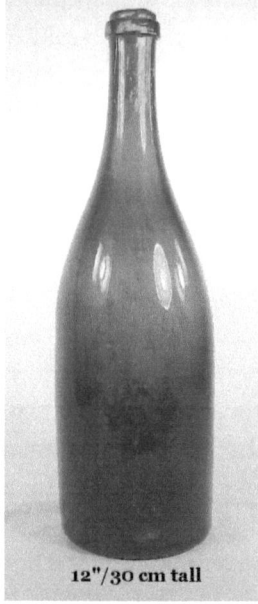
12"/30 cm tall

FIGURE 3.9. Examples of 19th-century green glass bottles used to contain wine. Left—Bordeaux-style. Right—champagne-style (also used for wine, beer, and cider) (Lindsey 2021a). Both types were uncovered in features associated with 472 and 474 Pearl Street.

ceramic. Newspapers reported the discovery of such stills in residential areas, such as one owned by two Irishmen on Houston Street in 1878. Neighbors claimed they thought the owners had been making vinegar (*NYT* 1878:8). There is no direct evidence of whiskey distilling, such as large amounts of grain or remnants of stills, in the archaeological deposits at 472 or 474 Pearl Streets, however. Several residents were involved in the liquor trade, including a liquor store on the ground floor of 472 Pearl Street, so residents had easy access to whiskey, whether or not it was made on the premises.[29]

Wine bottles would have been convenient receptacles for Irish popular cures containing whiskey as an ingredient, including cough syrups typically produced yearly by Irish women for their families (see Chapter 7) and some of the previously described herbal fever mixtures. Wine bottles also could have held recipes from specialized healers. There were several types of popular healers in Ireland, including seventh-born sons, herb doctors, priests, and bonesetters—all of whom were either always or typically male—but wisewomen were frequently sought out and particularly associated with bottles. Wisewomen, such as the famous Biddy Early (1798–1874) from County Clare, reportedly preferred to store and distribute their remedies in dark glass bottles. Early supposedly kept a bottle with her all the time. It was said that she could see "the future and anything else she wanted to know" in it, including how to cure people and animals (NFC 1938[560]:464–466; NFCS 1938[596]:126; Brew 1990; O'Regan 1997:6). Some curing women received training in making medicine from other family members. Others, such as Early, were said to have been instructed by the fairies, humanlike supernatural creatures said to occasionally intervene in human affairs (see Chapter 7).

Jonah Barrington (1832:34), a member of the Irish Parliament and a judge, defined wisewomen as, "The class of old women . . . held in the highest estimation, as understanding the cure (that is, if God pleased) of all disorders. Their materia medica . . . [consisted of] of bushes, bark of trees, weeds from churchyards and mushrooms from fairy grounds; rue, garlic, rosemary, birdsnests, foxglove, etc. . . . I never could find out what the charms . . . were. They said they should die themselves if they disclosed them to anybody."[30] He also described a wisewoman he encountered, named Jug Coyle, who "sat in a corner of the hob, by the great long turf fire in the kitchen, exactly in the position of the Indian squaw, munching and mumbling for use an apronful of her morning's gatherings in the fields." Figure 3.10 shows an early 20th-century photograph of an older Irish woman who evokes Barrington's description of Jug Coyle. This photograph was likely staged, but the woman's position seated next to the hearth and pipe smoking portray her as someone who had attained respect in her community. Many years of life experience brought older Irish women knowledge and higher status in their communities. During his ethnographic study of rural Ireland in the 1930s, Conrad Arensberg (1937:211) was similarly told by locals that "wise women are always old."

Irish physicians felt that Irish laypeople trusted wisewomen more than physicians. In an article in *Harper's Weekly*, for example, an Irish dispensary doctor quoted a conversation he overheard between some villagers. A man quipped, "Doctors is well enough when there's nothing sarious; but I wad recommend you, when he's that bad, to do nothing till Mrs. Featherstone [the wisewoman] has seen him" (*Harper's Weekly*

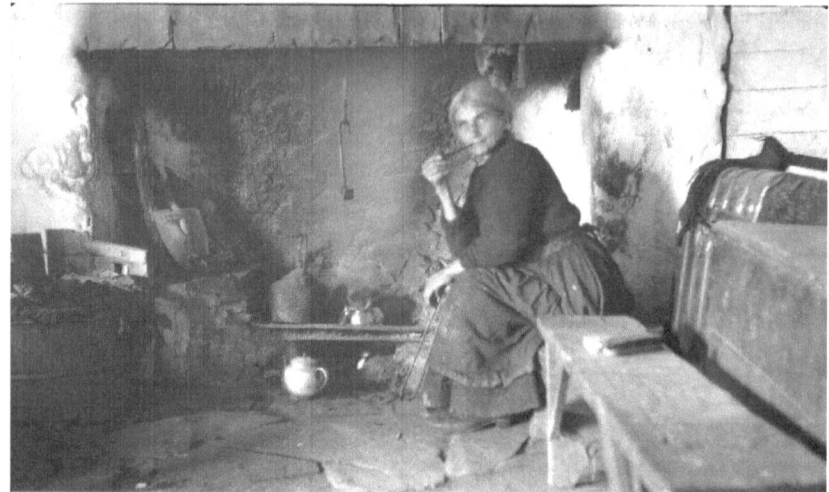

FIGURE 3.10. "Interior of house of M. Breathnach, Maam Cross, Co. Galway." A photograph of an Irish woman smoking a pipe by her hearth, Galway 1935. Courtesy of the School of Irish, Celtic Studies, Irish Folklore and Linguistics, University College Dublin and the National Folklore Collection.

[*HW*] 1879:806). Most Irish women would have had some wisdom about how to cure common ailments, even if they were not regarded as "wisewomen," because of traditional Irish gender roles and modes of transmitting knowledge of healing and assisting in childbirth from women of one generation to the next. Tending to ill and injured family members was part of women's traditional role, and age and experience often brought wisdom.

In the physically and emotionally challenging context of immigrant life in New York City, women with healing knowledge would have been even more important to the community than in the Irish countryside. As Jan Pacht Brickman (1983:70) points out in the case of midwives, healers "almost always foreign-born and living in the community, lay in the buffer that immigrant groups maintained against an already overwhelming cultural shock" (cited in Borst 1999:436). Historical records are, nevertheless, nearly silent about Irish wisewomen, or the healing activities of Irish women more generally, in 19th-century New York City, with the exception of some attention to the healing work of Irish-born nuns (see below and Chapters 5 and 7). It is not surprising that female healers would have kept a low profile outside of the Irish community, given Americans' negative opinions of practices they deemed to be foreign or superstitious. Within the Irish community they would have been known by word of mouth, and Irish-owned drinking establishments and groceries were places where such information could be found out.

U.S. Census records indicate there were a large number of older Irish women living in the tenements at 472 and 474 Pearl Street between 1850 and 1870. Of about 350 different individual residents during this period, 23 were Irish women over the age of 50, then considered to be an advanced age, and many had been widowed.[31] Census takers rarely noted an occupation for these women, even though it is unlikely that they did not do anything to support themselves and the contribution of Irish women was "a matter of survival for their families" (Groneman Pernicone 1973:158–161).[32,33] These older women almost certainly possessed knowledge of at least some popular Irish remedies and would have been accustomed to preparing cures for their families, a practice they very likely continued in New York City, as Mrs. Huxley did for her grandson (Chapter 1).

An example of a woman in the Five Points who likely provided healing, at least for her family, was Mary Twoomy. She lived at 472 Pearl Street in the household of Morris and Mary Callahan and their children. The 1855 New York State Census records her as a 60-year-old "grandmother" with no occupation, while the 1860 Federal Census lists her as 73 years old. The family resided at the same address from 1855 to 1870, adding two more children by 1870. The survival of six children from the same family in the Sixth Ward during this time was not a foregone conclusion. Mortality rates for immigrant children were high because of epidemic and endemic disease rife within the neighborhood (Blackmar 1995:57). New York Orthopaedic Dispensary Patient Records ([NYODPR] 1870–1873) also indicate that deaths of multiple children in Irish immigrant families were not uncommon. The fact that the Callahan children survived past five years old suggests that either they were lucky or they had special access to successful preventive and/or healing measures. It is possible that the medical wisdom of their grandmother, Mary Twoomy, contributed to the children's survival.

It is also possible that Mary Twoomy had been recognized in the neighborhood as a wisewoman. Given Irish social norms, women like Mary would have been obligated to help neighbors in need in New York City, which would have enabled her to contribute to her family and to build social capital. Although most Irish traditional healers would not accept monetary payment for their aid, most accepted gifts of food or liquor (O'Regan 1997:6; Buckley 1980:17, 33–34). The numerous wine bottles archaeologists found in Irish contexts at the Five Points, therefore, could index both healing activities and reciprocity for healing. Wine would have been an appropriate gift for a wisewoman that enabled her to prepare more healing remedies to aid others, reusing the bottles to multiply positive effects in the community.

Unfortunately, it is impossible to know for certain exactly how and why Irish residents of 472 and 474 Pearl Street used the wine and whiskey bottles archaeologists found in their buildings' cesspool and privy. However, combining information about Irish traditional uses of these substances with the pattern of other artifacts in the deposit, the ages and genders of associated residents, and the social and historical context of Irish immigration, raises the strong possibility that at least some were acquired by Irish women to remedy illness in their families and/or community. Considering these bottles in this way draws attention to underappreciated strategies of Irish women, who made up an increasing proportion of Irish immigrants as the century continued. Producing home remedies, many of which were alcohol based, was likely a "hidden industry" (McGowan 2000) that simultaneously benefitted women, their families, and their communities. It is to such women that newly immigrated Irish probably turned to first for help when they fell ill.

Interpreting the alcoholic beverage bottles at the Five Points as remains of Irish medicine also highlights conflicting Irish and American conceptions of alcohol and complicates the stereotypical understanding of Irish relationships with alcoholic beverages. From Americans' perspective, drinking whiskey, and perhaps even wine, was dangerous for those with sanguine temperaments, which they assumed characterized nearly all Irish immigrants. The excitement that this substance produced made them even more susceptible to typhus fever and other effects of overheating (see Chapter 3). From Irish immigrants' perspective, drinking alcoholic beverages was strengthening and helped to eliminate fever-causing poisons.

Of Priests and Wakes

Despite the best efforts of famine-era Irish immigrants to cure typhus by drinking whiskey, wine, or wisewomen's cures—or seeking the help of physicians at hospitals and dispensaries, for that matter—, these remedies are unlikely to have been very effective. Because of typhus's acute nature and Irish appreciation of the severity of epidemic fevers, it is likely that as a next step, some sought out a Catholic priest for healing or last rites. Catholic priests played many important roles in Irish society, as teachers, counselors, political leaders, advocates, and healers, as well as religious leaders. In Ireland, both Catholics and Protestants sought out Catholic priests for healing, particularly after treatments prescribed by other healers had failed (Gillespie 1998).[34] Although there would be little to no archaeological evidence of such practices, historical evidence demonstrates that Irish immigrants carried their faith in the healing powers of priests to England and America. According to the *New York Times* (1879:12), for example, a woman of Irish parentage in West Hoboken, New Jersey, reported that Father Victor, famous for his miraculous healing throughout the region, cured her of paralysis in 1879 with a relic bone of St. Vincent de Paul. As late as 1893, Father Thomas Adams, born in Ireland—like many Catholic priests in the U.S. at the time—in County Kerry and a priest in the St. Vincent de Paul Parish in Brooklyn, was frequented by members of the Irish American community for his miraculous healing power, according to the *Brooklyn Daily Eagle* (1893:10) and the *New York Times* (1908:9). Related to typhus, in particular, historian Lynn Hollen Lees writes that Irish immigrants in mid-19th-century London called upon priests when an epidemic disease threatened their community. They also flocked to confession, believing that being in a sinful state could make a person more vulnerable to an epidemic illness, and sought priests to relight hearth fires, believing that would drive away the epidemic (Lees 1979:168–170, 187).

Most Catholic priests in Ireland, England, and America nevertheless proclaimed that they had no special healing powers (Lees 1979:168–170, 187). The Catholic Church in the U.S. and England tried to discourage such beliefs, because of how they fed nativists accusations of Irish superstitiousness and irrationality and hindered the acceptance of Catholics

(Lees 1979). The Brooklyn Diocese defrocked Father Adams for his healing practices, although they later reinstated him in response to popular outcry and a change of bishop (*Brooklyn Daily Eagle* 1893:10). Neither the Church hierarchy nor Protestant nor nativist scorn persuaded Irish immigrants to disregard the healers and healing methods in which they deeply trusted when they needed them most, however. As will be discussed further in subsequent chapters, religious men and women were often at the bedsides of sick and dying Irish patients, providing spiritual and nursing care. They volunteered at immigrant quarantine hospitals when few others would and staffed Civil War hospitals and newly established Catholic hospitals.[35] Their work, as well as the demands of Irish patients, over time changed hospital care in New York City.

Priests were also important visitors at wakes. Epidemic typhus was a serious illness that caused the death of many Irish immigrants. Those who succumbed in a tenement would at least have had a chance of receiving the proper rituals for a good death—last rites and a wake—which were not guaranteed to those who died in public institutions. The wake was, and still is, an important communal mourning ritual. The Irish considered it to be an obligation to the dead, who would reciprocate with blessings, and an occasion to heal the social rupture caused by their death, to make new social alliances, and to strengthen old ones. It could also be an opportunity for personal healing; there were a number of cures associated with the bodies of the deceased and materials at wakes, including transferring an illness from one of the guests to the deceased.[36] Like drinking alcoholic beverages, which was typically part of wakes, this Irish practice that Americans found to be so objectionable in how it exemplified and inflamed Irish sanguine temperaments was of critical importance to Irish immigrants and communities, especially during this period of such loss.

Conclusion

Typhus fever afflicted many Irish immigrants of the famine era, as well as some who arrived in the following decades. This deadly disease was only one of many dangers to which they were exposed in the journey from their homeland to the U.S. The crowded lodging and poorhouses in which they took refuge before their departures as well as the ships that carried them to North America were sources of infection and danger, especially for those already weakened by hunger and sorrow. Their ordeals did not cease upon sailing into New York harbor. There they encountered uncomfortable inspection if not quarantine or hospitalization. In city institutions in a culture foreign to them, some, such as William Smith, received rough and disheartening treatment. Others at New York Hospital were subjected to harsh treatments that would have made little sense to them from well-meaning but prejudiced and helpless physicians. Those who fell ill from the fever in the city after passing inspection found themselves at the mercy of strangers on the street, some of whom were benevolent, but most were terrified at the sight of a newcomer with the fever. If they were luckier, they found refuge in a tenement surrounded by family or fellow countrymen and women.

Removed from the healing power in sacred places of their native land, they or their brethren who cared for them, sought customary curative substances and healers. In the urban environment of New York City, predominantly rural Irish looked to the trusted and the familiar. Drinking whiskey and seeking wisewomen and holy men were key strategies transplanted from the "old sod" to a place with little sod at all. Within this context, I have argued that alcoholic beverage bottles found in association with Irish tenements on Pearl Street in the Five Points should be considered as possible evidence of healing and the several older Irish women who lived there should be considered potential healers. Historical records, meanwhile, attest that Irish Catholic priests and nuns in America also tended to immigrants' physical and spiritual wellbeing.

Even if they were unable to cure typhus fever, these remedies—from the mundane to the miraculous—and the care of trusted healers brought immigrants some measure of much-needed relief in an unfamiliar and challenging new environment. The Irish ethic of mutual obligation informed immigrants' expectations of their neighbors in New York City and encouraged the ill or injured to seek help from friends and neighbors. When disaster struck in the form of illness, familiar people and familiar substances formed the first line of defense. Both distrust of hospitals and physicians and trust in home remedies and neighbors accounts for observed delays between when Irish immigrants fell ill from typhus fever within the city and when they resorted to hospital care.

Unfortunately, Americans interpreted the persistence of these practices among the Irish, along with typhus fever itself, as additional evidence that the Irish were naturally and immutably sanguine in humoral temperament and distinct from phlegmatic White Americans. These categorizations were not value-neutral, but instead provided so-called scientific support for naturalizing stereotypes and prejudice. The next chapter will center upon the kinds of work Irish immigrants were able to find in New York City and how their clustering in manual labor and service positions as well as the physical effects of labor on their bodies was interpreted by Americans as additional evidence of natural Irish difference.

CHAPTER 4

Fractures

Work, Injuries, and Irish Difference

ON A SWELTERING DAY in August of 1867, a match seller named Mary was admitted to Bellevue Hospital and diagnosed with "insolatio," or what today would be called sunstroke. The physician noted in her case record that the 32-year-old Irish-born woman had

> lost her right lower limb in this hospital nine years ago. While selling matches with her child . . . she was attacked about 11:30am, fell down and was found unconscious by a policeman . . . who helped revive her. She became conscious . . . about 1pm. Pain in head and cramps in belly and soreness. About 4 pm . . . took 2 drinks of whiskey "to strengthen her" . . . to get to her friends on 29th St. There she had some medicine called "diarrhea mixture" which gave her but little relief. Was troubled all night with great pain in the head and abdomen and diarrhea. Did not sleep. Brought to hospital at 1:30 pm. (BHMCB 1867:233)

In the hospital, Mary was treated with a cold bath to bring down her body temperature, sodium bicarbonate to decrease her nausea, and potassium bromide and iodide to quiet her bowels. A few days later she was discharged as cured from the sunstroke. Yet, while physicians treated Mary's immediate symptoms and gave her a much needed few days of rest, they were unable to address the underlying causes of her ailment: the social and economic conditions that compelled her to labor to exhaustion for a pittance each day. Her previous injury further added to her suffering. Mary's loss of a limb and her reputation as an Irish immigrant mother limited her employment opportunities. She had little choice but to take up the lowly and arduous occupation of selling matches on the street. In this painful struggle for survival, Mary was not alone. Hard work and injury played central roles in the lives of Irish immigrants during the middle of the 19th century.

Labor historians have highlighted the important contributions that Irish immigrants made to organizing labor and the railroads, canals, buildings, and more that Irish lives were sacrificed to build. Relatively few studies have focused on the embodied experiences of the immigrant laborers themselves. A growing number of historical archaeological and bioarchaeological studies have shed new light on how living and working conditions affected the health of working people, however (Howson 1987, 1993, 2013; Beaudry 1993; Ford 1994; Mrozowski et al. 1989; Reinhard 1994, 2000; Yamin 2000[1 and 2]; Blakey and Rankin-Hill 2004; Linn 2010, 2014, 2022; Geber and O'Donnabhain 2020; Lupu and Ryan 2022; Warner-Smith 2022). This chapter, and the next, contributes to this growing area of research and investigates the embodied experiences of Irish immigrant men, women, and children from the 1840s through the 1870s through the lens of the work-related injuries and sicknesses to which they were so vulnerable.

In this chapter, I argue that working-class identity was not simply inscribed upon immigrants' bodies but was embodied by them: work activities, conditions, and accidents physically transformed bodies. These injuries made them more susceptible as a group than native-born Americans to becoming living material for surgical modification and experimentation. Combined, labor and surgeries sculpted Irish immigrant bodies into what appeared to many native-born Americans to fit their stereotypes of the Irish as naturally sanguine brutes, best—or maybe only—suitable for the role of manual laborer on the urban stage. Physical appearance continued to affect how Americans categorized and treated Irish immigrants. As the numbers of injured Irish steadily increased, their broken bodies came to the center of debates about the appropriateness of anesthesia in surgery and the ethics of relieving pain in others, especially in cases of amputation and other painful procedures for women, such as Mary. These debates, along with the actions of Irish immigrant nurses, physicians, and Civil War soldiers, contributed to the beginnings of a shift in some Americans' perceptions in the late 1860s toward appreciating Irish immigrants as fellow sensitive and sensible humans.

Irish Expectations and the Injurious Realities of Labor in New York City

It has often been said that prior to their arrivals in New York City, Irish immigrants believed that "America was so rich that *anyone* could prosper there" (Miller 1985:487). This is an exaggeration, but many did anticipate better conditions and more opportunities for prosperity in the U.S. than in Ireland, certainly during the famine. Historian Kerby Miller's (1985, 1993) extensive study of immigrant letters found some reluctance to contradict this positive image of the U.S. but, more often, practical advice to family and friends about real conditions and limiting their expectations. Bridget Tunney warned her friends in Cork in 1855, for example, that "it is not so very easey to get Muney heer as we all [thought] . . . you have to work hard to make one pound" (Miller 1985:319). Would-be immigrants were sensitive to this news and information about downturns in the American economy, resulting in decreases in Irish immigration during recessions. Even those who were well informed and held moderate expectations were still surprised by how hard they had to work to get by in New York City, and how limited their opportunities and how dangerous available jobs were. This section sketches out an overview of the kinds and conditions of work most Irish immigrants performed from the late 1840s through the 1870s and how their involvement in mostly manual laboring and service positions was viewed by many native-born Americans as confirmation of stereotypes.

Most Irish immigrants of the famine and post-famine era arrived with little to no savings and needed to find employment right way in order to sustain themselves and their families. New York City was expanding rapidly and there was a great demand for labor. This demand, combined with help from previously immigrated friends, enabled many newly immigrated men, women, and children to get to work quickly, but mostly in manual labor and service. As Irishman Thomas Mooney (1850:84–85) described, in New York,

> Irishmen . . . do almost all the rude and heavy work: they are generally employed in buildings . . . they are found portering on the quays, repairing, cleaning, and watching the city; sawing wood, carrying packages; serving as waiters, hostlers, barkeepers . . . owning or driving carts, cabs, hackney coaches . . . trafficking in the vegetable and fruit markets; at work in the

tailoring "sweating shops" . . . digging foundations or blasting rocks uptown, mending the streets, digging sewers, and laying water or gas pipes, attending the merchant's auctions in Pearl-Street, and buying an odd damaged bargain . . . [which they] peddle . . . in the suburban districts of the city.

Historian Carol Groneman Pernicone's (1973:100) analysis of the Sixth Ward in the 1855 New York State Census and Tyler Anbinder, Cormac Ó Gráda, and Simone Wegge's (2019a) study of Emigrant Savings Bank records in 1855 support this description of the range of Irish immigrant men's occupations. Both studies found nearly half of Irish immigrant men in their samples worked as unskilled manual laborers, about a third worked in skilled or semiskilled labor such as the building trades, about 5% in storekeeping, 5% in service, 5% in sales or clerical work, 2% in petty enterprises, and only about 1% in government and 1% in professions such as physician or lawyer.[1]

The vast majority of Irish men thus worked in jobs requiring manual labor, and Irish men came to dominate day-laboring jobs. They remarked that pay for such work in New York City was better than that in Ireland or England, but the cost of living was high, chances for advancement low, and the work difficult and often dangerous. The *New York Times* and the *New York Tribune* estimated in the early 1850s that $11 per week was the absolute minimum required to support a family of four, while the average unskilled male laborer only earned about $1 per day (Groneman 1977:35). The increasing rationalization and mechanization of American labor created many permanently unskilled and semiskilled jobs, even within trades, where traditionally apprentices and journeymen had worked their way up to master craftsmen by learning all phases of production. The division of labor was helpful for unskilled Irishmen in the short term, because they could find work, but harmful in the long term because hires were not taught the skills that would enable them to rise up in the ranks (Roney 1931:31). Irishmen already skilled in a trade often had trouble finding such work, especially if they were older. Historian Richard Stott noted that the number of these positions was shrinking, most available positions were taken—and often protected—by native workers, and American business owners preferred to hire younger employees, who they believed could work harder. In 1855, more than one-third of Sixth Ward manual laborers were over the age of

40, despite their nearly universal desire to do work in less strenuous and better-paying occupations (Stott 1990:61). At 472 and 474 Pearl Street, most of the few older male residents between 1850 and 1870 who were above 40 years of age worked as laborers.[2]

Women's jobs were even more dependent upon their stage of life than men's, due to women's roles as primary caretakers for children. Groneman (1977:36) found that nearly half of all employed unmarried women in New York City's Sixth Ward in 1850 were engaged in domestic service, for which there was growing demand, as private servants, hotel servants, cooks, laundresses, nurses, etc. African American women had previously dominated these occupations, but Irish women accepted lower wages. Additionally, American-born women increasingly regarded domestic work as degrading, and domestic service was redefined as immigrants' work (Stansell 1986:155–157). Live-in domestic servants, who preferred to be called "help," earned between $4 and $8 a month plus room and board (Groneman 1977:36, Stott 1990). Because their costs of living were paid for, these jobs were attractive to many young single women or widows, permitting them to save money and/or send some home as remittances (Diner 1983:71; Anbinder et al. 2019a:1614). The hours of domestic servants were long, work was hard, and freedom was limited; turnover rates were high (Stansell 1986). The majority of the other half of employed single women in the Sixth Ward in 1850 worked in the sewing trades (Groneman 1977:36). In factories women were able to earn about $5.50 a week, significantly more than the average of $2 a week that women received for piecework at home, but less than their male counterparts. A *New York Tribune* contributor described the gender pay gap in 1853: "A woman may be defined as a creature that receives half price for all she does, and pays full price for all she needs. . . . She earns as a child—she pays as a man" (Groneman 1977:37).

Married women more often worked from home at jobs that included piecework sewing, laundry, and/or hosting boarders, which were compatible with their "second shift" of domestic work and childcare (Hochschild and Machung 1989). Groneman (1977:36) found that nearly 50% of women in the Sixth Ward over the age of 30 reported caring for boarders to 1855 New York State Census takers; however, Groneman argued that the practice was even more widespread, since it was usually only reported by women who took in multiple boarders or ran boardinghouses. Other Irish women earned money in a number of "petty enterprises," such as selling food or matches, working as wet nurses, or taking care of other people's children while they worked (NYODPR 1872:344; Groneman 1977; Quiroga 1984). Some engaged in prostitution, one of the better-paying options for women (Stansell 1986; Gilfoyle 1992; Yamin 2005). Others performed activities not well captured by historical records but seen archaeologically at the Five Points, including rug and bone button making and toolmaking from scavenged materials (McGowan 2000) and possibly homemade whiskey and/or medicine production (Chapter 3).

Children also helped with some of these home industries. The idea of childhood as a distinct period of life sheltered from adult responsibilities was emerging during this period. Until recently, scholars assumed it to be restricted to the middle and upper classes, who could afford to support noncontributing children (Fitts 1999). Working-class parents supposedly "expected their children to 'earn their keep'" (Stansell 1986:53). Archaeological evidence at 472 and 474 Pearl Street of children's dolls, tea sets, jacks, and mugs painted with children's names suggest that Irish parents also recognized childhood as a separate phase of life, however (Brighton 2000:27). Historical evidence shows Irish parents went to great lengths to send their children to school and to create lives for them that were better than their own.[3] Such records show Irish immigrant parents did not necessarily expect or desire their children to labor, but often desperately needed them to do so. Historical records show that Irish children as young as five or six worked in factories, peddled goods, sold newspapers, scavenged, cared for younger siblings, and/or helped parents with their work (Stansell 1986:50–54; Baldwin 2012). Boys of 16 years of age began work in trades; by 18 they labored as adults. Some girls, such as 11-year-old Catherine Garvey at 472 Pearl Street, began work as seamstresses at even younger ages (USBC 1850). The wages children were paid were paltry, however, even if they could produce as much as an adult (Brace 1873:326).

Anbinder et al. (2019a:1617, 1621) show that more Irish immigrants were able to pull themselves out of poverty by the mid-1850s than had previously been acknowledged, and interestingly, that laborers often put away more savings than tradesmen, if they transitioned to self-employment. Those who remained tied to their trades or locked in day laboring did not fare as well, and women were generally less able to amass higher balances than men of any occupation. Putting away savings was important for many reasons, but most relevant to this chapter is how necessary savings were for survival because of the conditions of manual laboring and service in 19th-century New York City. Day laborers could not always find consistent work, especially during the winter when industries slowed because of the weather. Prices of goods also rose whenever the Erie Canal and Hudson River froze and made transport more difficult (Stott 1990:115–120).[4] Lost wages due to unemployment from a layoff or from sickness or injury could be devastating, especially when combined with the costs of medical treatment. According to Stott (1990:115), savvy workers expected to be without work two to three months of the year and planned ahead, stocking up on goods and savings.

Work, whenever they could get it, was both a bane and a blessing for most Irish immigrants. In letters and diaries, as well as in remarks to physicians, they emphasized long hours of exhausting work with few breaks or safety precautions. A nearly deaf 29-year-old Irishman diagnosed with pulmonary tuberculosis, for example, explained to a physician at New York Hospital that he was exhausted from refining silver 16 to 20 hours a day over a furnace (NYHMCB 1852:C533). Longshoremen sometimes worked shifts that could last as long as three days straight loading and unloading extremely heavy cargo from ships, work "of the most arduous kind," according to the *New-York Daily Tribune* (1852:4). Nurses' hours were unceasing. James Duffe (1853), an Irish-born nurse at New York Hospital from 1844 to 1848, underscored his never-ending work by finishing many of his diary entries with "so this ends this day's work for work we may call it without end." Such endless work was not exclusive to Irish men. It was not uncommon for domestic servants to work 15-hour days, seven days a week, and to be "on call" at night (Groneman 1977:36).

In the rural areas where many famine-era Irish immigrants to New York originated, work was often long and difficult, but tasks and their duration varied by type and season. Work was also broken up by weddings, wakes, fairs, and holidays, but in America, only three holidays were officially observed a year: Christmas, New Year's Day, and July 4th (Stott 1990:132). Rural Irish sense of time was preindustrial; it was oriented to season, religion, and community. In American and European cities, as many scholars have noted, time was measured differently. Historian E. P. Thompson (1967:56-97) underscored how industrial capitalism imposed a new "time-discipline" that transformed not only labor habits but also the rhythm of their daily lives and reduced their ability to attain relaxation.[5] Irishman James Burn (1865:11) shared this impression, writing that in America, "work, work, work is the everlasting routine of everyday life."

Not only were the long hours wearisome, but the pace of work in America was disturbing to Irish immigrants. Stott (1990) relates that American workers were known for their fast-paced work, referred to as a "railroad pace." Irish workers objected that such a pace was morally reprehensible. In contrast to "American moulders [who] seemed desirous of doing all the work required as if it were the last day of their lives," for example, Frank Roney (1931:179-180) was accustomed to a system where workers spread out labor so as to ensure all were paid. Roney continued, "I did not and would not descend to their level. . . . I never hurried and always suppressed any disposition . . . to take work away from others." Rural Irish community-based ideals were significant in keeping many immigrants alive and well in New York City, as I will describe in the next chapter, but they directly conflicted with American every-man-for-himself capitalism.

The frenetic speed of work, wearisome hours, combined with dangerous working conditions led to high rates of accidents, as will be detailed later in this chapter. Irish immigrants had a clear view of these dangers. Roney (1931:180) described his horrified reaction to a New York City foundry in 1867, for example:

> I peered into the semi-darkness and saw men, bare-headed and bare-footed, almost nude, racing back and forth, handling between trips, small wooden tools most dexterously. . . . I had never seen or heard of a foundry like it. To see men half nude, exerting themselves as these were doing in a place imperfectly lighted, black and dirty, and perspiring on this hot morning, was a revelation to me. If this was moulding in America, then I decided it would be better for me to return to Ireland and go to prison.[6]

The callousness of bosses and employers concerned with maximizing profits and seemingly unconcerned about their workers also struck Irish nerves.[7] As a canal laborer described, his bosses "only give you twenty-one minutes to eat . . . scream, threaten, and shout at you while forcing you back to work" (Miller 1985:270). Edwin Godkin (1895:64), the Irish-born founder of the New York City newspaper *The Nation* (named for the well-known Dublin newspaper) opined that "the presence of an exacting, semi-hostile, and slightly contemptuous person" was the reason that domestic service was "extraordinarily full of wear and tear."

While American reformers were beginning to acknowledge by the 1860s that inadequate housing and poor sanitation directly led to high rates of immigrant mortality from disease, they were relatively blind to work-related injuries. Historian Elizabeth Blackmar (1995:58) points out that the same citizens who embraced housing and health reform opposed an eight-hour workday and labor unions. Until the 20th century, there was no city, state, or federally mandated workers' protection, compensation, or disability leave. Injured workers had little recourse, even if an employer's carelessness caused their injury. Historian Christopher Tomlins (1988:378) argues that American courts and lawmakers did not want to interfere with the growth of capitalism or the boss-worker relationship that had been guided by paternalism, but capitalist wage labor had already severed the traditional obligations of employers to their employees.[8] Additionally, most native-born American bosses and business owners did not have social ties to the newly arrived and many seemed to regard them as infinitely replaceable. James Dever, a farmer's son from County Donegal, expressed how this felt to him. He lamented that as "laboring men" Irishmen were "thought nothing of more than *dogs* . . . despised and kicked about . . . being compelled to labor so severely, up before the Stars and working till darkness, nothing but driven like horses" (Miller 1985:318).

Lack of legal protections, combined with long hours of fast-paced and strenuous labor led directly to the large numbers of Irish immigrants who sought aid at, or were brought unconscious to, city hospitals. Injured or sick workers with little savings had little choice but to appeal to charity—of their employers, friends, neighbors, public hospitals, and/or other organizations. Instead of blaming bosses or pushing to change laboring conditions, however, many New Yorkers faulted Irish immigrants themselves and accused them of draining public funds (Berger 1946:176; Hirota 2017:51, 59). Anti-Irish prejudice and capitalist desires clouded the judgment of the American public. As described in Chapter 2, native-born working-class Americans also generally resented competition from Irish workers, their support for the Democratic Party, their Catholicism, and their supposed unwillingness to assimilate. All of this animosity hampered workers' ability to unite and force improvement of laboring conditions. It also contributed to views of the Irish as a different people unfit for citizenship.

The supposed humoral temperament of Irish immigrants that typhus fever (see Chapter 2) highlighted to native-born Americans during the height of the famine, and during subsequent post-famine outbreaks, also simultaneously influenced and supported opinions of many native-born Americans of all classes that Irish immigrants were best suited for menial labor. Their supposed superabundance of blood was thought to make them emotional, irrational, and less civilized in character as well as brawny in body. According to the then popular Fowles *New Illustrated Instructor in Phrenology and Physiology* (1859), for example, people with the phenotypic traits of the sanguine type ("coarse red hair" suggesting emotions that were "excitable," ruddy complexions revealing "hearty animal passions," and dark eyes bespeaking "sensuality") "should never turn dentists or clerks, but seek some outdoor employment." They "would be contented with rough, hard work [rather] than with a light or sedentary occupation . . . for they require a great amount of outdoor air and exercise" (quoted in Knobel 1986:123–124). This idea that the Irish were naturally created for hard work was not only directed at men (Figure 4.1). Americans imagined Bridget, the stereotypical Irish domestic female servant, as brawny, animalistic, and unfeminine; Opper's cartoons for *Puck*, including Figure 2.4, are among the most vivid caricatures. As the Irish-born Unitarian minister Henry Giles (1869:42) stated, for Americans "Irish means . . . a class of human beings whose women do our housework and whose men dig our railroads."

Even some native-born Americans who treated Irish workers well and commended their ability to work hard (Berger 1946:176) only furthered the stereotype that strenuous labor was naturally agreeable to them. Historian Dale Knobel (1986:78–79) pointed out that "whatever contributions they made to the nation's material growth were [seen as] derivative neither of intention nor of character nor of skill; they were simply

Fractures 141

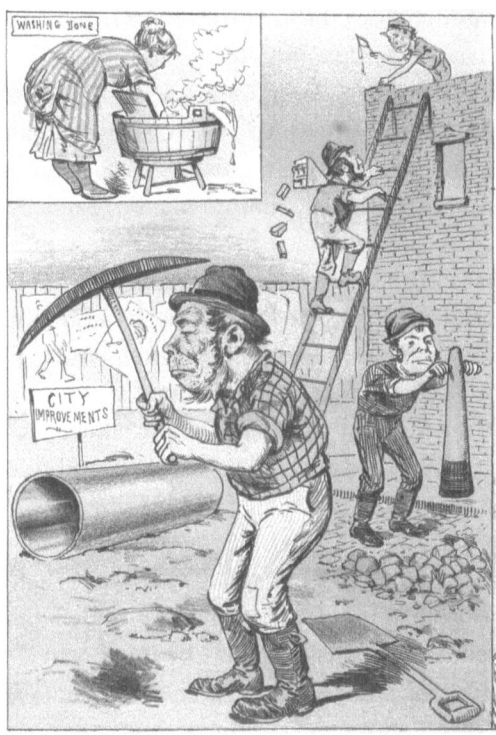

FIGURE 4.1. Left half of an illustration titled "American Gold" by Frederick Burr Opper. Published in *Puck* (1882:194), it depicts stereotypical Irish male and female laborers. Courtesy of Michigan State University Museum.

the products of the immigrant's most elemental brawn and brutality—directed to constructive purpose by others. . . . American ethnic imagery fastened . . . frequently upon the way in which the Irishman's body could be employed as a pack animal." New Yorker and Whig politician George Templeton Strong, for example, described Irish workers excavating his cellar in 1848 as "twenty 'sons of toil' with prehensile paws supplied them by nature with evident reference to the handling of the spade and the wielding of the pickaxe and congenital hollows in the shoulders wonderfully adapted to make the carrying of sod a luxury instead of a labor" (cited in Knobel 1986:87). Bioarchaeologist Alanna Warner-Smith (2022:191), citing labor historian Ava Baron (2006) and 19th-century literature and culture scholar James Salazar (2010), notes that by the early 20th century, the ideal muscular, White male body was contrasted with "the 'natural' laboring body that men from the lower orders of racial and immigrant groups were 'born with'" (Baron 2006:149).

Such descriptions and treatment of Irish laborers as pack animals in life and as specimens for scientific research in death (see more below) was dehumanizing and commodifying. Medical anthropologist Lesley Sharp (2000:293) observed that the English similarly commodified workers by referring to them as "hands." The English at least selected a body part that is distinctly human and has long been recognized as such in debates about human evolution. Associating Irish laborers with pack animals, bred to carry heavy loads on their backs, identified the Irish with the back, a part of the body that is easily injured by heavy loads, frequently leading to stooped posture. As medical anthropologists Nancy Scheper-Hughes and Margaret Lock (1987:18) note, in the U.S., "the backbone has great cultural and ethnomedical significance." Paraphrasing Erwin Strauss (1966:137), they explain that "the expression 'to be upright' has two connotations to Americans: the first, to stand up, to be on one's feet; and the second, a moral implication 'not to stoop to anything, to be honest and just, to be true to friends in danger, to stand by one's convictions.'" Some Americans interpreted stooped posture common among Irish and other workers as a reflection of naturally uncivilized sanguine character and, relatedly, moral laxity.

Many of these ideas about the physical and moral differences between Irish immigrants and native-born Americans existed only in the minds of 19th-century Americans. Nevertheless, I will show that real physical disparities did exist which bolstered prejudice. These physical differences were not a result of natural humoral divergence, as some Americans contended, however, but were caused by the ways that human bodies respond to activities and conditions. Strenuous work, repetitive tasks, unsafe working environments, injuries, violence, diet, and disease internally sculpted and externally marked many Irish laborers' bodies in ways that were distinct from the bodies of the American middle and upper class, and even from those of the American working classes.

Sculpting and Scarring Laboring Bodies: Work-Related Injuries among Irish Immigrants in New York City

In her survey of archaeological studies about bodies, archaeologist Rosemary Joyce (2005) found that two approaches were most common: the bioarchaeological approach, which examines the physical remains of bodies as artifacts bearing information about diet, health, and physical activities, and the political/symbolic approach, which focuses on bodily surfaces and how bodily ornamentation and modification practices signal identities including gender, class, age, and ethnicity. This study takes a third approach, considering the body above and below the skin and the interrelationships between the interior and the exterior and the biological and the social. Each shapes the other. How an individual interacts with the physical world—what one eats, what activities one performs, how one presents one's body, etc.—is, to a large extent, the product of culture and society. The body can be considered a form of material culture (Sofaer 2006; Novak and Warner-Smith 2020) that embodies social advantages or disadvantages, as medical anthropologists have long argued (Kleinman 1986:194–195; Farmer 1996, 1999).

Most 19th-century observers attributed difference in bodily architecture to complex interaction between humoral constitution, environment, and heredity. German orthopedist Julian Wolff first showed in 1892 that physical activity and injury play a far larger role in shaping the body than had been previously supposed. He demonstrated that in addition to changes in musculature and fat tissue, which had long been noticed, living bone also changes. His premise, that bones of healthy individuals respond to activities and remodel themselves to resist force, is now referred to as Wolff's Law. With habitual muscle exertion, bones become thicker and places where muscles attach via tendons become more rugose to maximize mechanical advantage. Bioarchaeologists today observe a variety of features, including the dimensions, shape, and surface texture of bones, to discover what kinds of activities a person habitually performed, how hard they worked, and evidence of injuries and illnesses (Munson Chapman 1997; Larsen 2000; Wilczak et al. 2004:204).[9] If archaeologists could locate and excavate the skeletons of mid-19th-century Irish immigrant laborers, they would likely find bodies that were distinct from those of native-born Americans, particularly those of the middle and upper classes. Habitual labor would have sculpted more muscular and thus stronger-boned Irish bodies, if they were in good health and had an adequate diet, making manual labor generally easier for them than for white-collar workers, who were less accustomed to physical exertion and had not developed the bodily architecture to support it. Thus the Irish laborer's body could, in some cases, have been better suited to manual labor, but not for the reasons related to humoral theory that native-born Americans suggested.

In comparison to native-born American working-class bodies, however, the bones of most Irish laborers would not have been quite as long or as robust and would likely exhibit more signs of stress and injury, because of the conditions of their lives in both Ireland and the U.S. In Ireland, diets insufficient in protein, iron, vitamin D, calcium, phosphate, and other necessary vitamins and minerals due to famine and poverty—which was by no means limited to the period of the Great Famine—would have weakened bones and led to osteoporosis and/or rickets, which make bones more susceptible to fracture. Malnutrition and/or sickness during childhood would have interrupted bone growth, visible as Harris lines (dense lines parallel to the growth plates of long bones visible on radiographs), and resulted in shorter stature. Shorter height of working-class Irish immigrants is supported by historical data. Irish prisoners transported to Australia in the early 19th century and Irish immigrant enlistees in the American Civil War averaged an inch or two shorter than their English and American-born counterparts (Hughes 1987:195; Stott 1990).[10] Shorter stature would have given Irish laborers less mechanical advantage for some tasks than longer-limbed individuals, making labor more strenuous. Once individuals gained access to a better diet in the U.S., and they were able to put on more muscle and fat, their shorter heights might have given some the stockier appearance that was an aspect of the Irish stereotype.[11] Laboring year after year in strenuous jobs put more wear and tear on Irish bodies, leading them to experience greater rates of osteoarthritis, joint degeneration, fractures, bursitis, and other chronic and acute injuries to their soft and hard tissues. In contrast, their American-born cohort moved more quickly up the occupational ladder and into less physically threatening work.

Two recent bioarchaeological studies of the Irish-born individuals in an anatomical collection created by physical anthropologist George S.

Huntington between 1893 and 1921 support these hypotheses. The collection was enabled by the passage of the 1854 "Bone Bill" which permitted the bodies of "all vagrants, dying unclaimed, and without friends" in public institutions to be used for dissection in medical schools or other study. The bill reduced graverobbing from cemeteries to meet the demands for corpses but was premised on the idea that paupers owed a debt to society that they should repay with their bodies. Kristen Pearlstein (2015) found that Irish-born individuals in the collection, some of whom were born before and during the Great Famine, exhibited higher prevalence of osteoarthritis than the German and Italian-born individuals. Alanna-Warner Smith (2022:3) examined the Irish-born individuals' skeletons as a "cumulative record of an individual's life," teasing out the long-term effects of famine in Ireland and labor in Ireland and New York City. Among many interesting findings, she discovered that the individuals who had immigrated as adults were shorter in stature than those who immigrated as children, likely due to undernourishment in Ireland. She also found increased robusticity of men's upper bodies and of women's upper and lower bodies correlated with longer time spent in the U.S., where they performed more physically demanding work. Warner-Smith additionally found evidence of a number of injuries, including healed fractures and worn-down surfaces of patellar (kneecap) bones, corresponding to injuries frequently reported among Irish immigrants in mid-19th-century hospital records, as I will show in the next section.

The physical changes that the combination of diet, work, and living conditions in Ireland and the U.S. produced in Irish immigrants' bodies were embedded within stereotypes of the Irish as brawny, stooped, and uncivilized. Famine, illness, and injury were not just marked on the exterior of Irish immigrants' bodies, they were woven into their very structure. The resulting visible features communicated meaning to others. Medical anthropologist Arthur Kleinman (1986:194–195) elaborates upon the causes of many bodily differences: "The body feels and expresses social problems. . . . The body mediates structure and cultural meaning making them part of the physiology." Irish immigrants in the 19th century, like many other working-class individuals in the past and the present, embodied the social inequalities of their day. The next section will flesh out how labor in New York City sculpted and differentiated the bodies of Irish immigrant men, women, and children from their more fortunate American-born counterparts.

Work-Related Injuries among Irish Immigrants in New York City

In his fascinating study of workers in 19th-century New York City, historian Richard Stott (1990:185) asserts, "Though many native New Yorkers regarded immigrants, especially the Irish, as simian brutes, there is no objective evidence of a physically degenerated working class." While it is true that the Irish were certainly not simian brutes, I argue that there is ample evidence in hospital records of greater rates of work-related illnesses, injuries, disfigurements, disabilities, and deaths among Irish manual laborers than among laborers born in the U.S. or in the German States. These work-related injuries brought Irish laborers into more frequent contact with surgeons, moreover, whose attempts to restore their broken bodies sometimes led to further trauma and bodily modification. This section reviews evidence in hospital records of work-related physical trauma and correlations between particular occupations and injuries common among the Irish in mid-19th-century New York City, as well as the hazards of hospitalization.

New York Hospital led the city in admissions for traumatic injury because of its downtown location on Broadway between Duane and Anthony Streets in close proximity to areas of industry and working-class residences. Seventy-five percent of the surgical cases brought to New York Hospital occurred locally (Larrabee 1971:211). The remaining quarter stemmed from further afield, including construction projects, such as the Erie Railroad; wars, including the Mexican-American War and the Civil War; and the longstanding contract that the hospital had with the Port of New York to care for seamen. By the 1850s, nearly all acute surgical cases in the city went to New York Hospital (Weir 1917:22). According to historian Eric Larrabee (1971:211), New York Hospital survived competition with newer hospitals, including St. Vincent's (est. 1849), the Jews' Hospital—later called Mt. Sinai (est. 1855), the German Dispensary—later Lenox Hill (est. 1857), and St. Luke's Hospital (est. 1858), because of its outstanding surgical reputation. Surgeons at New York Hospital had plenty of opportunity to hone their skills, especially on the bodies of Irish immigrants.

Annual reports from New York Hospital from 1845 until 1852, the last year that the reports tallied diagnoses by patients' place of birth, show that more than 50% of patients treated for the leading injury diagnoses at the hospital were Irish born. These diagnoses include: contusion, *coup de soleil* (sunstroke), fracture, *injuria* (injury), *ustio* (burn), and *vulnus* (wound). Table 4.1 shows how, in 1849, the percentage of patients treated for each kind of injury who were Irish born began to rise steeply, such that by the early 1850s, approximately 60% to 90% of patients admitted for these injuries were Irish. These figures are even more stunning considering that the Irish made up only 26% of the city's population in 1850 and 28% in 1855, according to federal and state censuses (Diner 1996:91).

In 1850 and 1851, Irish-born individuals made up more than 70% of patients admitted for fractures and more than 80% admitted for sunstroke, for example. These extremely high rates reflect the dangerous and strenuous jobs in which most immigrants were forced to labor and might also indicate that malnutrition-related bone weakening was present among famine refugees arriving during those years that made them more prone to fractures. Comparing the number of Irish-born patients treated for fracture at New York Hospital to the number of Irish-born residents of the city suggests that in 1845, roughly 1 of every 1,260 Irish-born

TABLE 4.1. Percentage of Patients Admitted to New York Hospital for the Listed Ailments Who Were Irish-Born (1845–1852).

	1845	1846	1847	1848	1849	1850	1851	1852	Average 1845–1852
Contusions	49	47	49	55	57	50	61	60	54
Coup de Soleil (sunstroke)	64	n/a	56	67	57	81	83	91	71
Fractures	48	55	54	50	71	72	73	66	61
Injuria (injury)	57	41	55	50	61	60	65	69	57
Ustio (burn)	44	58	47	59	72	62	65	72	60
Vulnus (wound)	40	51	53	57	45	54	53	58	51

Note: This table shows the percentage of the total number of patients admitted to New York Hospital yearly between 1845 and 1852 for contusions, sunstroke, fractures, injuries, burns, and wounds who were Irish-born.

Sources: Data from NYHAR (1846–1853).

residents of the city was hospitalized for a fracture at New York Hospital alone, whereas by 1850, when far more famine refugees had arrived, the rate increased more than two and a half times to about 1 per 483.[12] These trends clearly show increasing negative impacts of hard and dangerous labor on Irish bodies.

Medical and surgical case records provide more details about individuals and occupations.[13] Table 4.2 presents a sample of the injuries most common to Irish individuals laboring in specific occupations from the case records of New York Hospital (Medical Casebooks for 1847–1853 and 1865; Surgical Casebooks for 1848, 1851–1853, 1861–1862, 1865), Bellevue Hospital (Medical Casebooks 1866, 1867, and 1874), the New York Orthopaedic Dispensary (1870–1873), and the medical casebook of Dr. Peter S. Townsend (1847). The majority of the sample are Irish men treated at New York Hospital. Cases of women and children and from other institutions are noted. Injuries that were stated in the case record as having been caused by work, or seem likely to have been, are included.

Physicians rarely recorded the occupations of female patients or if their injuries were caused while laboring. Working-class women had little leisure time, whether they worked outside or inside their homes, or both, however, so the majority of injuries and sicknesses they suffered could be considered work-related. Cases in which women were burned by lamps, for example, could have occurred at a factory, while working at home on piecework, caring for children or boarders, or even while catering to clients in a brothel. Similarly, it is impossible to tell if women treated for injuries from what they reported to physicians as accidents or domestic violence were, in fact, from other kinds of assaults. Historical records and archaeological evidence show that some Irish women worked in prostitution, for example, and interpersonal violence and venereal disease were significant occupational hazards (Stansell 1986; Gilfoyle 1992; Wood Hill 1993; Yamin 2005). Injuries related to prostitution are virtually absent in hospital records; social stigmas encouraged women to hide their participation in this field, and only penitentiary hospitals openly treated women for venereal diseases. The majority of women treated at New York City hospitals for work-related injuries were domestic servants who were either under 25 or over 40 years of age. Women with children appear to have more frequently sought outpatient treatment at dispensaries or self-medicated, likely so as not to leave their children without care.[14]

TABLE 4.2. Sample of Work-Related Injuries among Irish Immigrants at New York City Hospitals (1847–1874).

Occupation	Ailment
Bleacher	Jaundice
Boatman	Diarrhea—multiple cases Fever—multiple cases Pneumonia—multiple cases Phthisis (Pulmonary TB) and coughing up blood (NYHMCB 1850: C759) Rheumatism—multiple cases
Bricklayer	Rheumatism
Brewery Worker	Ascites, linked to drinking of 2 to 4 gallons of beer per day (NYHMCB 1848:C58)
Domestic Servants (female)	Amenorrhea, possibly from hard labor—multiple cases Back injury, from "hard work" (NYODPR 1871:154) Bronchitis—multiple cases NYH and BH Chemical burn, from cleaning beds (NYHSCB 1852:C847) Delirium tremens (alcohol withdrawal) (BHMCB 1867:259) Fracture of arm, "fell on ice" (NYHSCB 1862:C166) Fracture of finger, "caught under box" and surgical amputation (NYHSCB 1862:C127) Fracture of thigh, "fell off coal box" (NYHSCB 1862:C122) Gangrene of foot, then leg, and surgical amputation at mid-thigh (NYHSCB 1852:C771) Heart palpitations, "after carrying loads of coal upstairs" (BHMCB 1867:100) "Housemaid's knee" (inflammation of knee) (NYHSCB 1852:C24) Iron-deficiency anemia—multiple cases "Insanity"—several cases BH, linked to alcohol consumption "Malingering" (BHMCB 1867:189, 233, 334) Pleuritis, working in "damp basement" (NYHMCB 1852:C412) Pneumonia—multiple cases Rheumatism—multiple cases Phthisis (Pulmonary TB)—multiple cases Ulcer on toe, "from wearing a shoe that is too tight" (NYHSCB 1848:C1810)
Dressmaker (female)	Phthisis (Pulmonary TB): "she has been obliged to work very hard and live poorly and she has not had sufficient food and has gradually lost flesh strength and appetite" (BHMCB 1874:265)
Drivers/ Coachmen	Back injury, from "jolting of truck" (NYODPR 1871:126) Frostbite, from driving without gloves, then surgical amputation (NYHMCB 1852:C461) Sunstroke, followed by possible brain damage and admittance to insane asylum (BHMCB 1874:196)

150 Fractures

Juvenile Factory-Workers (one girl, two boys)	Fracture of arm, caught in machinery (NYHSCB 1852:C633) Laceration of arm, caught in machinery, then surgical amputation (NYHSCB 1852:C9) Laceration of fingers, caught in machinery (NYHSCB 1848:C1480)
Farmers	Chronic inflammation of knee Hydrocele (an accumulation of fluid in the testis), from a fall (Townsend 1847:34)
Firemen	Crushed leg and surgical amputation (NYHSCB 1852:C543) Crushed fingers and surgical amputation (NYHSCB 1862:C103) Fractured leg Fractured skull
Gardener	Gangrene of the foot, "from wearing a boot that is too tight" and surgical removal of dead tissue (NYHSCB 1852:C369)
Hatter	Mercury poisoning
Horseshoer	Fracture of leg, caused by excited horse (NYHSCB 1848:C1229)
Hotel Servants (male) at Astor Hotel	Diarrhea, from "eating scraps of guests' food" (Townsend 1847:21) Erysipelas and wound of hand, from a rusty nail (Townsend 1847:19) Erysipelas and wound of hand, from a knife (Townsend 1847:20) Scalp wound, from a "lamp globe falling on it" (Townsend 1847:21)
Laborers (type unspecified)	Back injury, from lifting (NYODPR 1872:290) Back injury, from fall from building Back injury and paralysis, from fall from moving truck (NYODPR 1872:382) Burn—multiple cases Chronic synovitis Contusion—multiple cases Crushed fingers, by hay machine (NYHSCB 1848:C1837) Debility—multiple cases Dislocation of hip Dyspepsia Fracture of arm—multiple cases, including falls from heights and blows from heavy objects Fracture of leg—multiple cases, including attacked by bull (NYHSCB 1852:C169); knocked down by a horse and run over by cart (NYHSCB 1848: C1272); fall on railroad tracks (NYHSCB 1861:170); several subsequent surgical amputations Fracture of skull—"attacked by a bull"—and surgical removal of cranial bone (NYHSCB 1861:C165) Fracture of toe Fracture of wrist and surgical amputation Hernia—multiple cases Intermittent fever (malaria?) (BHMCB 1867:156) Lacerations—multiple cases Laceration and fracture of arm, from machinery and surgical amputation (NYHSCB 1848: C1127) "Malingering" (BHMCB 1867:273) Poisoning, from "handling green coffee bags" (NYHMCB 1865:C469) Sprain

Laborers (type unspecified), *continued*	Sunstroke, from laboring on hot days—multiple cases Wound of face, from explosion—multiple cases Wound, "struck by brass hose coupling," leading to necrosis of the skull (BHMCB 1874:165)
Laborer at Foundry	Nosebleed, "says he had been in stooping posture over a heated furnace" (NYHMCB 1848:C1573)
Laborers on Railroad	Burns, from explosions—multiple cases Contusion Destroyed cornea, from explosion (NYHSCB 1848:C1336) Fever Lacerated face, from explosion Intermittent fever (malaria?), from working on Panama Railroad (NYHMCB 1852:C449) Pneumonia
Laborer at India Rubber Plant	Lead poisoning, from "white lead used in rubber-making" (NYHMCB 1865:C352)
Laborer at Tannery	Destruction of eye and ulcer of cheek, from "hairs from the hides in his eye" (NYHSCB 1848:C1604)
Laundresses (female)	Back injury (NYODPR 1871:164) Bursitis of ankle: "about 6 weeks ago after a hard day's scrubbing a swelling appeared . . . and became so painful that she could not walk" (BHMCB 1867:277) Wound of hand, needles broke off into hands (NYHSCB 1848:C124, 1852:C161)
Lead Worker (female)	Ascites and lead poisoning (NYHMCB 1850:C727)
Longshoremen	Amputation of fingers, caught under a heavy barrel (NYHSCB 1862:C127) Contusion—multiple cases Fractured arm Hydrocele (an accumulation of fluid in the testis), fell on a plank (NYHSCB 1862:C251)
Mason	Sunstroke, from working on a hot day (NYHMCB 1852:C804)
Match Seller (female)	Sunstroke, from working on a hot day (BHMCB 1867:233)
Mechanic	Amputation of fingers, accidentally sawed off (NYHSCB 1861:C132)
Nursemaid (female)	Bursitis, from a fall and continuing to labor (NYHSCB 1852: C24)
Oystermen	*Delirium tremens* (alcohol withdrawal) (NYHMCB 1848:C65) Fracture of radius, from fall (NYHSCB 1861:C155) "Stabbed in an oyster saloon" (NYHMCB 1848:C1243)
Painters	Lead poisoning (BHMCB 1867:437) Dysentery and ptyalism (excessive salivation) Malingering (BHMCB 1867:172)
Peddlers	Head injury, from a "barrel that fell off a roof" (NYHSCB 1848: C1820) Diarrhea, from consuming fruit he sold (NYHMCB 1852:C4501)

Porters/Carters	Fracture of clavicle Fracture of skull and radius, "fell from hayloft" in a dispute (NYHSCB 1861:96) Rheumatism
Saloon Owners	Carcinoma of the stomach *Delirium tremens* (alcohol withdrawal) (NYHMCB 1865:C105) Rheumatism, "habit of drinking freely"; 10 drinks per day (NYHMCB 1852:C403)
Seamen	Concussion Contusion—multiple cases *Delirium tremens* (alcohol withdrawal)—multiple cases Fractured leg—multiple cases Fractured skull, from fall—multiple cases Pneumonia Intermittent fever (malaria?) (BHMCB 1867:25)
Soda Water Vendor	Lead poisoning and colic (NYHMCB 1852:C113)
Soldiers (from Mexican-American and Civil Wars)	Diarrhea Gunshot wound "Irritable Stump," from previous amputation (NYHSCB 1848:C1562) Remittent Fever (likely malaria)
Tapemaker (female)	Bronchitis
Tinner/Coppersmith	Contusion, "fell off a roof while working" (NYHSCB 1848:C1564)
Waiter	Lead poisoning and colic (NYHMCB 1852:60)

Note: This table is organized by patients' occupations as recorded by physicians. Citations are provided only for detailed New York Hospital entries and those from other hospitals.

Sources: Case records of New York Hospital (Medical Casebooks for 1847–1853 and 1865; Surgical Casebooks for 1848, 1851–1853, 1861–1862, 1865), Bellevue Hospital (Medical Casebooks 1866, 1867, and 1874), the New York Orthopaedic Dispensary (1870–1873), and the medical casebook of Dr. Peter S. Townsend (1847).

These case records show that work-related injuries among Irish immigrants resulted from a variety of factors including: sudden accidents, habitual hard labor, working conditions and hazardous substances, and work-related violence. Both acute and chronic injuries plagued male and female Irish immigrants, but acute injuries were especially prevalent among laboring men. These records also reveal the treatments they received, which often further shaped and scarred their bodies.

ACUTE INJURIES FROM ACCIDENTS AT WORK

Acute injuries were most frequent among men who worked carrying heavy loads, including longshoremen, seamen, and porters, and men who worked on railroads, canals, and in other construction (Figure 4.2). An Irish immigrant highlighted the vulnerabilities of these occupations for Irish workers in a letter home: "How often do we see such paragraphs in the paper as an Irishman drowned—an Irishman crushed by a beam—an Irishman suffocated in a pit—an Irishman blown to atoms by a steam engine—ten, twenty Irishmen buried alive in the sinking of a bank—and other like casualties and perils to which honest Pat is constantly exposed, in the hard toils for his daily bread" (Miller 1985:267).

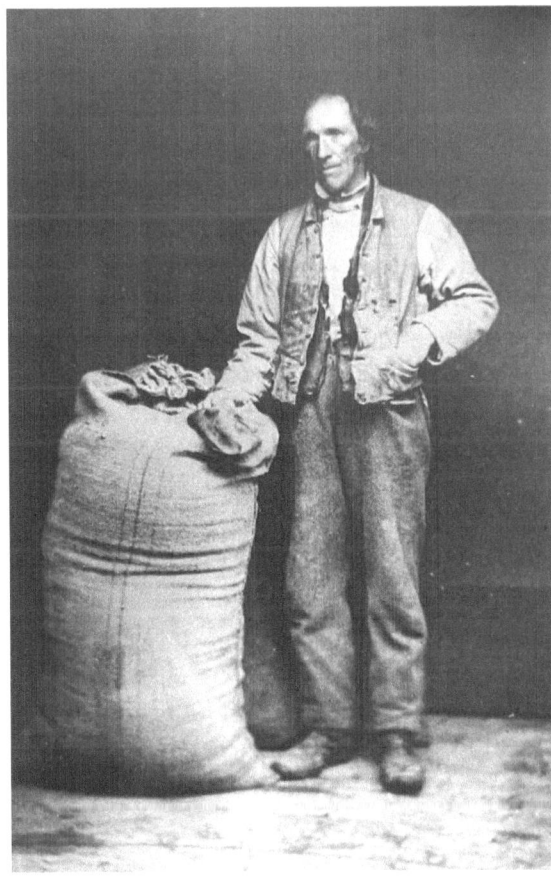

FIGURE 4.2. Early albumen print of a mill worker at Jerpoint, County Kilkenny, circa 1860. "Note the size of the sack, packed with grain that this man is used to lifting. Photography attributed to Rev. James Graves (a local Church minister)" (Sexton 1994:52–53). Courtesy of the Sean Sexton Archive.

Details of acute injuries in case records from New York Hospital confirm that this statement did not wildly exaggerate the real situation for Irish laborers, especially those involved in railroad construction. These men suffered from falls, explosions, and being crushed by heavy materials or equipment. Thomas, a 22-year-old fireman and railroad laborer, had his skull fractured and leg crushed when he was caught between two cars of the Long Island Railroad (NYHSCB 1852:C543).[15] Dr. George Hayward (1850:15) of the Massachusetts General Hospital in Boston remarked at how difficult it was to heal those injured by trains: "Everyone who has had frequent occasion to amputate for railroad accidents [knows that] a wheel of a locomotive engine or a railway car ... produces a compound and comminuted fracture of the worst kind."

Other railroad laborers were badly injured due to dangerous practices that would not be allowed under present-day labor laws. Hugh, a 35-year-old laborer, had his leg badly broken when an unshored bank he was excavating for the Erie Railroad collapsed, for example (NYHSCB 1848:C1289). Irish writer John Francis Maguire (1868:168) details how Irish workers were told to cut through mountains to build the path for the Erie Railroad. "Crews were lowered down the mountain sides in baskets; after setting their charges and lighting the fuses, they were hurriedly dragged back up the mountain before the explosion." These explosions spewed bone-crushing boulders and buckshot-like debris. At New York Hospital, a surgeon recorded treating one crew member, 35-year-old Michael, for "burns to face, left arm, and hand from an explosion of powder while blasting four days [previous to admission] ... face, lacerated, filled with debris, eyes closed and bathed in pus, cornea of left eye appears to be destroyed (NYHSCB 1848:C1336). Physicians removed the debris from his face, applied cold water dressings, and carron oil (a mixture of limewater and linseed oil) to his burns. Although discharged from the hospital as "cured," Michael no doubt bore the scars of his injuries on his face and never again saw out of his left eye.

Burns were also frequent among women engaged in sewing or domestic work, whose clothes caught fire from lamps or stoves or from building fires, which were common in tenement neighborhoods where many edifices were still built of wood.[16] Even today serious burns are difficult to treat. Without the protective dermis, patients succumb to sepsis, and as I will detail below, 19th-century hospitals were hotbeds of infection. Survival rates for people with serious burns at New York Hospital in the 1850s were low. Cases such as that of Sarah, a 23-year-old Irish married woman, for example, were too frequent. Sarah was admitted for burns on the face, arms, upper back, and chest after her clothes caught fire 12 days earlier. Surgeons administered poultices and carron oil and dosed her with stimulating elixirs and wine, but she died five days later (NYHSCB 1848:C1143).

Even more common acute injuries than burns, especially among male laborers and female domestic servants, were fractures, wounds, and bruises caused by falling or by heavy objects falling on them or machines crushing them while working. Patrick, a 19-year-old coppersmith, for example, fell from a third-story roof and miraculously survived with only bruises (NYHSCB 1852:C608).[17] Twenty-eight-year-old laborer, Mark, fell and broke his leg when moving a barrel of fish into a cellar (NYHSCB 1862:C89). Another Patrick, a 25-year-old seaman, fractured his tibia and fibula when a 670-pound box he was sliding down a ramp slipped and fell on his leg (NYHSCB 1861:C180). James, a 26-year-old laborer, similarly had his leg broken by a load of cotton falling on it (NYHSCB 1848:C1321). Domestic servants also suffered from similar kinds of injuries. Seventeen-year-old Catherine fell off a coal box and fractured her thigh (NYHSCB 1862:C122), and 30-year-old Mary slipped on ice and broke her arm (NYHSCB 1862:C161). Surgeons at New York Hospital treated fractures by realigning the bone, a process that was often painful. Then, once swelling subsided, they applied a dressing and a plaster splint. They were able to treat minor fractures well, but more complicated fractures like Mary's arm and Patrick's leg often did not heal straight, causing them to suffer in the longer term from some level of pain, disability, and deformation. A few individuals in Warner-Smith's (2022:193) bioarchaeological sample who passed away in New York City's almshouse exhibited misaligned healed fractures of the tibia, which made that leg shorter and, at minimum, caused a pronounced limp.

Fractures and other wounds that pierced the skin, such as that of Jane, a 45-year-old servant who fractured and lacerated her fingers under a heavy box (NYHSCB 1862:C202), were even more problematic, because they exposed the individual to life-threatening infection that often forced physicians to amputate, which caused even greater complications. This scenario occurred as a result of many different kinds of injuries, but the most difficult cases involved accidents with machinery. As historian of medicine Martin Pernick (1985:218) discovered in his examination of case records from hospitals in New York City, Philadelphia, and Boston, "extreme tissue damage caused by industrial accidents made infection far more likely in such injuries than any other type of surgery." An example in the case records of New York Hospital is that of Pat, a 10-year-old calico press worker. The press broke and lacerated his arm so badly that the surgeon felt his arm could not be saved. Initially, Pat's "friends" (who were probably his family members) would not consent to amputation.[18] Pat's friends likely worried about the potential consequences of a working-class boy losing an arm. After a few days, as Pat weakened from loss of blood and infection, the surgeon convinced them to allow it, arguing that Pat's wounds were life-threatening and "he would resign all responsibility in the case" if Pat's friends did not consent. They did, and the surgeon amputated Pat's arm three inches below his shoulder (NYHSCB 1852:C9).

In this era before the germ theory and before systemic antibiotic drugs, surgeons could do little to stop infection except to apply mildly effective topical treatments or remove the affected part. Patients with open wounds to a limb or tumors, incurable ulcers, gunshot wounds, etc. stood a better chance of survival if they had the limb amputated. Common forms of infections in 19th-century hospitals included erysipelas (streptococcal skin infection), pyemia (sepsis usually caused by staphylococcus), gangrene, and tetanus (Walsh 1965:17). So great were infection rates in hospitals and so little were these diseases understood they were collectively known as "hospitalism" (Larrabee 1971:215). The architecture of the hospital, made of wood and plaster, different standards of personal cleanliness among physicians and staff alike, and lack of aseptic technique were causes of such high infection rates (Figure 4.3).[19] Operating instruments were poorly cleaned, and gauze and sponges were rinsed in water and soaked overnight in open buckets. The surgeon's "black coat was covered with blood and pus, his badge of prowess from years at the operating table" (Leitman 1991:479, 485, 487). People's fears of hospitals were justified; even minor injuries could become life-threatening. Some patients even voluntarily left

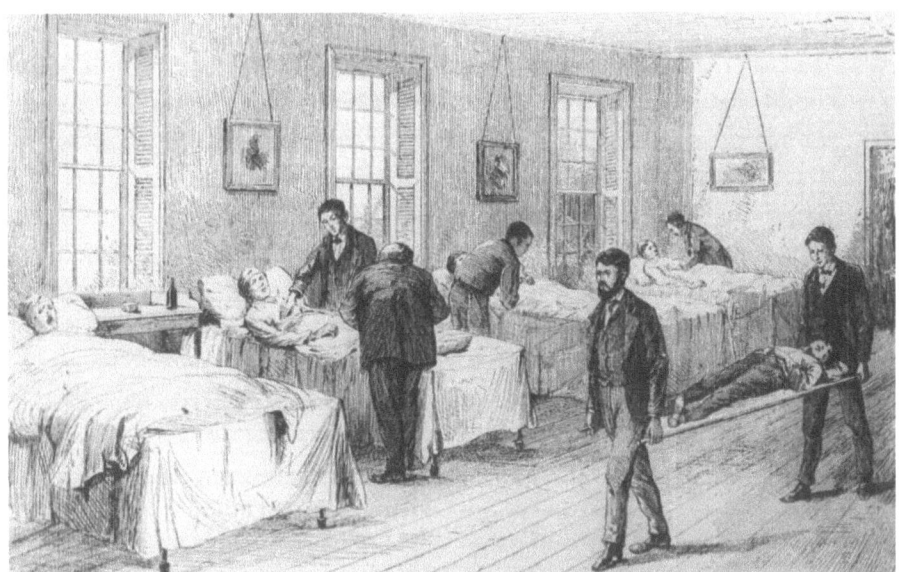

FIGURE 4.3. Sketch of a ward in the new New York Hospital building, ca. 1871 (National Library of Medicine). The wards of the new building were constructed to be easier to clean than those of the old building. Physicians and nurses still did not use gloves, gowns, or sterile techniques, however. Courtesy of the National Library of Medicine.

the hospital while still under treatment to avoid infections, including James, a 27-year-old Irish-born clerk, who a physician recorded "left early through fear of erysipelas" (NYHMCB 1848:C152). On another occasion, New York Hospital physician Dr. Parker advised an Irish patient, 35-year-old grocer Samuel, recuperating from an amputation at the forearm to leave to "get fresh air," because there was an outbreak of erysipelas in the ward (NYHSCB 1862:C276).

Surgery was relatively primitive, especially amputations, and often led to infection and death.[20] Sister Marie de Lourdes Walsh (1965:17) explains in her history of St. Vincent's Hospital that "amputation was often a vicious cycle: a germ-infected limb was removed to arrest the spread of infection, and the original wound-fever was followed by its counterpart, the dreaded hospital gangrene." The renowned Philadelphia surgeon Dr. Samuel D. Gross (1861:84)—who was immortalized by the first-generation Irish American artist Thomas Eakins in his famous 1875 painting "The Gross Clinic"—studied amputation mortality rates from the Crimean War and from English, French, and American hospitals. He found that more than one-quarter of patients died from amputations, with lesser chances of survival the closer the limb was severed from the body. Amputations at the hip were fatal more than 90% of the time, and amputations at the upper leg resulted in more deaths (71%) than those at the shoulder (25%).[21] Chaloner, Flora, and Ham's (2001:411) study of amputation at the London Hospital from 1852 to 1857 showed that mortality rates were even higher, likely because of higher rates of sepsis in the hospital than in the open surgical tents in Crimea. They found an overall mortality rate of 46%, and cause of death was attributed to sepsis in 50% of cases.

Deaths from even minor amputations of a finger were not unheard-of. At New York Hospital, for example, a 21-year-old laborer named James, who acquired frostbite while driving without gloves, had a finger amputated, then his hand, and then his arm, as gangrene from the initial procedure spread. This was all done without anesthesia, and James did not survive the ordeal (NYHSCB 1852:C461). Young Pat, the calico-press worker, fared better under ether. He survived his surgery and hospital stay, discharged "cured," but what became of him afterward is unknown. How surviving amputees fared after discharge is difficult to assess. Only one patient in the records surveyed returned years after an amputation. Mary, a 32-year-old match seller, mentioned at the beginning of this chapter, who was hospitalized for sunstroke years after a "lower limb" amputation, likely resorted to peddling because it was one of the few occupations available to her that was compatible with her altered locomotive abilities.

INJURY AND ILLNESS FROM HAZARDOUS WORK ENVIRONMENTS: ACUTE AND CHRONIC

Mary the match seller was not alone in suffering acute effects from New York City's extreme temperatures. Coming from Ireland's more temperate climate, many were unprepared for laboring in the heat of the city's summers or the cold of its winters. Traveler John White (1870:369) remarked that the Irish "hate the climate, most cordially; and, indeed, the moist mildness of Ireland is as bad a preparation as can be." In an 1849 letter to his family in Westmeath, Irishman Matthew Gaynor explained the climate was "troublesome," because it was "very cold in the winter [you] have to wear gloves and in summer you could roast beefsteaks out on the fences."

Hospital records contain many reports of Irish laborers, drivers, and vendors who nearly roasted themselves while working outdoors on hot days. Irish-born individuals were admitted to New York Hospital for sunstroke at a rate between 4 and 10 times that of American- and German-born individuals between 1845 and 1852 (NYHAR 1846–1853). To American physicians, the prevalence of sunstroke among the Irish, sanguine in temperament and thus already hot in nature, was probably not surprising. Mary the match seller was discharged from Bellevue as "cured," but others were not so fortunate. Some died and others were permanently injured. The case of Peter, a 26-year-old coachman admitted to Bellevue Hospital for catalepsy, a state of trance and bodily rigidity, stands out (BHMCB 1874:196). Peter had suffered from a sunstroke in 1872 that appears to have caused permanent brain injury. Afterward he had "peculiar conduct," characterized by neglect of his business, extreme melancholy, and wandering out at night, such that his family committed him to an insane asylum. After some time in that institution, he was malnourished, sickly, and unable to speak. His brother removed him, hoping to take him back to Ireland, but Peter was so weak he had to be admitted to Bellevue. What became of him was not recorded.

Laboring in New York City's cold and wet winters also caused acute injury, such as the frostbite James endured while driving without gloves, mentioned above, or chronic problems for those unable to afford proper clothing, shoes, and shelter. Ann, a 19-year-old domestic servant, and William, a 21-year-old gardener, for example, were both admitted to New York Hospital during the winter for foot injuries from wearing boots that were too tight; presumably they could not afford properly fitting pairs (NYHSCB 1848:C1810; NYHSCB 1852:C369). Both had parts of their foot tissue surgically removed, which likely made it more difficult to go about their work. Other immigrants were literally worn out over time from working in the cold without sufficient clothing and diets. Immigrant Thomas O'Reilly (1848:2) wrote in 1848 to a physician friend in Dublin, "It is true that the greater number of our countrymen die in a short time here they overwork themselves and the climate does the rest." Matthew, a 55-year-old laborer admitted to New York Hospital in

January of 1865, fit this description. The physician noted that he was a "small feeble oldish man who has not been well fed, clothed, or housed" (NYHMCB 1865:C334). Physicians treated Matthew for "debility" at the hospital for three months; afterward he was released "cured." Other hospitals suggest that some Irish immigrants became so desperate in the winter that they sought refuge there claiming illness. Case records show diagnoses of "impecuniosity" and "malingering" at Bellevue, while physicians at New York Hospital noted a few "miraculous recoveries" in the spring (BHMCB 1867:57, 172; Rosner 1979:119).

The constant necessity to labor for daily bread, combined with overexposure and malnourishment, led many Irish to fall victim to other diseases, especially tuberculosis, as I will explore in Chapter 6. Many were exposed to this disease at work and thus will be briefly discussed here. Hospital records show that younger and single seamstresses and domestics, as well as middle-aged or senior widowed female domestics and male laborers sought hospital care most frequently for pulmonary tuberculosis, usually after they had been ill for a long time. Margaret, a 50-year-old widowed domestic servant, "accustomed to living in basements" and whose diet was "made up largely of potatoes" sought relief at Bellevue in December after coughing for six months and experiencing night sweats for four weeks (BHMCB 1874:635). Similarly, Ann, a 41-year-old widowed dressmaker admitted to Bellevue for phthisis (pulmonary tuberculosis), had "been obliged to work very hard and live poorly and she [had] not had sufficient food." For "two years past she has had chills and night sweats... two weeks ago patient awoke at night with severe pain in right scapular region. She went to work the next morning but was obliged to go home from pain" (BHMCB 1874:265). And Mary, a 19-year-old domestic servant, also suffering from phthisis, believed that she became ill from "sitting in cold draughts when overheated at work." She experienced "pain in back and headache upon overheating herself after baking" (BHMCB 1874:93). Many perished from this dreaded disease, while others battled it for years and suffered its painful effects on the lungs, dramatic weight loss, visible skin lesions, and spinal deformities.

Hospital records show patients admitted for other diseases caused by their work environments as well. Nurses succumbed to typhus, typhoid, cholera, tuberculosis, and other communicable diseases spread in hospitals. Oliver, a 20-year-old Irishman, for example, was a nurse in one of New York Hospital's fever wards in 1848 until he too became ill; he recovered (NYHMCB 1848:C146). Railroad workers were afflicted with fevers rife in their camps. Twenty-two-year-old laborer John, whose name and age match that of a resident of 474 Pearl Street in the Five Points in 1850, was treated for fever he caught while working on the New York and Erie Railroad (NYHMCB 1848:C414). Workers of all kinds suffered from rheumatism, a catch-all diagnosis that could mean anything from simple joint pain, to an infection of the joint, to rheumatoid arthritis. Rheumatism was linked in the 19th century to cold and damp environments, while today doctors believe acute rheumatic disorders to be caused by infection, the chances of which would be higher while living and working in unhygienic conditions. Some of these same environmental dangers are still found in New York City today, while others emphasize how different the city was in the middle of the 19th century. Boatmen, sailors, and domestics occasionally presented with "intermittent fever," a diagnosis that was probably malaria. While other mosquito-borne illnesses do sometimes affect residents of the city today, malaria is no longer an endemic disease. Additionally, two Irish laborers were hospitalized for wounds sustained by being attacked by a bull in the city on two separate occasions (NYHSCB 1853:C169; NYHSCB 1862:C165). Large animals rarely roam New York City's streets today.

In the absence of protective labor laws some work environments were even more hazardous because of poisonous substances integral to the work. Laborers were provided with little protection or education about the disabling and disfiguring effects of substances such as mercury, lead, phosphorus, and silica. Glassblowers and stonecutters were often afflicted with silicosis, a painful and deadly lung condition caused by inhaling silica dust from stone and glassmaking materials (Kraut 1994). Hairdressers experienced high rates of lung disease from inhaling mineral powders used to whiten wigs (Hughes 1987:31). Girls who worked in match factories dipping matches into phosphorus often suffered from "phossy jaw," deterioration of their jaw often accompanied by brain damage, caused by inhaling phosphorus fumes.[22] While this condition is most well known from an 1888 strike of "matchstick girls" in London, it affected residents of New York City earlier as well. St. Vincent's Hospital's 1859 annual report lists one patient cured of "phosphorus disease of upper jaw," for example (SVHAR 1861:13). Workers in other industries suffered from other kinds of poisoning. Hatters notoriously bore the effects of poisoning and sometimes even mental illness from the mercury used in felting wool. A 41-year-old hatter named Dennis, for example, suffered "attacks" from mercury ten and four years prior to being admitted to Bellevue in 1864. At that point, he suffered from "nervous trembling—so severe lately he had to give up work" (BHMCB 1867:148). Irish workers often continued in these occupations, even after suffering from some ill effects, because these jobs were better paying than unskilled labor and possibly also because they took pride in their skills. Perhaps they also considered the risk of poisoning to be a lesser evil than the risk of being crushed, blown up, or used up like so many unskilled laborers.

The most commonly diagnosed work-related poisoning among Irish immigrants admitted to New York City hospitals from the 1850s to the 1870s was from lead. "Painter's colic," for example, appears as a category of disease in St. Vincent's Hospital's 1859 annual report; three patients at the small hospital were treated successfully that year (SVHAR 1861:17–18). Painters were not the only workers susceptible to lead poisoning, however. Metal founders, soda water makers, laborers in an India rubber factory, and lead workers were all hospitalized in New York City for the effects of lead poisoning. At the New York Hospital, 23-year-old Catherine, a lead worker, was admitted suffering from deafness and colic and "[did] not tell a straight story," while 23-year-old Nicholas suffered from colic, pains in arms and legs, and "complete loss of power of extensor and supinator muscles of forearm" from "working in India rubber in which process a good deal of white lead is employed" NYHMCB 1850:C727; 1865:C352. Nicholas, like several painters admitted for lead colic, had first treated himself with "a good deal of whiskey" to counteract the actions of the lead.

Physicians treated lead colic with liquor, too, and with strong cathartics, but appear to have made no attempt to convince their patients to pursue a lead-free line of work. With continued exposure to high levels of lead, these workers were likely to suffer from paralysis of the limbs, wasting of the body, deafness, mental impairment, convulsions, coma, and even death (Heywood 1999:84). Irish immigrants with anemia or a calcium deficiency caused by malnutrition or previous illness, moreover, would have been more susceptible to lead poisoning than other workers. As physician Audrey Heywood (1999:101) explains, inadequate amounts of iron and calcium increase the amount of lead that the body absorbs and retains.

High levels of lead in soils near factories and workers' residences have been found by archaeologists at Lowell, Massachusetts (Mrozowski 2006). It is likely the same could be found in some neighborhoods of New York City, because of the lack of separation between hazardous industries and residences in 19th-century cities. Given the connection now acknowledged between lead and developmental disabilities in children and cognitive impairment in adults, greater exposure of working-class Irish immigrants to lead is especially concerning. Lead and other industrial poisons in urban sites and factory towns posed great risks. Mental changes caused by chemicals such as lead and mercury might have contributed to violent confrontations at work and/or attempted suicides that caused injuries recorded in hospital records.

Disputes among workers or between workers and bosses sometimes made the workplace even more unsafe and led to more injuries and deaths. John, a 38-year-old Irish laborer, for example, sustained a fractured skull and radius after falling from a hayloft during an altercation (NYHSCB 1862:C96), while William, a 20-year-old oysterman, was stabbed in the side in an oyster saloon (NYHSCB 1848:C1243). John survived his injuries, but William did not. Historians have written about individual altercations among workers as well as large-scale fights between work-gangs on canals and railroads. In one case, Irish workers assaulted an American worker for working too fast, after repeated warnings that he should work slower to make the job last longer for everyone (Stott 1990:137). Irish work crews from different Irish counties sometimes fought each other for control of turf or prestige, and other times Irish crews fought with non-Irish workers brought in to break workers' strikes. Bruises, fractures, cuts, and even deaths were the outcome of these American donnybrooks. Stott (1990) and Shaw (1977) point out that Irish laborers' strikes were framed by native-born American bosses as "riots" to justify bosses' policies of ignoring workers' protests and using militias and police forces against them.

Domestic violence also manifests occasionally in the hospital records. Twenty-year-old Margaret's husband kicked her in the groin causing a severe contusion (NYHMCB 1848:C1356), 60-year-old Mary's "amiable husband" kicked her down the stairs breaking her leg (NYHSCB 1862:C76), 54-year-old Hugh received a scalp wound "from a blow of some sort of an iron dish in the hand of his wife" (NYHSCB 1862:C167), and 22-year-old Eliza fractured her arm and sustained a concussion from jumping out of a fourth-story window "to save herself from being beaten by her husband" (NYHMCB 1852:C1001). According to Christine Stansell (1986:78–80), fighting over how to allocate wages or divide labor in the household were the leading causes of domestic violence between men and women in 19th-century New York City. Emigrant Savings Bank records include notes that might have catalyzed a husband's rage, such as "Give him no money . . . , His Wife 2/27/60" and "Michael is drinking, his wife desires that he get no money, October 12, 1862" (Griggs 2000:45). Arguments and work-related accidents were exacerbated by the frequent practice of imbibing alcohol both on and off the job by most members of the working class (Rorabaugh 1979; Stivers 2000; Stott 1990). The liquor that laborers relied on to keep them feeling warm, to give them strength, to bring them health, and to dull their aches and pains also sometimes added to their suffering. Over time, managing painful labor with alcohol caused damage to the liver and the heart. Several older Irish immigrants admitted to New York and Bellevue Hospitals were literally worn out by years of the combination of hard drinking and hard work.

CHRONIC INJURIES AND DEBILITY

In the words of an Irish immigrant, "A man who labours steadily for ten to twelve years in America is of very little use afterwards . . . he becomes old before his time" (Miller 1985:319). Several case records of middle-aged Irish immigrants admitted to New York City hospitals support this observation. Physicians could not find any specific disease or injury afflicting them, and instead diagnosed them as suffering from "debility," "general malaise," or "exhaustion," the latter being perhaps the most accurate. Some recovered after a few months of rest in the hospital, while others declined. Irish patients over the age of 40 admitted to the city's hospitals for virtually any ailment fully recovered less frequently than their younger counterparts. Many Irish immigrants also sought care for chronic injuries, such as back pain, bursitis, and hernias, that had worsened because they had little choice but to continue to labor through the pain. Jane, a 27-year-old nursemaid, for example, was treated at New York Hospital for "housemaid's knee" (bursitis of the knee caused by kneeling and often linked to scrubbing floors) that had become very swollen over the course of two weeks. During that time, she continued "carrying and holding the child she was tending" (NYHSCB 1852:C24). What began as a minor injury turned into a major one, because Jane was unable to rest and allow her knee to heal. Chronic bursitis could cause changes to the patellar bone, something that Warner-Smith (2022:207–208, 219) noted in a number of Irish-born women in her bioarchaeological study sample, all of whom had worked in domestic service. Figure 4.4 shows a photograph of two women, likely inmates of the city's almshouse (Warner-Smith 2022:217–219), engaged in two of many physically demanding tasks that were required of female domestic servants throughout the 19th century: scrubbing on hands and knees and hauling heavy buckets of water.

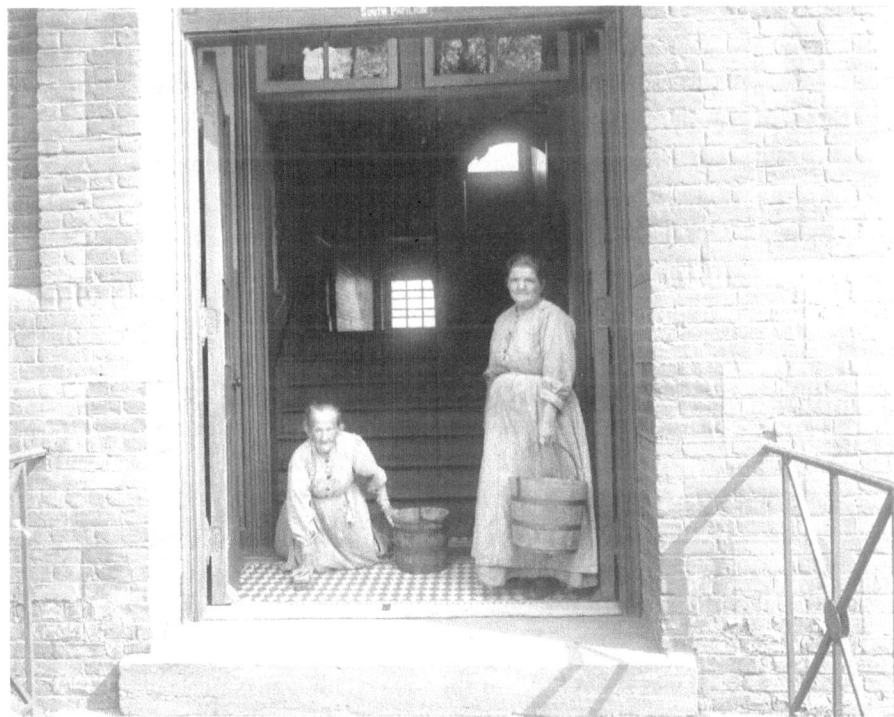

FIGURE 4.4. "City Home, Two women with wooden pails scrub the entry to South Pavilion," Blackwell's Island, ca. 1895–1905. Photograph attributed to Frederick A. Walter. Courtesy of the Municipal Archives, City of New York.

Men such as George, a 42-year-old laborer, also frequently suffered from repeated injury. George endured lasting pain from a back injury he initially sustained lifting heavy loads as a teenager that never had time to properly heal. "Ever since [he had] been liable to pain in the lumbar region when he made a sudden movement." Yet, "his usual employment" was "lifting coffee bags." He sought relief at the New York Orthopaedic Dispensary only after severe back pain and stiffness, which had begun two weeks previously, had made it difficult to walk and impossible to labor (NYODPR 1872:290). Chronic back injuries were also prevalent among seamstresses who were forced to sit for hours over their work or in front of sewing machines. This habitual work reshaped their bodies. Social reformer Virginia Penny (1863:310) claimed she could identify a seamstress on the street by the way she walked: "The neck suddenly bending forward, and the arms being, even in walking, considerably bent forward, or folded more or less upward from the elbows."

Hernias were another injury that frequently resulted from chronic labor and caused bodily changes. They appear only occasionally in hospital surgical records, because until later in the century, their surgical treatment generally yielded poor results (Leitman 1991:481). Hernias were, nevertheless, common among laboring men. According to historian Martin Rediker (1987), seamen were "peculiarly susceptible to hernia or the 'bursted belly,' as they preferred to call it" because their work required pulling and heavy lifting. The frequency of this condition among 19th-century New Yorkers is further supported by many advertisements for trusses, belts used to keep hernias from bulging, in newspapers including the *New York Daily Times* and *Harper's Weekly* (Figure 4.5).[23] Brands include Marsh's Radical Cure Truss (*New-York Daily Times* [*NYDT*] 1857a:5); Dr. Riggs Waterproof Trusses, "young cases cured" (*HW* 1861:159); Dr. Glover's Lever Truss (*HW* 1865:830); Bartlett Truss "free for servicemen" (*HW* 1873b:902); and Pomeroy's Trusses "the wire spring truss with oscillating pads" or "the elastic rupture-belt without metallic springs" (*HW* 1872:726).

Demand for treatment of hernias and skeletal injuries was so great in New York City in the middle of the 19th century that there were institutions dedicated to such endeavors. In 1863, Dr. James A. Knight, a general practitioner from Maryland, opened the charitable Hospital for the Relief of the Ruptured and Crippled in his own house on Second Avenue

Pomeroy's Trusses.

The WIRE SPRING TRUSS,

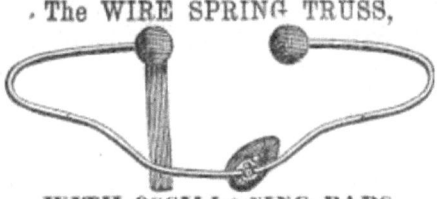

WITH OSCILLATING PADS.

The ELASTIC RUPTURE-BELT,

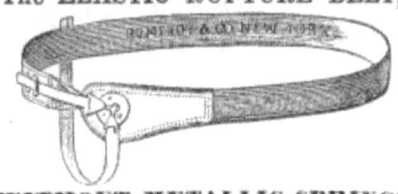

WITHOUT METALLIC SPRINGS.

Prices, when sent to correspondents, much lower than when fitted at office. Send for circular. Samples of above trusses, one of each, sent to any physician or druggist for $5. Address
POMEROY & CO., 744 Broadway, New York.
Pomeroy & Co. also apply, as a specialty, their celebrated Finger-Pad Trusses, and keep on hand or make to order the best Elastic Stockings, Knee-Caps, Belts, &c. Crutches, Shoulder-Braces, Suspensories, Abdominal Supporters, Club-Foot Shoes, Leg-Braces, and Surgical Appliances of every kind.

FIGURE 4.5. An advertisement for Pomeroy & Company's "wire spring truss" and the "elastic rupture belt," two braces for supporting hernias (*Harper's Weekly* 1872:726).

and Sixth Street, for example. Knight de-emphasized surgery, instead treating patients with sunshine, fresh air, diet, exercise, electrical stimulation, and rehabilitation. Case records from the New York Orthopaedic Dispensary show that many Irish patients had previously sought care at Knight's establishment. Knight's hospital expanded and moved uptown to 42nd Street in 1870, and then changed its name in 1940 to the Hospital for Special Surgery; it still exists today and is affiliated with New York Hospital and Cornell University Medical College (Hospital for Special Surgery 2021). The New York Orthopaedic Dispensary later became part of the Presbyterian Hospital in 1945 and moved to the Columbia-Presbyterian Medical Center in 1950. Irish immigrants, who suffered so disproportionately from work-related injuries, are partially responsible for the development of these healthcare institutions and for the many advancements in the treatments of injuries pioneered there (Larrabee 1971; Leitman 1991).

Scarred and Stooped Beasts of Burden?

These hospital and other historical records provide clues about the magnitude and types of work-related injuries among Irish immigrants in mid-19th-century New York City. What they show is that this group experienced a variety of injuries, including burns, fractures, and contusions, as well as general debility, at far greater rates than their American- or German-born counterparts. They reveal how these and other injuries frequently caused physical (and also sometimes mental) changes to Irish individuals that were visible to others.[24] Chronic back injuries caused stooped posture, fractured limbs led to limping gaits, burns scarred faces, lead poisoning produced paralysis, and mercury poisoning caused visible cognitive changes, for example. Hospital procedures seeking to mend injured workers sometimes caused further suffering and alteration, and even hastened deaths. Amputation of a limb was a procedure that could be lifesaving, by halting blood loss and infection, or life taking, from shock or sepsis. Even for those who survived, such as Mary the match seller or Pat the calico-press worker, however, the ordeal could be life altering. Neither Mary nor Pat would have retained the same chances of attaining good employment or advancement, for example.

One of the characteristics of urban life, as detailed by the renowned sociologist Louis Wirth, is the tendency of people to judge others by their appearance. Unlike in a village, where individuals are well acquainted with nearly all other residents on a personal level that enables them to move beyond appearance, in a city, there are far too many people for such intimacy with everyone. "The urban world," he wrote, "puts a premium on visual recognition. We see the uniform which denotes the role . . . and are oblivious to the personal eccentricities . . . behind the uniform" (Wirth 1938:12–14). The uniform that most Irish immigrants in 19th-century New York City wore was one fashioned by their daily toils, and it was one that they could not easily remove, because it was woven into their bones, flesh, and viscera.

To native-born Americans this uniform signaled that the Irish were best equipped to be manual laborers. It supported and exacerbated preexisting ideas that the Irish were a different and lesser group of humans that naturally possessed a different temperament and character. Complexions made ruddy by hard work in the elements or in hot kitchens seemed to reveal sanguine interiors. Muscular frames and stooped posture shaped by heavy lifting became evidence that the Irish were like beasts of burden or apes and that they lacked upright moral character. Scarred faces, instead of eliciting sympathy, became indicators of brutality. Even the well-meaning Ladies of the Five Points Mission (1854:33), who provided charitable services to the neighborhood, described Irish men there as "brutal men with black eyes and disfigured faces, proclaiming drunken brawls and fearful violence."

The physical effects of labor and injuries thus added further visual and tangible proof of Irish difference that reinforced and refined stereotypes. These effects influenced how Americans thought about Irish strangers they encountered on the city streets or in city hospitals or in their own homes as domestic servants. Included in assumptions about Irish brutishness was the notion that the Irish were less sensitive to pain, which to them might have been supported by so many instances in which Irish immigrants continued to labor despite injuries. This belief was so fully accepted that it sometimes led physicians to withhold general anesthesia from Irish laborers, even during the most painful surgeries.

Anesthesia and Irish Suffering: From Insensitivity toward Compassion

After driving a wagon without gloves for four hours on a cold winter day, James, a 21-year-old Irish-born laborer, mentioned previously, developed frostbite on his fingers and sought care at New York Hospital on January 25, 1852. The surgeons, then unaware of the importance of sterile techniques, punctured vesicles on fingers with unsterile surgical tools. James's little finger became gangrenous, so doctors amputated it on February 6th, without anesthesia. Two days later, James developed erysipelas, an acute bacterial skin infection, in his hand and extending into his arm. Surgeons responded by blistering his arm, causing it to swell. To reduce the swelling, they made an opening in the elbow joint, again without anesthesia. Soon James' whole arm became gangrenous. Surgeons applied a poultice on Feb 17th. Two days later, his arm hemorrhaged, and physicians applied a tourniquet to stop the bleeding. Later that day surgeons amputated James' arm at the shoulder without anesthesia. James survived the surgery, but afterward was "greatly prostrated." Surgeons administered brandy "freely," but James could endure no more, and he died early in the morning of February 20th (NYHSCB 1852:C461).

James's case is an appalling example of the kinds of treatments injured Irish laborers endured at even the best 19th-century American hospitals. His case illustrates not only the dangers of hospital infection, in the days before antiseptic procedures and antibiotics, but also the tortures of surgical treatments without general anesthesia. What is especially shocking about this case is that general anesthesia was readily available, inexpensive, and administered to other patients at New York Hospital while James was there. James was not offered this pain relief, which might have improved his chances of survival, because of his physicians' decisions that such relief was not necessary for him. They appear to have determined that James's ethnicity, class, gender, and occupation all pointed to a natural insensitivity to pain, making anesthesia unnecessary or even potentially harmful. James's physicians' calculations and American prejudicial ideas about working-class Irish immigrants, and especially male manual laborers, were mutually reinforcing.

Alcohol, opium, mandragora, and cannabis had been used as analgesics in surgical operations since antiquity, but anesthesia inducing complete unconsciousness and imperceptibility of pain was not accomplished until the surgical applications of ether and chloroform. Both were first applied to surgery in the 1840s. In 1846, Boston dentist William T. G. Morton famously first demonstrated that diethyl ether could be used relatively safely to render a patient unconscious and insensible to pain during a surgical operation (Figure 4.6). The following year, James Y. Simpson showed in Edinburgh that chloroform could produce the same result even faster and, arguably, more effectively. Within a few months of each discovery, each substance was used at hospitals in the U.S., Scotland, England, and France, but at no institution was the introduction of these new anesthetics complete.

Historian of medicine Martin Pernick (1983, 1985) found that many surgeons did not immediately embrace chloroform or ether for a number of reasons. They observed that administering either substance was not risk free; patients were sometimes inadvertently poisoned by too large a dose or suffocated when they vomited while under its influence. Until one or both could be administered without *any* risk, some argued

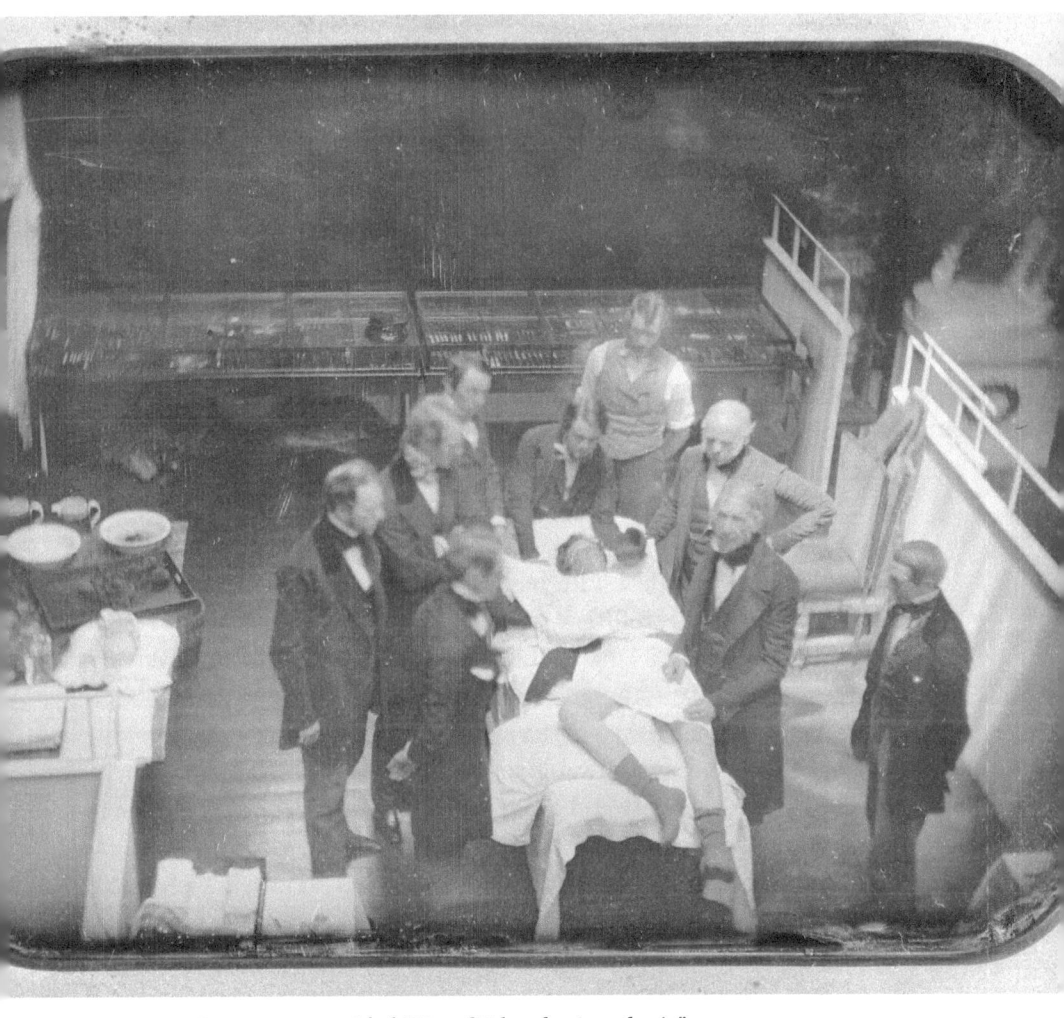

FIGURE 4.6. Daguerreotype titled "Use of Ether for Anesthesia" by Albert Sands Southworth and Josiah Johnson Hawes, 1847. Courtesy of the J. Paul Getty Museum, Los Angeles. Digital image courtesy of the Getty's Open Content Program.

that these anesthetics conflicted with their profession's foremost duty to preserve life. Many physicians also believed pain to be diagnostically valuable: those who suffered the most indicated that they possessed great vitality that bode well for their chances of recovery. Additionally, Pernick (1983:27) argues that anesthesia challenged surgeon's identities and reputations. They had been enculturated into a profession whose members distinguished themselves from "quacks" in part by their ability to remain levelheaded while their patients suffered. Medical students commented that the most difficult part of their training was learning how to perform lifesaving measures that required inflicting pain, an inescapable reality of surgery before the use of general anesthesia. The best surgeons were those who acted boldly and quickly: "When I was a boy, the best surgeon was he who broke the three-minute record for amputation," recalled the English physician Sir Clifford Albutt (Robinson 1946:79). Some physicians also rejected anesthesia on the basis of their own religious views that suffering was divine punishment for collective sin and/or spiritually refining.

A number of physicians in the U.S., particularly in New York City, readily embraced anesthesia, however. They argued that sparing surgical patients extreme pain was the proper course of action and part of the physician's duty because it would prevent more deaths from shock on the operating table than it would cause, because it would enable surgeons to attempt more delicate surgeries—potentially saving more lives and increasing the prestige of American surgeons—and because they felt pain was useless and dangerous to the pained (Pernick 1985). Valentine Mott (1862:5, 7–8), a celebrated New York surgeon who performed cases at New York Hospital, Bellevue, and St. Vincent's, and who trained many other physicians and surgeons, including John Griscom (1845), was an advocate of anesthesia and other pain relief.[25] Like Mott, most of those who supported anesthetics considered themselves to be "conservative" physicians, who advocated moderate instead of "heroic" treatments and who had trained in Europe. Many were concerned by the increasing numbers of severe injuries caused by mechanization, railroads, and massive urban building projects, and some were inspired by religious convictions about the value of caring for the sick and injured. Mott, who had trained in London and Edinburgh, and Griscom were both from Quaker backgrounds. Mott later converted to the Episcopal Church and became involved with the Roman Catholic St. Vincent's Hospital, where the Sisters of Charity emphasized humane care (Walsh 1965:12–17). There was also considerable pressure from patients, who demanded pain-free surgeries, and from alternative practitioners who lured away patients with the promises of pain-free healing (Pernick 1985:222, 234).

Even surgeons who supported the use of anesthesia did not always use it in practice, however. Pernick (1983, 1985) shows that physicians employed an early form of risk-benefit analysis specific to each patient, weighing the patient's chances of dying from the pain of a surgery without anesthesia with the chances of dying from anesthetic poisoning. The results of this "calculus of suffering," Pernick found, frequently deprived Irish immigrant male laborers and African Americans of the benefits of anesthesia. His examination of case records from the Pennsylvania Hospital (from 1853 to 1862) and Massachusetts General Hospital (in 1847) revealed that about 33% of painful surgeries at each hospital, including major limb amputations, were performed without anesthesia (Pernick 1985:4). In practice, surgeons at these hospitals administered anesthesia only for the most major surgeries, and more often for those whose identities intersected with some combination of the following categories: children, women, older adults, the wealthy, and the native born (Pernick 1985:191–194). At Massachusetts General, Pernick (1985:191) found that only 43% of laborers and sailors, occupations in which the Irish and African Americans were overrepresented, were given anesthesia, whereas 57% of all men otherwise employed received anesthesia.

Physicians' decisions, Pernick argues, were influenced not only by the ailment requiring attention but also by how they categorized each patient along a spectrum of civility. Dr. Silas Weir Mitchell (1910:13), the founder of American neurology, wrote in 1891, "In our process of being civilized, we have won . . . intensified capacity to suffer. The savage does not feel pain as we do; nor as we examine the descending scale of life, do animals seem to have the acuteness of pain-sense . . . often observed in regard to wounded horses on the battlefield." Nowhere was the difference in ability to bear pain thought to be more apparent than in the suffering of genteel White women giving birth, versus the virtually painless birthing experiences, according to the noted gynecologist Dr. Gunning S. Bedford (1863:4), of "savages" and "the poorer classes [of women] in our cities, fortified by constant exercise in the open air."

Surgeons thus often made the choice to withhold anesthesia from Irish and African American patients on the basis of presumed lesser civility and insensitivity to pain. Just as many Americans attributed the ability of Irish workers to continue to labor through injuries as an indicator of their natural incivility, rather than recognizing their determination in difficult circumstances, such surgeons credited natural insensitivity for the ability of members of this same group to (often but not always) bear excruciatingly painful surgeries.

Stereotypes about supposed Irish drinking practices and temperaments (Chapter 2) might have also played a role in surgeons' decisions to withhold anesthesia. Physicians observed that habitual drinkers were harder to anesthetize and required more anesthetic, which increased risks of side effects, including cardiac arrest. They were also more likely to awaken in the middle of a surgery and thrash about, injuring themselves or the surgeons.[26] The use of anesthetics on individuals who were actively drunk was prohibited at most hospitals (Pernick 1985:178–179). Case records from New York Hospital show that several laboring men who had suffered accidents were brought in under the influence of alcohol, oftentimes administered by their coworkers, or even policemen, in an attempt to revive or comfort them. A physician recorded, for example, that a patient named Richard, who had fallen off a cart and was in shock, was also "under the influence of alcohol that was given to him by a policeman after receiving the injury" (NYHSCB 1862:C206).[27] Physicians themselves sometimes administered liquor to patients to try to revive them, as in the case of James the wagon driver. Other times, physicians did not note drunkenness or suspicion of alcoholism, but might have made assumptions based on stereotypes of laborers, and of Irish laborers in particular, as heavy drinkers.

Conversely, how anesthetics acted upon patients was taken to indicate their drinking habits (Pernick 1985:178). If a large dose of ether was needed to render a patient unconscious, the patient was thought to be of intemperate habits, even if not inebriated at the time. This belief, I suggest, unfairly judged redheaded individuals, who are most numerous in Irish and Scottish populations, because of another effect of the genes that produce red hair. There has long been anecdotal evidence that redheads require more anesthesia to "knock out." Recent studies have come to the same conclusion with statistically significant results showing they require about 20% more ether than their non-ginger counterparts (Liem et.al. 2005). When 19th-century surgeons administered diethyl ether to redheaded Irish patients and observed they required more, this phenomenon reinforced Irish stereotypes. It also might have led to surgeons' assumptions about other Irish patients as habitual drinkers, regardless of their hair color, reinforcing inclinations to withhold anesthesia that they applied to laborers more broadly.

Some physicians and surgeons also expressed prejudiced personal views against the Irish that likely affected their calculations: a surgeon at Massachusetts General, for example, recorded in 1855 that an Irish patient was "importunate for delicacies; declaring that he was always accustomed to them. This last is hard to believe, he being an undoubted bogtrotter. May have as an addition to his bill of fare, a potatoe" (Pernick 1985:18). The label bogtrotter was roughly equivalent to savage, and as we learned from Dr. Townsend (1847) in Chapter 1, physicians of the day regarded the potato as the crudest of vegetables, suitable for the crudest of people. Another physician at New York Hospital remarked sarcastically that his patient, a 35-year-old Irish-born clerk, had "treated himself heroically with immoderate doses of alcoholic drinks" (NYHMCB 1853:C121). These kinds of outright prejudicial statements are rare, but physicians' actions of withholding anesthesia from Irish patients, as well as their differential treatment of Irish patients with typhus (Chapter 2), show physicians consciously and unconsciously incorporated prevailing social and cultural prejudices into their treatment decisions.

Irish Influences in Increasingly Compassionate Calculations at New York Hospital

Close examination of surgical casebooks from New York Hospital shows that in contrast to Massachusetts General and the Pennsylvania Hospital, surgeons in New York began to administer anesthesia routinely to Irish laborers in the 1850s. James's case, in fact, stands out as an unusual exception. This markedly different approach might be explained by several factors, including the greater influence of European practices and of conservative medicine in New York City, more competition from sectarian medical practitioners (especially German homeopaths), and the influence of particular individuals, such as Dr. Valentine Mott. It is also likely that Irish immigrants themselves played a role in how New York physicians understood patients' pain, both by their demands for care to meet their own expectations and by their adverse reactions to surgeries without anesthesia.[28]

On the one hand, the large numbers of Irish laborers who, like James, did not survive surgeries without anesthesia, showed surgeons that they miscalculated. Witnessing such deaths personally as well as reading reports from other influential hospitals might have convinced them that the benefits of anesthesia outweighed the costs for nearly everyone. Reports from the London Hospital, where Irish laborers composed a large portion of trauma victims, for example, showed that physicians there attributed about 20% of deaths after amputations between 1852 and 1858 to pain and shock (Chaloner et al. 2001). On the other hand, patients, both Irish and non-Irish, also demanded anesthesia. After ether became available, physicians noted that patients who had previously refused operations for years for tumors, for example, finally consented to having them removed with anesthesia (Pernick 1985:222).

Irish cultural ideals about appropriate care for the sick and injured additionally seemed to have more successfully infiltrated hospitals in New York City than in Philadelphia or Boston. Irish traditional obligations to provide care to anyone seeking it are deeply rooted in Irish history and myth. In the famous tale "The Cattle Raid of Cooley" from the *Book of Leinster* (12th century CE), for example, the two enemy heroes, Cuchulainn and Ferdiad, who struggled in hand-to-hand combat for several days, shared their provisions of healing herbs each night (Fleetwood 1983:4). The Brehon Laws, the statutes that governed life in medieval Ireland, obliged a man who had injured another, even if the other was a criminal, to provide care of a physician, shelter, food, and a substitute to carry on his labor (Ellis 1972:22; Fleetwood 1983:8). St. Patrick and St. Brigid, the patron saints of Ireland and moral exemplars, prioritized relieving the sick and the injured; they are credited with creating one of Ireland's first hospitals in 432 C.E. (Fleetwood 1983:12). By the 19th century, these ideals were still embedded in Irish popular medicine, in the practices of folk healers who rarely turned away anyone seeking help, did not require payment, and sometimes provided more of what might be categorized today as psychological counseling than medicine (Buckley 1980; Logan 1994).

Use of anesthesia and compassionate care, more generally, might have been supported not only by Irish patients who filled New York City's hospital wards but also by Irish-born caregivers in these institutions, whose numbers increased over time. There were several prominent Irish-born physicians in New York. Dr. William James MacNeven, for example, immigrated in 1805 after training in Germany because Penal Laws in Ireland prohibited Catholics from higher education. He had also been imprisoned in and liberated from Kilmainham Jail for his involvement in the United Irishmen (MacNeven 1842a).[29] MacNeven ran a respected medical practice with offices on Nassau and Mott Streets and was a member of nearly every society involved with helping other Irish immigrants, according to his daughter Mary Jane MacNeven (1842b). Additionally, he had two sons who became physicians and worked at New York Hospital and might have had influence over other physicians there.

There were also Irish-born nurses at New York Hospital, who might have successfully impressed views about compassionate care upon other staff and physicians. James Duffe, a nurse at New York Hospital's Marine Ward, noted in his diary his horror about how several doctors and nurses abused a female patient who had overdosed on laudanum in 1845. The treatment involved drenching her with cold water, "dragging her fore and aft the floor," pumping coffee into her stomach and out again, applying a "few sharp strokes of the rattan," placing her feet in boiling hot water "she was made to walk or rather kept upright on her poor flayed and bleeding feet," forcing brandy down her throat, slapping and shaking her (Duffe 1853). In contrast, Duffe treated his patients kindly. He remembered their names and their predicaments. He ran personal errands for them, such as making sure one discharged patient got a coat and another his clothes, and he sought out special equipment for patients that the hospital did not have, such as India rubber sheets (Duffe 1853:18, 20). These actions conform to Irish cultural obligations for treatment of the sick and Irish immigrants' expectations of care.

In response to such expectations and the healthcare needs of a growing Irish Catholic population in New York City, the Sisters of Charity founded St. Vincent's Hospital in 1849 on East 13th Street. This Catholic order of nuns was almost wholly Irish born, and the hospital was run by the Irish-born Sister Mary Angela Hughes, the biological sister of Archbishop John Hughes.[30] According to an 1849 advertisement in

178 Fractures

the newspaper the *Irish American,* St. Vincent's provided "tender and skillful nursing" and "kindest attention for which the Sisters of Charity are remarkable," even for the terminally ill, who were turned away by New York Hospital (Larrabee 1971:107). By the 1850s, St. Vincent's had gained a reputation among the Irish in New York as the best place to seek hospital care. Reporters from the *New York Freeman's Journal* in 1850 found the wards to be "remarkable for cleanliness and order . . . everything betokens the careful, kind and conscientious attention to the needs of the sick which so powerfully assists recovery from disease" (Walsh 1965:19).[31] In 1856, the hospital relocated to a larger building at 11th Street and 7th Avenue (Figure 4.7). Patients requested to be transferred to St. Vincent's from other city hospitals. Mary, the 19-year-old domestic servant admitted to Bellevue who attributed her phthisis to "sitting in cold draughts when overheated at work," requested she be brought to St. Vincent's, for example (BHMCB 1874:93).

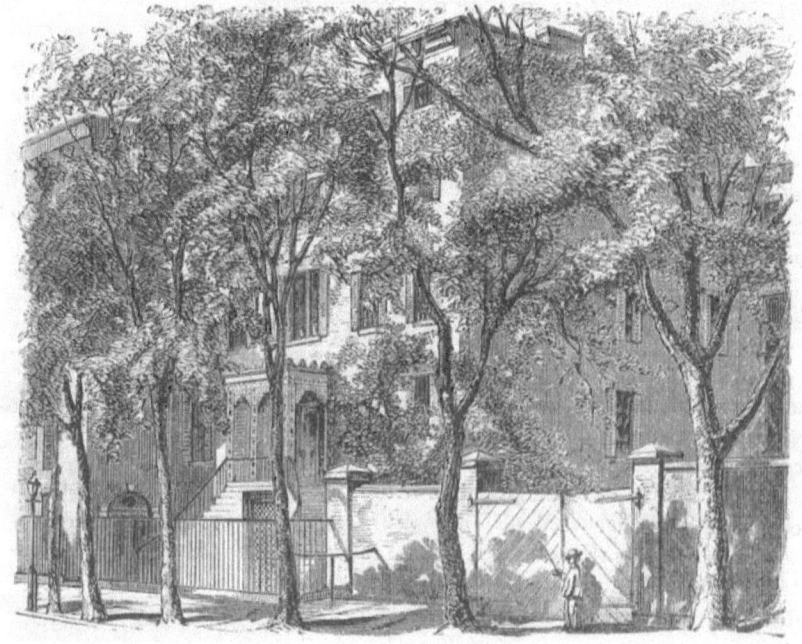

FIGURE 4.7. Illustration of "St. Vincent's Hospital, (under the charge of the 'Sisters of Charity,') corner of Eleventh Street and Seventh Avenue" (ca. 1856–1870). Courtesy of the New York Public Library Digital Collections.

Those involved with St. Vincent's, whether Irish Catholic or not, were influenced by the quality of the care the sisters provided. They were widely regarded as exemplary nurses; "even the most rabid bigots showed a grudging respect for the Sisters of Charity" (Oshinsky 2016:60). Valentine Mott was President of the St. Vincent's Medical Board and a consulting physician at the hospital, along with his son-in-law William Holmes Van Buren. Both performed complicated and pioneering surgeries at St. Vincent's. Both also held positions of prominence and influence in the city's other hospitals and leading medical schools.[32] Irish cultural ideas about compassionate care informed practices at St. Vincent's and likely intensified Dr. Mott's compatible views about pain, which he went on to disseminate. In fact, in the introduction to a series of essays prepared for the U.S. Sanitary Commission, Mott (1862:5–6) turned the tables on his fellow physicians, calling out those who withheld anesthesia from any patient as the real savages. He wrote, "*To prevent pain is humane.* No gentleman, not to say Christian, would needlessly inflict pain on any creature. . . . Only savages inflict upon their victims the horrors of torture."

Conclusion

Most Irish immigrants living in New York City from the 1840s through the 1860s worked in manual laboring or service positions that were extremely physically demanding and often dangerous. Others worked in skilled or semi-skilled positions that frequently exposed them to hazardous conditions or chemicals. These jobs had significant impacts on their health and reputations. From the 1840s through the 1860s, Irish immigrants suffered disproportionately from illness and injuries, both acute and chronic, and were overrepresented in city hospitals and dispensaries. Their overwhelming presence in these lines of work and in public institutions reinforced prejudiced ideas about the supposed Irish natural temperamental suitability for manual labor and proclivity toward pauperism. Such prejudice had ramifications not only on the streets in confrontations with native-born Americans but also inside hospitals in surgeon's calculations about whether to administer anesthesia in surgeries that could cause death from pain and shock.

Such assessments were probably not dependent—at least not wholly and not for every surgeon—upon blind anti-Irish sentiment. American surgeons, as well as other native-born Americans in New York, judged most Irish immigrants by what they could see upon quick glance. What they often saw were bodies that were, in fact, sculpted and marked by work and injuries: red faces, sometimes scarred, sometimes grimacing in pain, muscular bodies that often limped or stooped but were still usually capable of feats of great strength. Irish immigrants' courage, tenacity, and necessity to continue on through pain from injuries or a surgeon's scalpel (or saw) were not fully appreciated, and instead, many Americans read these achievements as additional evidence of natural Irish difference and incivility.

Over the course of the next few decades, ideas about essential Irish difference slowly began to dissolve. I suggest that debates about anesthesia and compassionate care played a role. Influential American-born surgeons, such as Mott, as well as Irish-born physicians and nurses, especially the Sisters of Charity at St Vincent's, and clearly suffering Irish immigrant patients themselves demanded pain relief and modeled humane care, highlighting the barbarity of American practices and attitudes. The next chapter will explore how Irish immigrants managed pain and injuries at home, drawing again upon material evidence from the Five Points excavation read through the lens of Irish popular medicine.

CHAPTER 5

Irish Remedies for Relief
Old and New Recipes

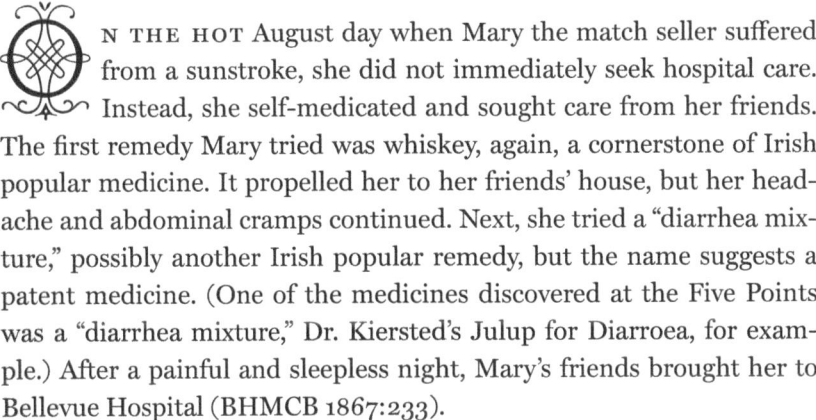

ON THE HOT August day when Mary the match seller suffered from a sunstroke, she did not immediately seek hospital care. Instead, she self-medicated and sought care from her friends. The first remedy Mary tried was whiskey, again, a cornerstone of Irish popular medicine. It propelled her to her friends' house, but her headache and abdominal cramps continued. Next, she tried a "diarrhea mixture," possibly another Irish popular remedy, but the name suggests a patent medicine. (One of the medicines discovered at the Five Points was a "diarrhea mixture," Dr. Kiersted's Julup for Diarroea, for example.) After a painful and sleepless night, Mary's friends brought her to Bellevue Hospital (BHMCB 1867:233).

How individuals perceive pain is complex and incompletely understood today, so it is difficult to fully appreciate how injured Irish immigrants in the 19th century, like Mary the match seller, experienced painful injuries or conditions and how they decided when to self-medicate versus when to seek care from others. Hospital records from New York and Bellevue Hospitals make clear that Irish immigrants often continued to labor while afflicted by painful conditions and that most did not immediately request treatment at hospitals, even those with injuries more serious than Mary's, such as severe burns and broken legs. What they did in between the time of injury and admission is only occasionally noted by physicians in case histories and how they fared after discharge even more rarely, but there are more clues in the archaeological record.

This chapter investigates Irish immigrants' strategies to manage and heal work-related injuries, drawing upon material remains of healing practices among the residents of 472 and 474 Pearl Street as well as hospital casebooks and other written records. My interpretation of both kinds of sources is informed by Irish folklore records and read through a lens of Irish popular approaches to healing. The first part of the chapter lays out the practices and ingredients popularly used in Ireland to treat pain and injuries. The second part shows that Irish immigrants used a variety of approaches to attend to their pains and injuries in New York, including self-medicating with popular Irish remedies and patent medicines and seeking out care from folk healers and professional physicians. They did not choose just any patent medicines or necessarily use them as advertised, however, but adopted types and brands that resonated with their own expectations of healing substances and ideas about how to use them. Aided by this variety of healing resources and their knowledge, as well as determination and necessity, many Irish immigrants labored on, despite injury. Many were also aware, however, that no matter how effective a remedy was in relieving pain or injury, it was only a temporary fix. To prevent further injury required altering their jobs or social positions. The last section discusses how archaeological remains suggest Irish immigrants also utilized bottled cosmetic products, along with other commodities, to take greater control over how others viewed them and thus to expand their opportunities.

Irish Popular Remedies for Relief: Ordinary and Extraordinary

The majority of Irish individuals who immigrated to New York City would have been well versed in popular remedies for minor injuries common to rural life, such as cuts, bruises, sprains, strains, etc., what we might today call basic first aid. Such remedies drew upon a wide variety of ordinary materials, easily accessible in rural areas. For problems deemed to be more serious, specialized healers with additional knowledge or skill and special places in the landscape were sought out. This section provides an overview of everyday remedies as well as more extraordinary ones, but even ordinary materials could have extraordinary effects when used in healing.

The kinds of remedies that most people in 19th-century Ireland first turned to in order to relieve pain and injury included whiskey or whiskey-based mixtures, ointments, liniments, poultices, cloths, and strings.

Whiskey, as noted in previous chapters, was considered a cure-all, and was also used to preserve and draw out the healing properties of other ingredients in medicinal herbal mixtures. Along with other liquors and ivy berries, whiskey was one of a few painkillers that the Irish took internally.[1] The majority of recorded cures for injury and pains were applied externally.

In Irish households, typically a mother or grandmother would prepare ointments, lotions, and liniments to be kept on hand for injury. Milk or buttermilk was the base for lotions to soothe burns. If a lotion was not on hand, milk or buttermilk alone or tea or linseed oil were recommended (NFCS 1938[45]:249; Logan 1994:104). The fat, or grease, of a goose or sheep; eel, olive, or cod liver oil; or beeswax served as the base of ointments, which were used to seal wounds and massage sore muscles and sprains.[2] An ointment for cracked hands from Wexford, for example, consisted of whiskey, milk, olive oil, and cod liver oil (O'Regan 1997:21). The oil from a conger eel, according to informants Jimmie McElroy and Con McAllister in Cushendall, County Antrim "had a wild bad smell, but it was great" for sprains (NFC 1953[1364]:52). Goose grease was the most frequently reported base for ointments in the folklore records surveyed. Mrs. Kenny of County Galway told a folklore collector, for example, that her family kept a jar of goose grease around the house for headaches, stiff joints, sprains, and swellings (NFCS 1938[45]:247).[3] Michael Kennedy, a farmer from County Kerry, said that to cure a swelling one should "get a lump of goose grease and rub it to the leg or hand" (NFC 1941[782]:357). The grease from a Christmas goose was often recommended (O'Regan 1997:21). Arensberg (1937:75) notes that during marriage negotiations the potential groom's family traditionally served a goose to the potential bride's family. It is likely that such connections with sacred holidays and family alliances was thought to enhance the healing power of goose grease.

Liniments, also called balms, are mixtures made to rub on the skin for relief of sore muscle or joint pain. They typically contain quickly evaporating chemical ingredients or counterirritants and were used in professional medicine and manufactured as patent medicines during the 19th and 20th centuries. Homemade Irish versions included paraffin oil and kerosene (after their discoveries in the late 1840s and early 1850s) and turpentine, and appear to have only been applied externally, although one remedy for toothache from County Carlow was to hold hot turpentine in the mouth for as long as possible (NFC 1935[265]:597). Whiskey was also applied externally to relieve headaches, earaches, toothaches, and congestion.[4]

Poultices were masses of softened and sometimes warmed substances applied to wounds, bruises, and sprains and left on like a bandage. They were prepared at the moment of need, when the ingredients would be freshest, and the substances used depended on the desired action. To simply encourage a wound to heal, a poultice of a common grass or bread was sufficient.[5] To promote coagulation, Irish informants told folklore collectors that they used cobwebs, smartweed, or plantain leaves (*Plantago major*, St. Patrick's leaf, or *slánlus* [health plant] in Irish).[6] To prevent blood poisoning (infection), they used plantain, tobacco, a mixture of salt and sugar, or a mixture of oatmeal and nettles.[7] Sometimes they washed the area with urine first.[8] To provide topical relief for sore injuries they applied many plants, including comfrey, chickweed, dock, ivy, ragweed, blackberry, and willow bark.[9] Comfrey roots were said to be especially good for bruises and broken bones. They were washed, grated, applied, and left to fall off.[10] The curative and numbing properties of topical applications of tobacco, lily root, and elder were also recognized.[11] An informant in County Wexford told a folklore collector in 1935 that he had suffered from a painful varicose ulcer that would not heal, for example, but "then he remembered a cure his mother had for every sore: 'an Elder leaf. Just hold it . . . to the fire in your hand until the juice begins to leave it. Then lay the side facing the ground on the sore, or the wound. I cured several people with it" (NFC 1935[54]:191).[12]

Home healers also exploited the therapeutic effects of warm and cold, applying warming poultices of mustard or warmed cabbage leaves, or heated potatoes or bran wrapped in a cloth to sore backs or other injured body parts.[13] For cold therapy, they recommended cold seaweed, immersion in cold springs or the sea, or lying on cold stones.[14] Like 19th-century physicians in the U.S. and Europe, Irish laypeople utilized methods to produce counterirritation (localized inflammation) to relieve conditions such as rheumatism, bursitis, headache, and backache. They applied nettles, mustard, and horseradish, as well as bream fish oil, and pitch.[15]

Several of the abovementioned ingredients contain chemicals shown to have verifiable effects. For example, certain species of willow contain salicin, a chemical with pain-relieving and anti-inflammatory properties similar to aspirin (acetylsalicylic acid), which inspired the latter's development (Desborough and Keeling 2017). Plantain's ability to stop bleeding in "a matter of minutes" is well known in many parts of the world; it and some species of ragweed have been shown to have antibacterial properties (Allen and Hatfield 2004:247; Woods-Panzaru et al. 2009:14). Comfrey is rich in allantoin, which promotes healing in connective tissues by encouraging proliferation of new cells (Allen and Hatfield 2004:208). Sugar and salt have long been used throughout the world to treat wounds. Anthropologist Bernard Ortiz de Montellano (1990), writing about Aztec applications, cites scientific studies that found the combination of the two to be more effective against most common bacteria and better at promoting wound healing than modern antibacterial ointments.

Trusted remedies also appealed to psychological processes that are important in pain relief (see Chapter 1). Their administration sometimes included techniques that further increased patient confidence, such as making the sign of the cross and/or saying the name of the Trinity over wounded areas. Some employed tangible objects that, from a present-day perspective, seem to work only by psychology alone. Nuts or pieces of potatoes carried in the pocket were said to cure or prevent rheumatism, for example. John Barbour (1897), an early contributor to the British journal *Folklore*, wrote, "Believe me . . . the Irishman trusts in a potato in his trouser-pocket as a guard against rheumatism." Another example is the practice of tying a string around a sprain, with the promise that when the string fell off the limb would be cured (NFCS 1938[345]:7). This appears to be a clever way of biding time for the body to heal itself. Other examples include wrapping or touching afflicted areas with a cloth; those associated with Catholic feast days were especially recommended, including a *Brath Bridhe* ("St. Brigid's Cloth," a piece of white cloth put on a bush on the eve of St. Brigid's Feast Day) or a cloth dipped in the blood of an animal killed on the eve of St. Martin's Feast Day. Alternatively, a cloth that touched a deceased person or red-colored flannel were used.[16]

Some of the ingredients and techniques used in Irish cures, especially for serious or intractable injuries, involved special, and sometimes visually spectacular, places in the Irish landscape, such as natural rock formations, holy wells, and soil from priests' graves.[17] A coffin-shaped stone in Bannow Bay in the southeast of Ireland, for example, was said by informants in Wexford to cure a "person suffering from backache or headache;" if he "lies in that coffin . . . he is to be cured" (NFC 1935[54]:78). Figure 5.1 shows "St. Bridget's Chair" along the rugged coast of County Donegal, which was said to protect anyone who sat there from accident or sudden death (Hardy 1840:4). There were also numerous reports of people cured of various injuries, including lumbago and palsy, by making pilgrimages to holy wells (see Chapter 7) and drinking and/or washing with the water; sometimes multiple visits were required (NFCS 1937[598]:434).

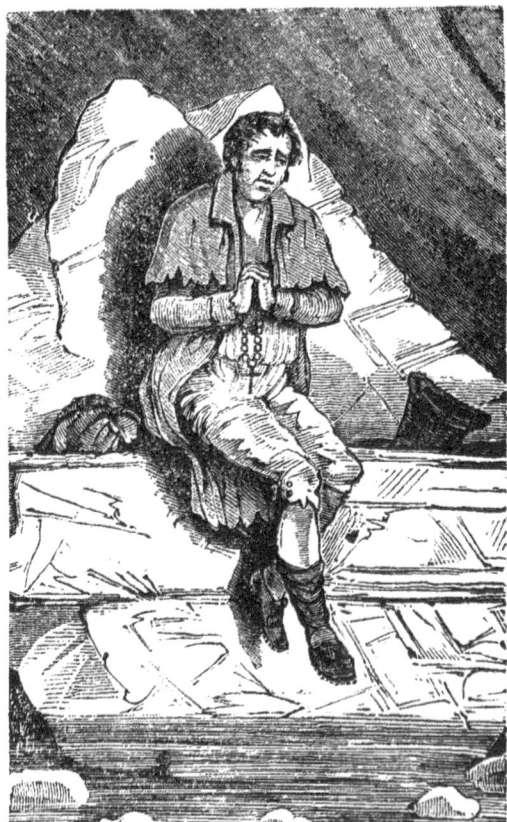

St. Bridget's Chair stands close to the water's edge, and in which, it is said, whoever once sits, is ever after preserved from accident or sudden death. *See page 4.*

FIGURE 5.1. Illustration of St. Bridget's Chair, a natural rock formation near the sea in County Donegal believed to have special powers (Hardy 1840).

Certain special individuals were also sought for more serious problems. A person who had licked a frog nine times on nine consecutive days was said to have the power to cure burns with his tongue or saliva.[18] Particular families were said to possess charms for stopping bleeding, such as the Curtis family of Corofin, County Clare (Westropp 2000:43). Blood from someone with the surname Keogh was said to cure St. Anthony's fire (erysipelas) in Wicklow, Kildare, Carlow, and Dublin (O'Connor 1943:278–279; Logan 1994:70). In Clare and Longford, the blood of a Walsh was recommended (NFC 1930[80]:12; NFCS 1937[598]:98). It was said that a child born feet first could cure back pain (lumbago) by walking on the back of the afflicted (Blake 1918:223). Certain people, usually women, possessed a cure for "heartache" or "heart trouble" or "heart fever," which seems to have described physical chest pain and/or emotional "heartache." The healer placed a cup filled with oatmeal on the patient's chest and a few minutes later checked to see how much meal had gone. If most of the meal was gone, the healer said the heart was badly damaged and "took the medicine." The patient was required to rest and have this procedure performed every day for nine or ten days to complete the cure.[19] Time and this frequent personal attention likely had benefits, even if the meal did not.

Bonesetters were also sought out for skeletal injuries more serious than could be handled in the household. Usually passed down in families, bonesetting was an art that was highly valued, and good bonesetters were well respected.[20] According to Patrick Logan (1994:90–93), they knew better techniques and were more skillful in their execution than 19th- and early 20th-century orthopedists. Bonesetters understood the main principles used by physicians today: extension and counterextension (pulling the broken bone fragments apart), coaptation (putting the bone back into place), and fixation (making sure the bone stays properly realigned). They were able to deal with complicated fractures and dislocations using these methods.[21] Once they had properly aligned the broken bone, bonesetters applied splints and casts made from materials such as sally rods (willow branches) bound with calico. Strong but flexible sally rods enabled the splint to be closer fitting, more comfortable, and more supportive than a plank splint. For breaks accompanied by considerable swelling, bonesetters made a temporary cast and replaced it with a harder cast after about ten days when swelling reduced. Harder casts were made of bandages soaked in fine soot or flour and egg white or five parts burgundy pitch to one part hard resin. Sometimes the resin was applied directly to the skin while warm and strengthened with cotton bandages (Logan 1994:94; NFCS 1938[920]:78; NFCS 1939[917]:58).

Like surgeons before general anesthetics, bonesetters were renowned for being able to set bones quickly so as to minimize pain to their patients. A story from County Louth illustrates one bonesetter's clever technique. A man with a broken arm set by a doctor that did not heal properly sought out Brian Reilly, a well-known bonesetter. Initially, Mr. Reilly told the man that he could not help him. Then, as the man was leaving, Mr. Reilly shook the man's hand through his gate and refractured his arm. Mr. Reilly then reset the man's arm, and it healed correctly (NFC 1974[1838]:161). To realign dislocated shoulders bonesetters reportedly employed a similar technique, although without the element of surprise; they had patients rest an arm padded on the underside over a half door and pulled down on it (Logan 1994:92).

While primarily focused on broken bones, some bonesetters used their skills in skeletal manipulation to heal back pain and other related complaints. It was reported to Lady Gregory (1920:157), for example, that a female healer cured a woman in Limerick of a pain in her side by hanging her on a branch of an apple tree. The healer swung the woman and then had her lie in the grass and said a prayer over her. After nine visits she was cured. Although most reported bonesetters were male, female bonesetters were not unknown (NFC 1955[1389]:203). Bonesetters achieved esteem locally and nationally in Ireland. Several made their way into Irish politics. The County of Clare is particularly famous for its bonesetters, two of whom, Joseph Sexton and Patrick Burke, had seats in the Dáil (the Irish Parliament) (Logan 1994:96). Good bonesetters likely developed such positive reputations because the effects of their therapies could be relatively dramatic. Setting a broken bone properly can instantly diminish pain and encourage a full recovery without deformity, so that patients could resume normal activities more quickly and avoid lasting traces of injury.

Evidence of Irish Popular Remedies for Relief in New York City

Evidence of specialized Irish healers active in 19th-century New York City is scant. Their practices would not leave much of a material trace, and social censure by both Americans (for "superstitious" practices) and the Irish (for shameless self-promotion) would have discouraged them from advertising their services in newspapers or directories. Instead, they would have been known through word of mouth. One record from New York Hospital might contain evidence of a bonesetter. When Patrick, a 40-year-old laborer who fell from a ten-foot-tall ladder and struck his right foot on a block, upon "attempt[ing] to rise he found that he was badly hurt and called a fellow Irish workman who pulled upon the foot until the bones 'snapped into place.'" Patrick or his friend appears to have had some knowledge of bonesetting skills (NYHSCB 1848:C1287). The presence in New York City of individuals with surnames associated with bonesetting in Ireland suggests the possibility that some bonesetters had immigrated to New York City. Examples include Tully and Lane in census records of the city's Sixth Ward and Tully, Lane, Acton, and Donaghy in Emigrant Savings Bank records (Yamin 2000[3]; Anbinder et al. 2019b).[22]

More discernible than evidence of specialized healers are some of the strategies that nonspecialist Irish men and women employed. These are occasionally noted in records from hospitals and private physicians, and even more tantalizing are the material traces of healing left behind at sites occupied by Irish immigrants. The archaeological deposits associated with the Irish tenements in the Five Points, 472 and 474 Pearl Street, contained a number of artifacts and floral and faunal remains that were used in Ireland to cure musculoskeletal pain and minor wounds.[23] As noted in Chapter 3, the presence of such ingredients does not guarantee that Irish residents used them for healing, as they have other nonmedicinal uses, nor does the absence of a substance used in Irish popular medicine indicate conclusively that residents did not use it, since archaeological deposits are always incomplete records of past materials and activities. Presence of ingredients does confirm, however, that immigrants could and did access those potentially healing substances. Census records indicate that the Irish inhabitants of 472 and 474 Pearl Street were employed in service and skilled, semi-skilled, and unskilled occupations requiring manual labor and thus would have had a regular need for relief from pain and injury. See note for a list of their occupations.[24]

Floral and Faunal Evidence

Floral and faunal remains uncovered at archaeological sites are usually interpreted as indicators of diet or surrounding environment. Given the prevalence of medicinal remedies made from plants and animals in Ireland and the fact that in most cultures the boundary between food and medicine is highly permeable, it is important to consider the possibility that floral and faunal remains could also be traces of healing. Within archaeological features associated with the Irish-inhabited tenements at the Five Points—Feature J (a stone-lined cesspool at 472 Pearl Street with two layers, one with a TPQ of 1850 and the other of 1870) and Feature O (a stone-lined privy at 474 Peart Street with one layer, with a TPQ of 1860)—archaeologists discovered evidence of a number of plants and animal parts used in Ireland to treat injuries and pains, specifically. They are presented in the following list along with which ailments they were used to heal in Ireland in parentheses. "Applied" indicates they were placed directly on the affected part, often as a poultice.

FLORAL AND FAUNAL MATERIALS USED IN POPULAR IRISH MEDICINE TO REMEDY PAIN AND INJURIES IN DEPOSITS ASSOCIATED WITH 472 AND 474 PEARL STREET

Floral—from Features J (TPQs of 1850 and 1870) and O (TPQ 1860)

- **Blackberry/raspberry** (leaves applied to burns, cuts, sores, swelling, swollen feet, ulcers; berries eaten or teas made from various parts of plant drunk for cough, diarrhea, indigestion, kidney problems)[25]
- **crabgrass and foxtail grass** (a variety of grasses applied to blisters, corns, and cuts)[26]
- **dock/sorrel** (leaves applied to burns, bruises, cuts, stings, swellings, rheumatism; also decoction of leaves or roots drunk for blood purification, liver complaints, and worms)[27]

Irish Remedies for Relief   191

- **elder** (bark, roots, or pith applied to burns, boils, cuts, erysipelas, eye trouble, inflammations, ringworm, sores, warts; infusions of various parts drunk for colds, coughs, dropsy, epilepsy, gout, jaundice, kidney trouble, indigestion, a cure-all)[28]
- **fig** (fruit applied to aching or wounded gums or eaten for stomach ulcers)[29]
- **goosefoot** (decoction of stems drunk for rheumatism)[30]
- **mint** (leaves eaten or infusions drunk for anemia, cold, cough, headache, indigestion, jaundice, measles, whooping cough)[31]
- **ragweed** (applied to abscesses, burns, cuts, rheumatism, sciatica, sprains, swollen joints, warts; decoction drunk for colds, coughs, hives, jaundice, sore throat)[32]
- **wheat** (bread applied to boils, cuts, infected wounds)[33]

Faunal—from Features J (TPQs of 1850 and 1870) and O (TPQ 1860)

- **chicken bones** (the blood of a black chicken sacrificed on St. Martin's Eve put on a cloth and applied for pain relief or to stop bleeding)[34]
- **fish bones** (fish and eel oil applied for sprains, cracked hands, rheumatism, earache, and deafness)[35]
- **goose bones** (goose grease applied for burns, headache, pains, rheumatism, sprain, swelling, colds)[36]
- **rabbit bones** (skin of a hare worn on one's back for pain relief; fur used as a styptic; hare soup for colds and to increase fertility)[37]
- **pig bones** (bacon and pork fat applied for corns, cuts, and sprains)[38]
- **sheep/goat bones** (milk and fat applied for burns, cracked hands; sheep liver applied to black eye; goat milk drunk for asthma, consumption, jaundice, kidney trouble; sheep milk drunk for diarrhea)[39]

Note: Floral and faunal materials discovered at 472 and 474 Pearl Streets were compiled from Milne and Crabtree (2000) and Raymer et al. (2000). Each type of floral or faunal remains were found in all three deposits, unless noted. Popular Irish medical uses for each are indicated in parentheses. Selected citations are in endnotes.

Many of the healing plants discovered could have been gathered from vacant lots and in between bricks and pavement (e.g., crabgrass, dock, ragweed), others could have been purchased at one of the nearby markets (e.g., blackberry, fig, wheat), and others could have been grown by residents themselves (e.g., mint) (Lobel 2014; Baics 2016). Archaeologists found remains of almost two dozen clay flower pots in deposits associated with 472 Pearl and five in deposits associated with 474 Pearl, suggesting that some residents cultivated plants (Yamin 2000[1]:Appendix A). Similarly, the fish and animal types discovered could have been easily acquired in New York City, by fishing, from markets, or through local animal husbandry: chickens, geese, pigs, sheep, and goat were all raised in and near New York City, often by Irish immigrants, to the dismay of many health reformers (McNeur 2014).

A comparison of the floral remains found in association with tenements inhabited by Irish immigrants with those found in association with tenements inhabited by German immigrants at the Five Points highlights some plants as exclusive to the Irish contexts, including mint, dock, and ragweed (Raymer et al. 2000).[40] According to Allen and Hatfield (2004:270, 306–307), dock was used medicinally more extensively in Ireland than elsewhere in Europe, while medicinal use of ragweed (also called ragwort and *buachalán*) is almost exclusive to Ireland.[41] Dock is a plant that even young Irish children knew about; they used it to soothe nettle stings, cuts, and burns (Logan 1994:67–68). The presence of these particular plants *only* in Irish contexts supports interpreting them as traces of Irish medical practices, rather than as traces of weeds that simply grew in the Five Points neighborhood.

Medical case histories of work-related injuries also support the idea that Irish immigrants used some of the plant and animal remains unearthed at the Five Points medicinally. A number of laborers admitted to New York Hospital arrived with poultices already applied to the site of their injuries, including a few mentioned in the previous chapter: the gardener whose foot became gangrenous from wearing a boot that was too tight (NYHSCB 1852:C369), a laborer admitted for synovitis of the ankle (NYHSCB 1853:C114), and a laborer whose eye was damaged at a tannery (NYHSCB 1848:C1604). Unfortunately, physicians rarely recorded what ingredients the poultices contained. One specified that 27-year-old Bessie "ha[d] been applying 'fat pork and chicken grass'" to her knee, which had been swollen for three weeks after a fall (NYHSCB 1848:C1718). It is likely that "chicken grass" was chickenweed (or chickweed) (*Stellaria media*), a weed that is found throughout Ireland and used in poultices to cure cuts,

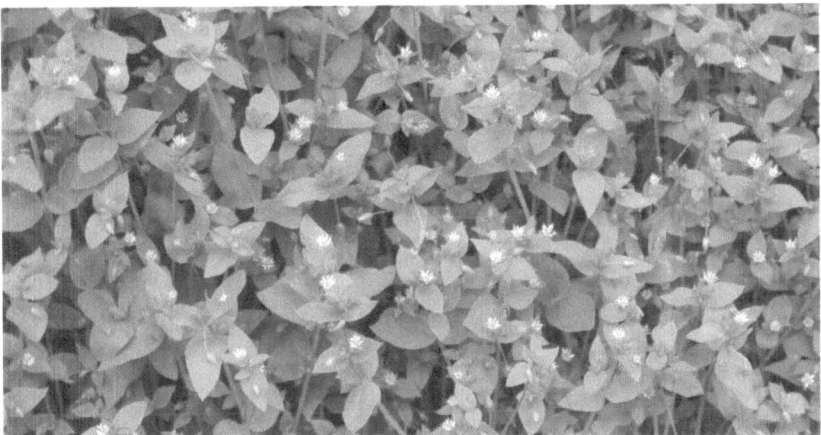

FIGURE 5.2. Photograph of the common chickweed (*Stellaria media*), a plant used by the Irish to poultice wounds in Ireland and America. Courtesy of the Virginia Tech Weed Identification Guide (2022).

burns, sores, rashes, earaches, headaches, and "pain in the side," and to reduce swelling (Figure 5.2).[42]

An example of a plant that figured prominently in Irish popular medicine, but was not found by archaeologists at the Five Points for reasons of preservation, is the potato. It was used to remedy many ailments, including burns, heartburn, rheumatism, sores, sore throat, sprain, swelling, warts, and whitlows.[43] Historical sources confirm that Irish immigrants continued to use potatoes as a health-promoting food in the U.S.; recall Dr. Townsend's dismay in the case of little Huxley McGuire from Chapter 1 (Townsend 1847; Diner 2001). An article in the *Atlanta Constitution* in 1872 advocated the healing properties of water in which potatoes had been boiled, which was used in Ireland to treat chilblains and warts. The newspaper suggested it would also cure rheumatism. The same article cited another remedy using potatoes: "*Charlotte Bulletin* says, 'This we can vouch for ourselves; that a raw Irish potatoe, carried in the pocket, will cure rheumatism. We can point to over twenty individual cases, some in this city, laugh as anyone may.'" Irish popular remedies made their way into the popular medicinal kit of wherever the Irish settled in the U.S. from the Northeast to the South to Appalachia to the West Coast (Hilliard 1966; Hand 1981).

In addition to relying on familiar plants used in Ireland, archaeological remains at the Five Points suggest that Irish immigrants incorporated unfamiliar plants native to the U.S. in cures, such as jimsonweed, and pokeweed.[44] Material resemblance to familiar plants and intelligence gained from non-Irish neighbors probably enticed the Irish to try these new plants. Even in heavily Irish neighborhoods, such as the Five Points, Irish immigrants were in frequent contact with non-Irish neighbors, and they almost certainly learned of the popular remedies used by people from other ethnic groups. Jimsonweed and pokeweed were both valued by Americans for healing in the 19th century. Social historian Herbert C. Covey (2007:100–101) reported that African Americans smoked jimsonweed, also known as thorn apple (*Datura stramonium*), for coughs, ate it for worms, and knew it to be a powerful narcotic and hallucinogenic. It is still smoked for coughs in southern Appalachia today, and people there made a poultice of the blossoms to treat wounds and relieve pain in the 20th century (Krochmal et al. 1969:108; Covey 2007:100–101).[45] Pokeweed (*Phytolacca americana*), also called American nightshade, was used by practitioners of American folk medicine as a sedative for gout, pneumonia, rheumatism, and typhoid fever and by Native Americans as a poultice for skin diseases, sores, ulcers, and tumors (Covey 2007:106). According to historian of medicine John K. Crellin and botanist Jane Philpott (1989), pokeweed was also well regarded by professional physicians in the 19th century; for a time it was thought to be a cure-all.[46] Popular medicine is flexible and typically easily incorporates new ingredients and techniques, when compatible with the logic of the medical system. In Ireland, people used a wide variety of substances, including poisonous weeds, to treat illness and injury. There is no reason to assume that they would not have easily adopted pokeweed and jimsonweed on their own terms, as well as other new substances they deemed to be useful.

Evidence in Artifacts: Whiskey, Tea, Tobacco, and Oil

In Ireland, substances that crossed the boundaries between popular healing, social drugs, and official medicine, including whiskey, tea, and tobacco, were used for healing pain and injuries. At the Five Points, utilization of these substances by Irish immigrants is evidenced not by the presence of these substances themselves, but by the vessels used to contain or consume them. As discussed in Chapter 3, many wine and some whiskey bottles were found in Irish immigrant contexts at the Five Points, and it is possible some residents used their original contents or homemade whiskey (*poitín*) or other popular cures subsequently stored in them to treat typhus fever. It is also possible that some residents sought out strong liquor contained within them to relieve pain and injury, given these other applications of whiskey and *poitín* in Ireland. Historical records support this continued use in the U.S. Miller (1985:320) notes, for example, that "Irish emigrants arrested for mid-century drunkenness in Pittsburgh attributed their habit to the uncongenial weather, to a lack of proper food and clothing, or to a need to assuage both the physical pain caused by work accidents and the psychological anxieties stemming from unfamiliar situations." At Bellevue Hospital, 27-year-old Elizabeth confessed to physicians that she had been "drinking freely" to ease her suffering from the pain of tuberculosis (BHMCB 1867:67). A case record from New York Hospital suggests Irish immigrants continued to use whiskey as a topical remedy as well.[47] Laborers tried to revive their fellow Irish co-worker who had been poisoned by handling bags of green coffee by rubbing whiskey on his chest (NYHMCB 1865:C469).[48]

Tobacco is another social drug that Irish immigrants continued to use in New York City. Many smoking pipes in the archaeological deposits evidence tobacco use among residents of 472 and 474 Pearl Street (see Figure 3.4), which is not surprising given that tobacco smoking was so prevalent among workers on both sides of the Atlantic (Reckner and Brighton 1999; Reckner and Dallal 2000; Brighton 2005). In New York City, the stimulant and appetite suppressing properties of tobacco helped Irish immigrants to keep up with the "railroad pace" of American labor. Applied topically, tobacco's analgesic, antibacterial, and antifungal properties helped to remedy the pain and injuries caused by such demanding work (Pavia et al. 2000:674–675). Tobacco smoking also helped to soothe grief; it was important in Irish mourning rituals (see Chapter 6).

The presence of many teacups and teapots in Irish contexts suggests continued tea consumption in New York City (Brighton 2000). Like liquor and tobacco, tea had important social uses in Ireland in providing hospitality to guests, and its simulant properties also helped to propel labor. Tea was consumed on a daily basis, if it could be afforded, and popularly used to soothe burns, headache, sore eyes, and styes.[49] It is probable that these uses endured in New York City, and recent research has shown that both green and black tea (*Camellia sinensis*) have antimicrobial properties (Hamilton-Miller 1995). Tea, like tobacco and whiskey, was also used by professional physicians in Ireland and New York City for convalescing patients. Dr. Townsend (1847), for example, prescribed tea for Huxley McGuire.

Also found in deposits associated with 472 Pearl were two olive oil bottles that suggest possible enduring use of this oil for burns, cuts, and sprains among Irish immigrants (Yamin 2000[1]: Appendix A-42). Two patients admitted to the New York Hospital suffering from burns applied another kind of oil also used in Ireland to their injuries: carron oil (NYHSCB 1852:C461, C585). Made from a mixture of olive oil or linseed oil and limewater, it was supposedly named for the Carron Ironworks in Scotland where the combination was much used by workers (OED 1989a).[50] Physicians at New York Hospital also prescribed it for patients (NYHSCB 1848:C1143, C1330, C1336, C1759). This mixture was also called lime-liniment; patent medicine liniments uncovered in the Irish deposits at the Five Points are discussed in the next section.

In summary, Irish immigrants brought with them to New York City knowledge of many remedies for healing the kinds of ordinary pain and injuries they would have encountered in Ireland, such as burns, bruises, cuts, sprains, muscle aches, and back pain. The majority of ingredients in these cures would have been available in New York, and some were found in the archaeological deposits associated with Irish residences in the Five Points. Continued use of some remedies by Irish immigrants was also occasionally noted in physicians' records. Some cures incorporated ingredients with effective analgesic, antimicrobial, or other healing properties verifiable by present-day scientific studies. Others brought relief primarily through the meaning response. These tried-and-true remedies helped many Irish immigrants to continue to labor on in physically demanding jobs, despite aches, pains, and injuries.

Nevertheless, many Irish immigrants were severely injured by new and different working conditions in the U.S, including the intensity of American labor, exposure to dangerous chemicals, accidents involving machines and railroads, more frequent workplace altercations, and more (Chapter 4). These assaults to the body and spirit were well beyond what most had experienced in Ireland in the rural places to which Irish popular medicine had been adapted. In severe cases some sought care at dispensaries, physicians' offices, or hospitals. Others likely consulted specialized Irish healers such as bonesetters. Others appear to have tried new local healing plants they learned about from non-Irish neighbors. And still others looked to the extremely popular and widely available over-the-counter remedies of the day: patent medicines.

New Additions to the Irish Popular Medical Kit: Patent Medicines for Pain and Injury

Patent medicine is a term that was first used to describe proprietary medicines made under "patents of royal favor" in 17th-century England and that was later used to describe proprietary, over-the-counter medicines, whether or not they were patented. In the 19th century, these unregulated liquids, powders, pills, and ointments became immensely popular in the U.S.[51] A variety of different types of people created and sold these concoctions, including professional physicians, trained pharmacists, sectarian doctors, folk healers, quacks, and con men. Some had a genuine interest in helping others, and some had a genuine interest in making money. While 19th-century patent medicines have since earned a negative reputation as useless nostrums or "snake oil," they varied in quality and effectiveness. Many were reasonable choices given the state of professional medicine and other available options (Linn 2022). Based on this premise, in this section I propose a new method of interpreting these curious commodities and apply it to the patent medicines uncovered at 472 and 474 Pearl Street, revealing new ideas about Irish immigrants' strategies to manage injuries.

The Appeal of Patent Medicines

The categories of prescription medicine and patent medicine are often presented as distinct, but in the 19th century, they frequently overlapped, in shared ingredients and even in shared products. Like prescription medicines, most patent medicines contained active ingredients that could ease pain, alter perception, or produce other reactions then thought to improve health. Hooper's Pills, containing aloes, produced catharsis, for example. A major component of Turlington's Balsam, tincture of benzoin, acted as an expectorant and has been shown to have topical antimicrobial action (Jones and Vegotsky 2016:40; Marsalic et al. 2007). Both of these brands, as well as many others, made their way into official pharmacopeias. Physicians prescribed them by name at New York Hospital (NYHSCB 1852; Remington and Wood 1918). Turlington's Balsam was still listed as a synonym for tincture of benzoin in *The Dispensatory of the United States of America* as late as 1955 (Griffenhagen and Young 1959). Other patent medicine brands that did not cross over to professional medicine nonetheless contained ingredients used by professional physicians. Hostetter's Bitters, for example, contained Peruvian bark (also called Jesuit's bark or *cinchona*), which contains quinine that has efficacy against malaria, and the purgative senna was a major component of Pitcher's Castoria (Oleson 1896:519–520; Young 1961:129).[52] Godfrey's Cordial and Mrs. Winslow's Soothing Syrup, both popular "child pacifiers," contained opium, still regarded as an optimal painkiller, although now known to be highly addictive and potentially fatal if misused.[53]

Patent medicine sales expanded exponentially in the U.S. from the middle to the end of the 19th century, and they were popular among the wealthy and the poor, the native born and immigrants, and men and women (Adams 1912:3). They appealed to consumers for a number of reasons. They offered much-desired alternatives to the painful and often ineffective treatments of professional physicians. At prices ranging from 50 cents to a few dollars, they were significant expenses for working people, but roughly a third the cost of a physician's visit. They allowed individuals to self-medicate at home and keep their ailments private, if so desired. Those that contained addictive substances, such as alcohol or opium, kept customers coming back for more. Others that contained effective ingredients and delivered at least some of the actions that they promised earned good reputations for doing so. Recommendations from physicians, pharmacists, and newspapers also added to the appeal of patent medicines. Patent medicine sales were important to drugstores, because during this period physicians often directly supplied their patients with medicines. Pharmacists were critical to communities as more accessible sources of medical advice and materials than physicians, and they often held considerable influence. Many were immigrants who were well-trained in pharmacy and who served their own ethnic communities, translating between cultures and medical sectors (Dykstra 1955; Howson 1993:147–148).

The popularity of patent medicines can also be attributed to producers' sophisticated advertising strategies that by mid-century had already pioneered many of the mainstays used today, including testimonials, claims of secret or exotic ingredients, assurances of safety and efficacy, catchy slogans, and distinctive bottle shapes and/or colors and labels to help customers remember their brands.[54] Newspapers were eager to publish advertisements for patent medicines because they relied on advertising to stay in business (Laird 1998:74).[55] Patent medicine producers also gave away free samples, cards, posters, calendars, and trinkets such as rulers, shoehorns, playing cards, and paper dolls with company names on them (Figure 5.3).[56] They hired street-criers, organized shows, and even sponsored baseball teams, such as the Rochester Hop Bitters. This advertising predisposed consumers to experience benefits through placebo effect/meaning response, if not via chemically effective ingredients (Lupu 2022). Many injuries and illnesses improve with time as

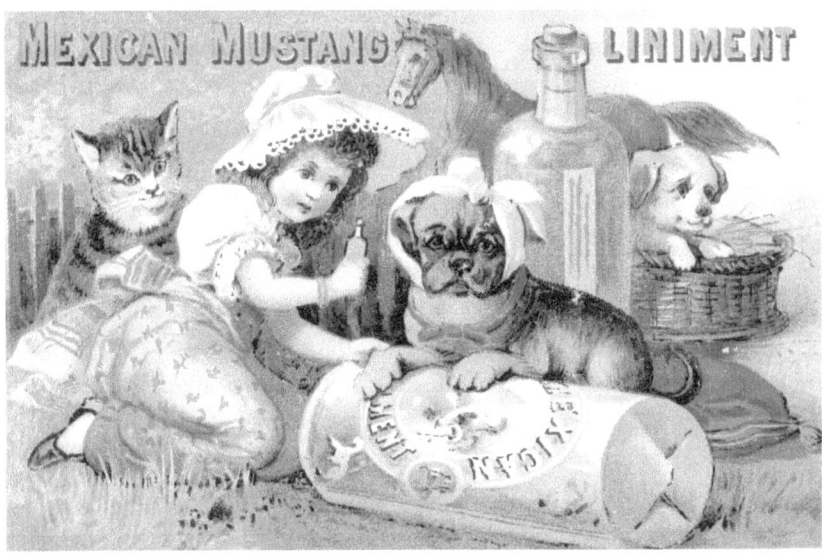

FIGURE 5.3. A trade card from the second half of the 19th century for Mexican Mustang Liniment advertising its safety for people and animals. Courtesy of the National Library of Medicine.

the body heals itself, but consumers frequently credited these medical mixtures for their recoveries.

Archaeologists found numerous patent medicine bottles in Irish immigrant contexts at the Five Points showing that some patent medicines appealed to Irish immigrants as much as and maybe more than their American-born counterparts. Dispersed from their homeland and extraordinary sources of healing in the Irish landscape, some Irish immigrants looked to patent medicines for relief. A close examination shows that did not choose just any patent medicines, however, but ones that appealed to them to fit their needs and that resonated with their own perspectives about healing.

Interpreting Patent Medicines

Patent medicine bottles are artifacts that have long been challenging for archaeologists to interpret. Even putting aside the critical point that any bottle could have been reused to hold any number of liquids and even assuming that a bottle embossed with a patent medicine's name was purchased by a consumer for the medicine it contained, it is extremely difficult to determine what ailment the consumer hoped to alleviate with it. Advertisements and labels claimed broad curative powers, exact contents of the medicines are often unknown, and we cannot travel back in time to interview consumers about their motivations.

In previous studies, archaeologists have responded to these problems in various ways, which I will simplify into three different modes of investigation. First, some archaeologists have focused upon trends of relative consumption of patent versus prescription medicines to ascertain residents' relationships with official medicine (Brighton 2008, 2009). Second, many have examined the advertised claims of all the patent medicines found at a site to discover trends that suggest residents' main concerns (Larsen 1994; Bonasera and Raymer 2001). Sometimes they are lucky enough to have historical records that confirm residents' illnesses or causes of death (Gallagher 2006). Third, some have investigated histories and dominant social meanings of specific brands of patent medicines and their marketing to understand the issues consumers hoped to remedy (Jones 1981; Larsen 1994; Jones and Vegotsky 2016; Lupu 2022). These are all important steps, but another one is crucial.

What also must be considered are the needs and perspectives of consumers—especially if they are from different cultural or social groups than patent medicine producers—and how they likely understood different types and brands of patent medicines, considering not only advertisements but also the material qualities of the medicines and their containers.

Medical anthropologists and public health officials have long noted that medicines and other health-related items are frequently interpreted by consumers differently than their producers intend and that advertisements alone are unreliable indicators for how products are used in practice (Van der Geest et al. 1996). This dissonance is not unique to cross-cultural situations, but it is more frequent. In Nigeria, for example, Etkin et al. (1990) observed that the Hausa administered different medicines for what they considered to be different stages of a disease. In a Guatemalan village, Logan (1973) found that locals used pharmaceuticals based on their own categorization of the drug as "hot" or "cold" and which they thought was appropriate for a particular illness. In East Africa, Luise White (2000:99) found that the local symbolic meanings of the color red led individuals there to believe red and pink pills were more effective than pills of other colors. De Craen and colleagues (1996) found consumers in the U.S. and Europe also made assumptions about medicines on the basis of their color; they were confident that red, yellow, or orange pills would have a stimulant effect, and linked red specifically to cardiovascular functions, while they anticipated blue or green pills to have sedative effects. In each of these cases, the material qualities of the medicines affected how people perceived them.

Historian Timothy Burke's (1996:163–172) study of the consumption of hygiene-related commodities in Zimbabwe shows that new products with material similarity to known home remedies are often more readily adopted. Vaseline, a foreign product patented by the American chemist Robert Chesebrough in 1872, became a popular and more convenient substitute for oils and lards that locals had long used to cleanse and beautify their skin. Using this Western commodity also had symbolic importance in communicating wealth and "civility" in this colonial context. Laurie Wilkie (1996, 2003) similarly found that African American women in the South adopted patent medicines and hygiene-related commodities that were materially similar replacements for ointments and mixtures that they would have otherwise prepared at home. They, too, chose Vaseline, for example, as a more convenient and time-saving version of ointments they already used. These examples highlight the importance of cultural perspectives, users' needs, and material qualities in interpreting medical choices.

Patent/Proprietary Medicines at the Five Points

The archaeological deposits associated with 472 and 474 Pearl Street stood out from those associated with non-Irish residents in the neighborhood in containing a greater number of medicine bottles, and patent medicine bottles especially.[57] Stephen Brighton's (2008) study of the proportion of ethical (prescription) versus patent medicine bottles suggests Irish residents chose to self-medicate with patent medicines instead of seeking prescriptions from physicians more often than their German-born neighbors at 22 Baxter Street in the Five Points or American-born families in Greenwich Village.[58] Brighton interpreted this as evidence that Irish immigrants were more reliant upon over-the-counter remedies and suggested this was because they had become alienated from professional medicine after receiving callous, prejudiced treatment at city institutions. Michael Bonasera and Leslie Raymer (2001:59–60) proposed that Irish residents more often chose patent medicines because of their lower cost compared with a physician's visit and because some residents were so desperately ill or injured that they would try anything. While alienation, cost, and desperation are all important, this section also considers Irish immigrants' ethnomedical perspectives and how they might have responded to advertisements and the material qualities of the medicines and their containers. Taking all of these factors into account, I suggest that Irish immigrant residents utilized the majority of the patent medicines discovered by archaeologists to relieve painful and often chronic injuries.

Of the medicine bottles found in the three deposits associated with 472 and 474 Pearl Street, 26 were identifiable by embossments or by distinctive bottle shapes. These can be classified into 12 different types of medicines on the basis of major contents or function, as determined by their names and advertisements. The types are: anti-diarrheal medicine, balsam, bitter/tonic, child pacifier, cod liver oil, cough/respiratory medicine, liniment, magnetic cure, ointment, sarsaparilla, (medicinal) schnapps, and urological medicine. These are shown in Table 5.1, which compares the types (and brands in parentheses) of patent medicines found at 472 and 474 Pearl Street with those found in Irish contexts in Paterson, New Jersey, in non-Irish contexts in the Five Points (two brothels and one German-occupied tenement), and in two contemporary non-Irish sites in Greenwich Village in New York City, 25 Barrow Street and 93 Amity Street (home to native-born Americans and English and Scottish immigrants). Three additional types of medicine, castor oil, catarrh powder, and indigestion medicine, were found in the comparative contexts and are thus included in the table, bringing the total number of types of medicines represented to 15. Table 5.2 provides the complete name of each brand.

Of the 12 types of medicines identified at 472 and 474 Pearl Street, four were commonly advertised to relieve injury or musculoskeletal pain: balsams, liniments, magnetic cures, and ointments. With the exception of magnetic cures, these types of patent medicines' advertised applications were complementary to the uses of materially similar substances in Ireland. It is thus likely that Irish immigrants considered using them similarly to their advertisements. The material qualities of another five types of the medicines that were found—bitters/tonics, child pacifiers, cod liver oil, sarsaparilla, and schnapps—suggest Irish residents could have employed them to treat pain and injury, applications that diverged from their advertisements.

TABLE 5.1. *(following pages)* Patent Medicine Containers: Numbers, Types, and Brands Identified at the Five Points, Paterson, and Greenwich Village—in Irish, German, and American Contexts.

Note: The Greenwich Village sites are 25 Barrow Street and 93 Amity Street; in the caption headings, Scot = Scottish, Eng = English, and American = native-born American. Bold numbers = total number of bottles containing the type of medicine specified in each row within each archaeological context. Abbreviated medicine brand names are in parentheses; see full names in Table 5.2. Asterisks indicate medicine bottles found in Feature J that are not clearly linked in the Five Points site report (Yamin 2000) with either the 1850 TPQ stratum or the 1870 TPQ stratum. I have grouped them into the 1850 layer based on their dates of production and advertisement. Brighton (2005:193) notes that the bottle of Hegeman's Cod Liver Oil was found in the 1850 stratum.

Type/ Function of Medicines	5 Points Feature J+Z TPQ 1850 Irish	5 Points Feature O TPQ 1860 Irish	5 Points Feature J TPQ 1870 Irish	5 Points Feature AM TPQ 1851 Irish	Paterson Features ca. 1850s Irish	Paterson Features ca.1860s Irish
Anti-diarrheal			1 (Dr. Kiersted's)			
Balsam	1 (Hyatt's)	1 (Turlington's)	1 (Hyatt's)			2 (Hyatt's)
Bitter/ Tonic	1 (Dr. Hostetter's*)	1 (Brown's)				3 (Atwood's, Plantation, and. Dr. Siegert)
Castor Oil						
Catarrhal Powder						1 (Dr. Birney's)
Child Pacifier	2 (Dr. Evans, Godfrey's*)					1 (Mrs. Winslow's)
Cod Liver Oil	1 (Hegeman*)					1 (Hegeman)
Cough Medicine			1 (JR Stafford's)			2 (Dr. Wistar's, Moore's)
Indigestion						
Liniment	1 (Mexican)	3 (2 Radway's, 1 Liquid O.)	2 (Mexican, Radway's)	1 (Liquid O.)	3 (2 Winant's, 1 Radway's)	
Magnetic Cures		1 (Christie's)				
Ointment	1 (Hunt's)					1 (Holloway's)
Sarsaparilla	1 (unidentifiable brand*)				1 (Dr. Townsend's)	2 (Bixby's, Scheuer)
Schnapps			6 (5 U. Wolfe's, 1 V. Oldner's)			
Urological Medicine			1 (Santal)			1 (Dr. Kilmer's)
Total Number of Containers	8	6	12	1	4	14

Sources: Howson (1987); Bodie (1992); Yamin (1999, 2000); Brighton (2005)

Paterson Features ca.1870s Irish	Paterson Features ca.1880s Irish	5 Points Feature AG TPQ 1841 Brothel	5 Points Feature AL TPQ 1860 Brothel	5 Points Feature AN TPQ 1860 German	25 Barrow Feature TPQ 1863 Scot, Eng, & American	93 Amity Feature ca. 1870s American
1 (Traveler's)						
2 (Atwood's and unknown)	5 (2 Atwood's, 1 Wild Cherry, 1 Dr. Chipman's, 1 Dr. Morse's)					
	1 (Pitcher's)					
						1 (Marshall's)
					6 (Mrs. Winslow's)	3 (Mrs. Winslow's)
1 (Marvin)						
1 (Hale's)	1 (Maple's)				1 (Nowill's)	1 (Jayne's)
	2 (Bromo-Seltzer)	5 (3 Henry's, 2 Essence)	3 (Henry's)	1 (Essence)		
1 (P. Davis)	1 (P. Davis)		1 (Liquid O.)		2 (Tobias's)	2 (Tobias's, Radway's)
	3 (Vaseline)				1 (unidentifiable brand)	
3 (2 Ayer's, 1 unidentifiable brand)		1 (Bristol's)		1 (probably Sand's)		6 (Ayer's)
					1 (U. Wolfe's)	
9	13	6	4	2	11	13

TABLE 5.2. Full Names of Patent Medicine and Cosmetic Brands Referenced in Table 5.1.

Atwood's Jaundice Bitters	Hyatt's Infallible Life Balsam
Ayer's Sarsaparilla	J. R. Stafford's Olive Tar
Bixby's Sarsaparilla	Jayne's Expectorant
Bristol's Sarsaparilla	Liquid Opodeldoc
Brown's Aromatic Essence of Jamaican Ginger	Maple's Compound Horehound Cough Syrup
Bromo-Seltzer	Marvin Bros. & Bartlett Cod Liver Oil
Christie's Magnetic Fluid	Mexican Mustang Liniment
Dr. Birney's Catarrhal Powder	Moore's Croup
Dr. C. W. Chipman's Health is Wealth Tonic	Mrs. Winslow's Soothing Syrup
Dr. J. Hostetter's Stomach Bitters	Nowill's Pectoral
Dr. J. B. Siegert & Hijos Angostura Bitters	Perry Davis Vegetable Pain Killer
Dr. Kiersted's Julup for Diarroea	Pitcher's Castoria
Dr. Kilmer's Swamp-root	Plantation Bitters
Dr. Marshall's Catarrh Snuff	Radway's Ready Relief
Dr. Morse's Celebrated Syrup 1846	Sand's Sarsaparilla
Dr. Townsend's Sarsaparilla	Santal de Midy
Dr. W. Evans Teething Syrup	Scheuer & Fleischer Cash & Grocer Sarsaparilla
Dr. Wistar's Balsam of Wild Cherry	Tobias's Venetian Liniment
Essence of Peppermint	Traveler's Star Companion
Godfrey's Cordial	Turlington's Balsam of Life
Hale's Honey of Horehound and Tar	Udolpho Wolfe's Aromatic Schnapps
Hegeman & Co. Chemists (probably cod liver oil)	V. Oldner's Aromatic Schnapps
Henry's Calcinated Magnesia	Vaseline
Holloway's Family Ointment	Wild Cherry Family Bitter
Hunt's Sovereign Ointment	Winant's Indian Liniment

Thus, a total of 9 of the 12 types of patent medicines found in association with Irish immigrant tenements at the Five Points, or about 75%, were likely recognized and used by Irish residents for healing injuries and their related pains, as will be explained further below. Counting the *number* of bottles of these types of patent medicines (23 of 26) further intensifies a focus on healing injuries; such medicines represent 88% of the patent medicine bottles found. This suggests that when Irish residents acquired these American over-the-counter medicines it was usually because they sought new remedies for the new and repeated pains and injuries they suffered as a result of living and working in New York City. The following discussion delves deeper into why Irish immigrants living in the Five Points might have selected the particular types and brands of patent medicines that archaeologists uncovered there almost 150 years later.

PREFERRED PATENT MEDICINE TYPES

Liniments are the type of patent medicine most represented in the Irish contexts at the Five Points. Archaeologists found seven bottles in total and at least one bottle in all three Irish-immigrant-tenement-related archaeological deposits (Feature J's 1850 and 1870 layers at 472 Pearl Street and Feature O's 1860 layer at 474 Pearl Street), as well as in a deposit associated with an Irish-owned oyster saloon and tenement at 110 Chatham Street (Feature AM, TPQ 1851). Some liniment brands were advertised as virtual cure-alls and recommended to be taken internally, but liniments were primarily understood by 19th-century Americans as pungent painkilling mixtures to apply to the skin to relieve muscle soreness, back pain, stiff joints, rheumatism, cuts, and burns. Most patent medicine liniments contained turpentine and camphor among other pungent and cooling or warming ingredients (Hiss 1900:183–185). As mentioned previously, folklore records indicate that turpentine was used for these ailments in Ireland, and a record from the New York Hospital indicates continued use after immigration, so a turpentine-based patent medicine might have seemed familiar.[59] The texture and odor of patent medicine liniments and the sensations they produced when applied topically would have likely appealed to Irish consumers for these uses and reminded them of occasions they or a family member utilized turpentine in Ireland. Furthermore, Liquid Opodeldoc, one of the brands found at 474 Pearl Street and at 110 Chatham Street (the oyster saloon) was an American version of an old British brand that Irish immigrants might have encountered prior to arriving in the U.S. Beginning in the 1820s, many Irish men labored seasonally in Scotland or England (Harris 1989:iii). Liquid Opodeldoc was a "soap liniment" (a solution of soap in alcohol) with pungent camphor and essential oils, and thus, like turpentine, it would have had a distinctive and memorable odor. For Irish immigrants, patent medicine liniments were familiar and convenient mixtures with which to soothe a variety of minor injuries and pains, and thus it might not be surprising that liniments were the most-represented patent medicine type.

Convenience and compatibility with Irish remedies might also help to explain why a resident of 472 Pearl Street in the 1850s acquired a jar of Hunt's Sovereign Ointment. Irish immigrants were well acquainted with using homemade ointments for chapped hands, wounds, sore muscles, and sprains. A patent medicine ointment possessed a similarly greasy texture. A busy mother might have found it more expedient to buy a jar of Hunt's Sovereign Ointment than to render the fat of a goose or an eel in a small tenement kitchen. It is also possible that a young Irish man or woman who had emigrated alone and had not been taught how to make an ointment was drawn to this this preparation that resembled what he/she remembered from home. Irish residents probably used ointments, such as Hunt's, either as bases for the addition of other healing ingredients or as stand-alone remedies.

Folklore records from Ireland indicate that greasy patent preparations, such as Vaseline and Vicks Vapo Rub, had been similarly easily adopted into the Irish popular medical toolkit by the early 20th century, likely because of their textural and odiferous similarities to traditional remedies. Schoolchildren in Galway in 1938 recommended rubbing Vicks (patented in 1890 and containing turpentine and camphor) on the chest for a cold and on the neck for a sore throat in the same sections where they listed older homemade remedies (NFCS 1938[35]:126, 140 Galway). After its introduction in 1872, Vaseline was used in Ireland like homemade ointments for chapped hands and cuts (NFCS 1938[773]:19–21; McClafferty 1979). Logan (1994:72) notes that "a mixture of equal parts of zinc ointment and vaseline is probably the best of all *folk preparations* for eczema [emphasis added]."

It should be noted that patent medicine liniments and ointments were also uncovered in *non*-Irish archaeological contexts in nearby Greenwich Village. Archaeologists found two bottles of Tobias' Venetian Liniment and one unidentifiable ointment at 25 Barrow Street (ca. 1860s), and one bottle each of Tobias' and Radway's Renovating Resolvent at 93 Amity (ca. 1870s) (Bodie 1992; Howson 1987; Ponz 2000). This supports the assessment by historians that for minor day-to-day injuries and minor illnesses, native-born Americans also frequently turned to these over-the-counter products (Young 1961).

Balsams are another type of patent medicine marketed to heal injuries and well represented by three bottles in Irish contexts at the Five Points. Balsams contained benzoic acid, derived from the resins of Central and South American balsam trees (Blasi 1974). Several proprietary medicines containing benzoin were manufactured in England by at least the 1740s, including Jesuit's Drops, Friar's Balsam, and Turlington's Balsam. Robert Turlington created Turlington's Balsam in England in 1744 and advertised it as a cure for many different kinds of ailments, from nausea to tuberculosis, and as a topical healing application for wounds and burns. Turlington's Balsam was very successful and sold in distinctive violin-shaped bottles to (unsuccessfully) discourage counterfeiters. In the 19th century, the formula of this patent medicine appears to have been simplified, and physicians used Turlington's Balsam primarily to disinfect wounds (Griffenhagen and Young 1959; Jones and Vegotsky 2016). Tincture of benzoin is still used as an antiseptic glue for Steri-Strips today. Turlington's as well as the brand Friar's Balsam was also available in Ireland, although probably not easily accessible outside the cities of Dublin, Galway, and Cork (Fleetwood 1983:111–112). One bottle of Turlington's was found at 474 Pearl Street.

This patent mixture and other brands of balsams, such as Hyatt's Infallible Life Balsam, found in both 472 Pearl Street deposits and in Irish contexts in Paterson, New Jersey, probably derived from an even older mixture of olive oil and benzoic acid from the aromatic sap of a Middle Eastern plant. This older mixture was used by monks to treat wounds and called "friar's balsam," after which one British patent medicine balsam was named. The original friar's balsam was itself likely derived from sacramental oil and incense (OED 1989b; Meehan 1907). Physician and folklorist Patrick Logan (1994:56, 74, 104) recorded four uses of friar's balsam (which he appears to use in a generic sense and not in reference to a particular brand), in Ireland. These include applying a mixture of friar's balsam and linseed oil to the skin for wounds, burns, and ringworm and adding it to boiling water in a tea kettle and inhaling the vapors for a sore throat.

For Irish immigrants in New York City who were Catholic, which were the majority, balsams might have been especially appealing. The characteristic smell of balsams might have evoked for them memories not only of using friar's balsam in treating wounds in Ireland but also of Church rituals. Such associations likely increased confidence in this type of patent medicine, which were found in association with Irish immigrant residences in the Five Points and Paterson, New Jersey, but not with German immigrant residences at the Five Points nor with the residences of English and Scottish immigrants or native-born Americans in Greenwich Village. This might suggest that Americans and English, Scottish, and German immigrants rejected balsams outright or sought out generic versions from physicians or druggists instead of patent medicine versions. Patent medicine balsams seem to have interested the Irish especially: Balsams were empirically effective in treating wounds, resonated with popular Irish medicine and religion, and were respectable medicines approved by professional physicians, but purchasing an over-the-counter version did not require an expensive or uncomfortable consultation.

Irish immigrants thus probably used the patent medicine liniments, ointments, and balsams found at the Five Points in ways that resembled some of these medicines' advertised applications because they converged with popular Irish applications of similar substances. Other medicines, however, they likely used in ways that were not advertised because these medicines materially resembled substances used differently in Ireland. Medicines that they likely used off-label, although not necessarily exclusively, include one bottle of Hegeman's Cod Liver Oil, found at 472 Pearl Street and dating to the 1850s, as well as eight bottles of medicines that can be grouped into a larger combined category of bitters/tonics/schnapps, represented in all three contexts associated with 472 and 474 Pearl Street. Cod liver oil was advertised as a strengthener and digestive system regulator and was widely prescribed by physicians for tuberculosis by the 1850s and later for rickets (with some popular medicinal antecedents—see Chapters 1 and 7) (Rajakumar 2003:e134, Grad 2004:106). In addition to these advertised uses, in Ireland cod liver oil was also used in ointments for cracked hands and chilblains (painful swelling of hands or feet from exposure to cold), and it is thus possible that the Irish would have used it for these purposes in New York City as well (Logan 1994:68; O'Regan 1997:21).

Bitters, tonics, and schnapps, as well as sarsaparillas, were all mixtures of alcohol and plants that materially resembled Irish popular whiskey and plant mixtures. Hostetter's Stomach Bitters (found in Feature J's 1850 layer) contained between 39% and 47% alcohol plus essential oils of anise and coriander, in addition to the Peruvian bark mentioned previously (Young 1961:130).[60] Udolpho Wolf's Aromatic Schnapps (found in Feature J's 1870 layer) was composed predominantly of gin. These medicinal liquors were advertised as anti-dyspeptics, diuretics, blood cleansers, restoratives, and stimulants, all applications for which Irish immigrants also used whiskey-based cures. Sarsaparillas were slightly different, composed of mixtures of alcohol and infusions of the roots of plants from the genus *Smilax*, and marketed more exclusively for blood purification. One unidentifiable brand of sarsaparilla was found in the 1850 layer of Feature J at 472 Pearl Street.

It is probable that Irish immigrants employed these medicinal liquors not only for the purposes advertised but also for other maladies for which they had used whiskey, such as general pain or headache relief and as a topical disinfectant and stimulant. Products advertised as blood purifiers, moreover, would have been particularly attractive to individuals hoping to prevent a cut or burn from infection, as the Irish understood an infection to be the result of poisoned blood. Irish residents at 472 and 474 Pearl Street might have chosen these patent medicines instead of whiskey mixtures because they found that whiskey mixtures were insufficient to counter the increased severity of injuries caused by labor in the U.S. They might have looked to these American remedies as appropriate for relieving the pain of American labor. Medicating with bitters and schnapps instead of whiskey was also considered by the American middle class to be more respectable. Utilizing these patent preparations thus might have enabled an injured immigrant to continue to labor, while avoiding arousing an employer's suspicion of intemperate habits.

The presence of two patent medicines containing opium—Godfrey's Cordial and Dr. W. Evan Teething Syrup—and syringes at 472 and 474 Pearl Street, further support the idea that Irish residents were seeking more effective analgesics than whiskey or traditional herbal remedies (Yamin 2000[4]). Godfrey's Cordial was another well-known English patent medicine with which Irish immigrants might have had prior familiarity. American-born New Yorkers appear to have preferred Mrs. Winslow's Soothing Syrup, a competing American brand, several bottles of which were found at the Greenwich Village sites. Both were marketed in the 19th century as teething aids and to reduce fretfulness and colic in infants, but adults also used these kinds of medicines for themselves (Adams 1912). An Irish laborer at 472 Pearl Street suffering from a serious injury or recovering from a traumatic surgery, such as an amputation, might have tried Godfrey's Cordial after failing to experience relief from other remedies. It is also possible that a resident used these medicines containing opiates to relieve painful pulmonary tuberculosis (see Chapter 7).

Opiates, in the form of opium-laced mixtures, laudanum, and morphine, were the strongest painkillers available. Opium was prescribed frequently by physicians in hospitals, including New York, Bellevue, and St. Vincent's Hospitals, and it brought relief to many patients, but not without risk. Opiates, as we know today in the midst of an opioid epidemic in the U.S., are highly addictive, and it is common for individuals to become dependent upon opiates initially prescribed by physicians. This was also a cause of addiction in the 19th century. For example, a 31-year-old Irish widow who was diagnosed at New York Hospital with debility and a fractured arm confessed to the admitting physician that "three years ago while a patient in this hospital she contracted the habit of taking opium and since then has been unable to break herself of it.

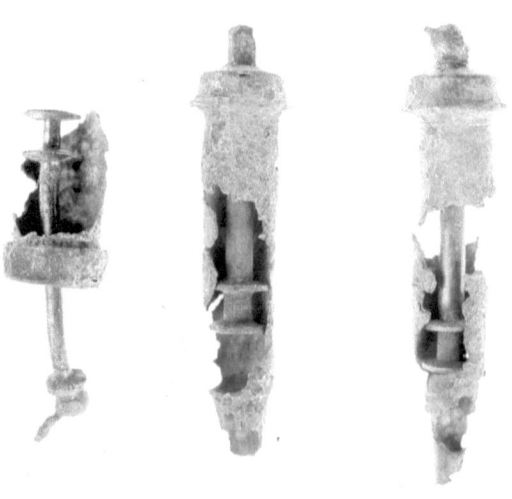

FIGURE 5.4. Metal syringes discovered at the Five Points. Images courtesy of Rebecca Yamin and the New York City Archaeological Repository: The Nan A. Rothschild Research Center.

[She] has used daily 3 pills, when she can't get it, [she has] diarrhea and general prostration" (NYHSCB 1862:C287). It is possible that a resident of 472 Pearl Street had similarly become addicted while hospitalized and looked to Godfrey's Cordial or Dr. W. Evan Teething Syrup, medicines advertised to be mild enough for babies, to support a habit or wean from dependence. Another individual in a similar predicament might have tried to inject morphine instead, using the syringes uncovered there (Figure 5.4).[61] In the 19th century, the primary use of hypodermic syringes was to inject morphine (Haller 1981b:1677).

PREFERRED PATENT MEDICINE BRANDS

The numerous patent medicine bottles found by archaeologists at the Five Points suggest that Irish immigrants sometimes employed patent medicines for relief of injuries and pain, instead of or in addition to other strategies, such as using homemade traditional remedies or seeking professional medical care. This discussion thus far has suggested a few reasons why they might have chosen patent medicines, including convenience, previous familiarity with a product or particular brand, the failure of other approaches to heal an injury or mitigate pain, recommendation by a trusted source, and the ability to medicate "respectably" and without missing work and thus wages. All these potential reasons, however, depended on the ability of the product to appeal to Irish ideas about healing. The types of patent medicines represented at the Five Points were not the only types that were available, but each of them, with the exception of a magnetic cure (Christie's Magnetic Fluid), had some kind of material resonance, especially smell and texture, with substances used in Ireland for healing injuries and pain. Similarly, the brands of patent medicines found were not the only ones available. Irish consumers had a number of different liniments or balsams, for example, to choose from, but they appear to have selected only a few brands. Examining the names and advertisements of particular brands provides further clues about what Irish residents sought from these medicines.

Before delving into the content of patent medicine advertisements, it is useful to consider how accessible they might have been to Irish immigrants in New York City. Literacy rates among adults in mid-19th-century Ireland were only about 50%, but there was a widespread practice of public reading of newspapers such that even people who could not read stayed informed. Newspapers were also shared among many people, and subscription rates reflect only a small portion of their actual circulation (McMahon 2015a:4, 17). In New York City, reading rooms also provided additional access to nonsubscribers. James Markey's Citizen House was located at 499 Pearl Street, only steps away from the 472 and 474 Pearl Street tenements, for example; it was advertised in the early 1850s as having reading rooms "kept well supplied with Irish and American newspapers" as well as "a good supply of the choicest Ales, Liquors, and Segars" (McMahon 2015a:87). Patent medicine advertisements containing images would have caught the eyes of even those who only viewed or listened to the paper, and images became more prevalent in advertising over time; but even the graphic layouts of text-only ads stood out on the page. It is also important to remember that although newspapers are the most accessible sources of advertisements for historians today, patent medicine producers advertised well beyond newspapers, and included ephemeral, non-textual modes of promoting their products, as mentioned previously.

Beginning with liniments, the type of patent medicine most well represented in Irish contexts at the Five Points, the brand Mexican Mustang Liniment stands out in being found in both the 1850 and 1870 layer at 472 Pearl Street but not at sites in Greenwich Village associated with native-born residents. Residents of 93 Amity Street instead preferred Tobias' Venetian Liniment and Radway's Renovating Resolvent. A reason Mexican Mustang Liniment (Figure 5.3) might have appealed to Irish residents was because it advertised that it was suitable for "man or beast." In rural Ireland, healers often treated both animals and people, sometimes with the same medicines (Logan 1994). To the Irish, successful trial of a medicine on animals suggested its safety, a reasonable principle still in use today. In a short satirical account of his experiences in the north of Ireland, published in *Harper's Weekly* (1879:806), a supposed dispensary doctor commented upon a patient's father who applied this principle. When he returned to check on Marianne Mulloy, the ill young woman, and found that her condition had not improved, he asked her father if she had taken the medicine he prescribed for her. "'Troth she did not, doctor,' the father replied with emphasis." When the doctor asked why, "Mulloy rose up, with an expression of indignation on his face, he said, 'Biddy, go fetch out that cat.' Biddy . . . opened the door of a cupboard . . . and there bounced out of it something like a half-roasted hare; an animal without a bit of fur on its body, and of a dull patchy slate-color. As it fled . . . old Mulloy pointed sternly toward it and said, 'No! by the blessing of Providence, we tried your powders upon the cat, and that's the way our Marianne would have been this day if she had taken what you sent her.'" Mexican Mustang Liniment's promise to be safe and effective for both men and horses probably would have appealed to most Irish parents, and to their children.

The appeal of the novel or exotic also could have been a powerful enticement for Irish immigrants. Van der Geest et al. (1996:168) point out that the "belief that medicines that come from afar are stronger than native ones is present in many cultures" including our own, where "pharmaceuticals from Switzerland and Sweden are metonymically endowed with the prestige of these countries' advanced technology; . . . this foreign aura is dexterously exploited in drug advertisements. Exotic ingredients provoke wonder." In its brand name, Mexican Mustang Liniment drew upon the mystique of the Catholic land to the south to provoke wonder and utilized appealing imagery of the horse, an animal greatly valued in Ireland.

Use of images or logos in patent medicine advertisements or on bottle labels helped them to be quickly identified by consumers and distinguished from other brands. These images also attracted attention and were often a part of the calculus customers used to determine whether to buy the product. Another liniment brand that was found at the Five Points was Radway's Ready Relief. Radway's depicted an image of an angel as part of its logo (Figure 5.5), which might have signaled to an Irish consumer that this medicine was sanctioned by a higher power, or that the producers must be God-fearing and honest. Symbols like an angel and a horse, because they were familiar to Irish immigrants and had positive associations, might have provided reassurance to Irish consumers.

Recommendation by a trusted source is another factor that could have enticed an Irish immigrant to spend a considerable amount of money on a patent medicine. In Ireland, folk healers' reputations were based on the results that they were able to deliver to their patients. Patients or their families spread word of success or failure that built the healer's reputation. Word-of-mouth recommendations about certain brands from other immigrants or from American-born neighbors and coworkers were thus likely to have a profound impact on the reputations of certain medicines and thus Irish immigrant purchasing habits. Radway's Ready Relief was popular among the native-born population, and it is possible that an American coworker or boss recommended it to an Irish laborer who used it at 474 Pearl Street.

In the absence of a recommendation from a known individual, it is possible that some Irish immigrants found testimonials—published affirmations by supposedly independent individuals attesting to the efficacy of the medicine that were often part of advertisements in newspapers—to be reasonable substitutes. Testimonials supposedly written by Civil War veterans, "respectable citizens," doctors, professors, lawyers,

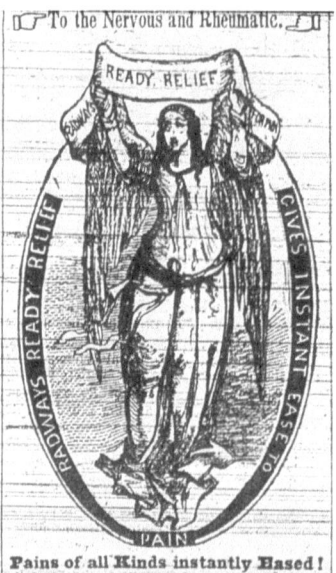
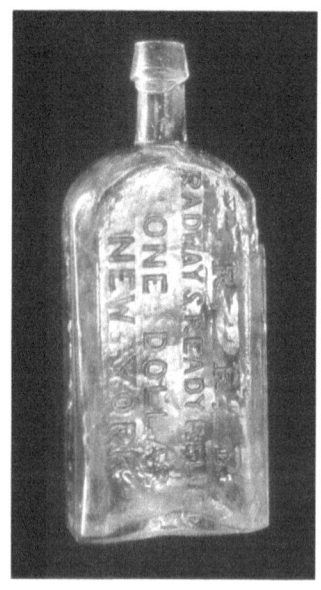

FIGURE 5.5. Left—Advertisement for Radway's Ready Relief showing an angel that might have appealed to Irish customers (Figure 199 in Bonasera 2000a:376). Right—Photograph of a bottle of Radway's unearthed from Feature O, 472 Pearl Street. Image courtesy of Rebecca Yamin and the New York City Archaeological Repository: The Nan A. Rothschild Research Center.

clergymen, and postmasters, some even with Irish surnames, appear in newspapers of this era. Hyatt's Infallible Life Balsam, which was the most popular brand of balsam among the Irish at the Five Points and Paterson, New Jersey, published a series of ads in the 1850s and 1860s featuring testimonials. These ads might help to explain residents' preference for this brand over the more established Turlington's Balsam.

In one 1863 advertisement (Figure 5.6), for example, Hyatt's Life Balsam claimed to cure "H. K. Chapman, belonging to Fourth Regiment, New-York Volunteers, of severe rheumatism of three years duration, after all other remedies had failed" and "Willet Jarvis, Esq., No. 277 Hicks-St., Brooklyn, of deep and terrible ulcers on the leg, after his physician had decided that amputation was necessary to save his life" (*NYT* 1863:5). Hyatt's thus attempted to sell itself as a remedy that could be effective even on the toughest cases, even when all other approaches failed, and even when painful surgery loomed. This advertisement could certainly have been attractive to someone like James, the laborer with the frost-bite-related amputations, or the family of Pat, the boy whose arm was lacerated by a calico press (Chapter 4). Similar miraculous cures are found sprinkled throughout Irish folk sources. A resident of County Mayo in Ireland, for example, was healed of an ulcerous wound on a limb scheduled to be amputated by a mixture prepared by an old woman living in the mountains (Logan 1994:111).[62] (See Chapter 7 for a continued discussion of the appeal and uses of Hyatt's Balsam.)

In addition to testimonials, the publication of an advertisement in a particular newspaper or journal probably added to (or subtracted from) a patent medicine's credibility. It is reasonable to assume, for example, that many Irish immigrants trusted Irish American newspapers, including the *New York Freeman's Journal and Catholic Register*, an Irish American weekly publication owned for a time by New York City Catholic Archbishop John Hughes.[63] Irish weeklies published information that was important to emigrants throughout the Irish diaspora, often reprinting articles from Ireland, Great Britain, Canada, and Australia. As McMahon (2015a:83) describes, they "offered a place for Irish people to virtually assemble once a week." Three of the patent medicine brands found at the Five Points were advertised in this newspaper in the 1850s and 1860s, Mexican Mustang Liniment (*New York Freeman's Journal* [*NYFJ*] 1854a:8), Udolpho Wolfe's Aromatic Schnapps (*NYFJ* 1854b:6,

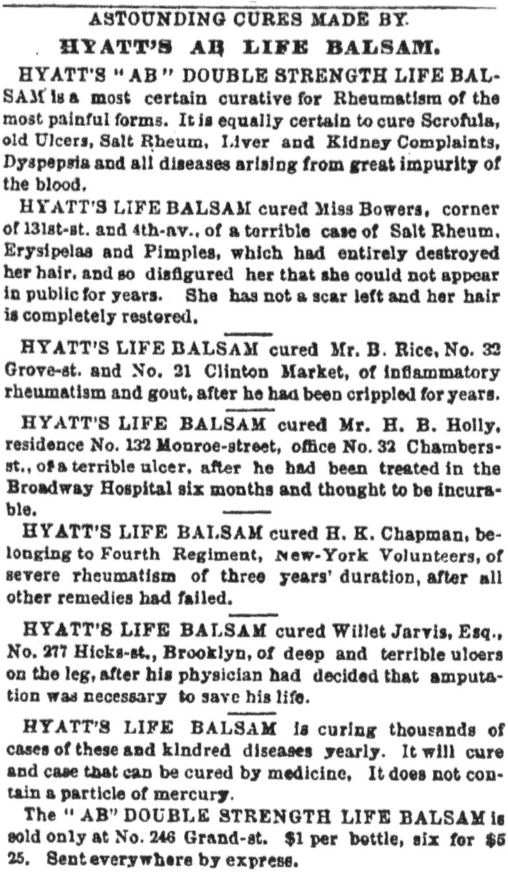

> ASTOUNDING CURES MADE BY
> **HYATT'S AB LIFE BALSAM.**
> HYATT'S "AB" DOUBLE STRENGTH LIFE BAL-
> SAM is a most certain curative for Rheumatism of the
> most painful forms. It is equally certain to cure Scrofula,
> old Ulcers, Salt Rheum, Liver and Kidney Complaints,
> Dyspepsia and all diseases arising from great impurity of
> the blood.
> HYATT'S LIFE BALSAM cured Miss Bowers, corner
> of 131st-st. and 4th-av., of a terrible case of Salt Rheum,
> Erysipelas and Pimples, which had entirely destroyed
> her hair, and so disfigured her that she could not appear
> in public for years. She has not a scar left and her hair
> is completely restored.
>
> HYATT'S LIFE BALSAM cured Mr. B. Rice, No. 32
> Grove-st. and No. 21 Clinton Market, of inflammatory
> rheumatism and gout, after he had been crippled for years.
>
> HYATT'S LIFE BALSAM cured Mr. H. B. Holly,
> residence No. 132 Monroe-street, office No. 32 Chambers-
> st., of a terrible ulcer, after he had been treated in the
> Broadway Hospital six months and thought to be incura-
> ble.
>
> HYATT'S LIFE BALSAM cured H. K. Chapman, be-
> longing to Fourth Regiment, New-York Volunteers, of
> severe rheumatism of three years' duration, after all
> other remedies had failed.
>
> HYATT'S LIFE BALSAM cured Willet Jarvis, Esq.,
> No. 277 Hicks-st., Brooklyn, of deep and terrible ulcers
> on the leg, after his physician had decided that amputa-
> tion was necessary to save his life.
>
> HYATT'S LIFE BALSAM is curing thousands of
> cases of these and kindred diseases yearly. It will cure
> and case that can be cured by medicine. It does not con-
> tain a particle of mercury.
> The "AB" DOUBLE STRENGTH LIFE BALSAM is
> sold only at No. 246 Grand-st. $1 per bottle, six for $5
> 25. Sent everywhere by express.

FIGURE 5.6. Advertisement for Hyatt's Life Balsam claiming "astounding cures" (*New York Times* 1863:5).

1860a:5), and Hegeman & Co. Cod Liver Oil (*NYFJ* 1860b:5). The presence of their ads in this Irish Catholic newspaper could have contributed to Irish residents' decisions to purchase these brands over others.

Nevertheless, it appears that almost twice the number of the patent medicine brands found at the Five Points were advertised in American newspapers such as the *New-York Daily Times*, which became the *New York Times* in 1857, and *Harper's Weekly* as in the *New York Freeman's Journal*. Brands found in the 472 and 474 Pearl Street deposits that were advertised in the *New York Times* include Radway's Ready Relief, Hyatt's Life Balsam, and J. R. Stafford's Olive Tar, some even on the same page (e.g., Radway's and Hyatt's [*NYT* 1857:5, 1858a:5, 1858b:5]).

Brands advertised in *Harper's Weekly* included Hostetter's Bitters, Stafford's Olive Tar, and Hegeman & Co (*HW* 1860:318, 1862:175, 1867b:479, 1867c:511). The companies that frequently advertised in these newspapers that primarily targeted native-born Americans had large advertising budgets with advertisements visible all over town.

Radway's Ready Relief stands out as a medicine that was advertised more frequently and conspicuously than other brands in the *New York Times*, with nearly one ad per week from 1857 to 1873; some of the ads take up a whole column. Only a handful of patent medicines were advertised in this newspaper as frequently during this period, such as Mrs. Winslow's Soothing Syrup and Ayer's brand products. Archaeological evidence suggests these advertisements were successful and that these products were generally popular. Mrs. Winslow's, for example, was present at 25 Barrow Street and at 93 Amity Street in Greenwich Village, sites associated with Scottish, English, and native-born American families; Radway's Ready Relief and Ayer's Sarsaparilla were present at 93 Amity Street (Bodie 1992; Howson 1987).

Conspicuous presence of ads and inclusion in a major American newspaper, such as the *New York Times* or *Harper's Weekly*, might have validated a product in the minds of Irish immigrants, implying it was trusted by native-born Americans who were more knowledgeable about American products. Paul Mullins (1999:25) has convincingly argued that African American families in 19th-century Annapolis, Maryland, purchased brand name goods to guarantee good quality as well as to reap the "greater symbolic worth of nationally recognized brands." As Mullins (1999:25) contends in the case of African Americans, visibly using brand-name goods could have also enhanced Irish immigrants' status among both fellow Irish immigrants and native-born Americans. The absence of some well-advertised, major American patent medicine brands in deposits associated with Irish residences at the Five Points, including Ayer's products and Mrs. Winslow's Soothing Syrup, nevertheless, indicates that medicines still had to appeal to Irish cultural views; being a popular American brand was not enough.

Lizabeth Cohen (1990) has also pointed out that particular shops were similarly trusted to provide quality goods and conferred social cachet to their patrons, in her study of African American shoppers' preferences for chain stores in 20th-century Chicago. Trust in a well-known chain store might help to explain why Irish residents at the Five Points and in Paterson, New Jersey, chose cod liver oil from Hegeman & Co. over other brands. Hegeman & Co. was one of the first chain drugstores, with at least four shops in New York City by 1859 at 161, 399, 511, and 756 Broadway (*NYT* 1859:5).

The personal relationships made with druggists (also called pharmacists, chemists, and apothecaries) working at Hegeman's or other drugstores could have enhanced trust in medicines they sold. In Irish and American cities, druggists were indispensable; in New York City by this time, they were also reasonably qualified. An 1832 law required druggists in the city to have attended sessions at the College of Pharmacy of New York City or to pass an exam or to have a diploma from another school (Duffy 1968:474). They performed a variety of functions including minor surgical procedures, filling physicians' prescriptions, and dispensing advice, herbs, chemicals, and patent medicines. Their shops, filled with herbs, powders, liquids, and devices, were veritable cabinets of curiosities, and patent medicine sales were important to drugstores, because during this period physicians often supplied their patients with medicines directly (Dykstra 1955:403). Irish immigrants would have found druggists to be more accessible than physicians, more knowledgeable about how to treat urban ailments than Irish folk healers, and possibly also subject to some important social rules as shopkeepers living in a community (Haller 1981a:268). Anthropologist Conrad Arensberg (1937) described how shopkeepers in Ireland were expected to extend credit to their customers, and customers were expected to never fully clear their tabs, such that both remained entangled in a series of exchanges that made them reliant on one another. It is likely that this system continued in New York City. Irish immigrants often needed to purchase items on credit, and because there were so many competing drugstores, the stores that could afford it probably found that extending credit earned loyal customers.

Oral historian Kevin Kearns's (1994:103–105) interview with Harry Mushatt, a chemist in the Dublin tenements in the early 20th century, attests to the importance of druggists among the tenement population there. Mushatt explained that "tenement people came from *all over* Dublin. They came to us because they really couldn't afford a doctor. The shop was never empty. We worked like slaves. Oh, there was a bond of trust. There was tremendous faith in us." Apothecaries like Mushatt were integrated into the community, subject to its scrutiny, but also trusted if they passed muster.

Historical records confirm that a few Irish-born druggists, including one woman, resided in the Sixth Ward.[64] They might have worked at one of the nearby drugstores, such as the Family Drug Store and R. Dillon's, located at 505 and 421 Pearl Street, respectively. The proprietor of the Family Drug Store, H. Drew, advertised in *The Citizen* (1854b:18) that he was a Licentiate of Apothecaries Hall, Dublin. Irish druggists would have known some Irish popular cures as well the professional pharmacy of the day, as an advertisement of R. Dillon's suggests: "physicians' and *family* recipes carefully dispensed [emphasis added]" (*NYFJ* 1854c:6). Druggists like these served as mediators between Irish popular medicine and American professional medicine and helped fellow immigrants transition from rural to urban life. Participating in the popular American demand for patent medicines was both a means and a symptom of this transition. Purchasing these remedies at a drugstore was not a simple economic transaction but an opportunity to build a relationship with this other kind of healer. It also showed fellow working-class American customers that the Irish too were sensitive to the pains and injuries of labor and that the Irish too sought many of the same medicines for healing.

NEW RECIPES FOR RELIEF IN NEW YORK

In summary, a combination of historical and archaeological records indicate that Irish immigrants in mid-19th-century New York City utilized a variety of approaches to treat painful everyday, and perhaps even more serious, injuries at home before seeking professional medical care. They continued to create popular remedies used in Ireland, or perhaps obtained them from a neighbor who knew the recipes or possessed special cures. Life in New York City was different than rural Ireland, however, and some of the resources relied upon in Ireland were unavailable, inconvenient, or insufficient. Irish immigrants integrated new, local healing resources and knowledge from non-Irish sources into their toolkits, including plants and patent medicines.

Patent medicines varied in quality and effectiveness but were incredibly popular and more affordable alternatives to physicians' prescriptions.

Free prescriptions were available at dispensaries and hospitals, but dispensary hours were limited—the New York Orthopaedic Dispensary, for example, was only open from 1:00 to 3:00pm on weekdays (NYODAR 1869:1)—requiring many to miss a day of work. Free treatment at hospitals came with the shame of accepting charity, the dangers of "hospitalism," and the possibility of being subjected, as nonpaying patients were, to experimental and/or painful procedures without (or even with) the benefits of anesthesia (see Chapter 4). How much medicine Irish immigrants at the Five Points acquired from dispensaries is difficult to assess archaeologically; dispensaries did not always dispense medicines in prescription medicine bottles. Rosenberg (1974b:36) notes that New York City's Eastern Dispensary was chronically short on funds and thus did not give patients bottles or written directions. Patients brought their own bottles or teacups to contain medicine. Historical records clearly show that many Irish immigrants did seek care at dispensaries and hospitals, but these records also show that they preferred to manage injuries at home. Most Irish immigrants went to hospitals only after they had exhausted other options or in cases of severe conditions when they were often brought by friends or authorities.

A close examination of the patent medicines found in association with the tenements at 472 and 474 Pearl Street suggests Irish immigrant residents chose types that were materially similar to substances used in Ireland to remedy injuries and pain, such as greasy ointments, liquor and plant-infused bitters, and pungent liniments. They likely used some as directed for applications they deemed compatible and others for purposes other than advertised but that resonated with Irish popular practices or fit new needs. They also appear to have selected particular brands of compatible patent medicine types that were attractive because of previous familiarity, culturally resonant symbols or testimonials, or recommendations from trusted sources, such as neighbors or druggists, or even newspapers.

The archaeological remains at the Five Points thus suggest that residents drew on a wide variety of medicinal substances to remedy illness and injury at home. Like their American-born and German-born neighbors, they treated conditions they felt they could manage themselves at home, but often with different substances or alternative applications. Another difference between most Irish immigrants and their non-Irish neighbors was the frequency and degree to which they were injured as well as the prevalence of chronic injury, all reflected in greater representation of patent medicines used for injuries and pain than those at non-Irish sites and in greater representation of Irish immigrants in New York City hospitals. No treatment—whether a home remedy, patent medicine, physician's prescription, or surgical operation—could permanently cure the suffering that Irish immigrants endured as a result of their social positions in the lowest echelons of the working class in New York City, however. There were only temporary escapes from pain, injury, and social stigma for those who had to work long hours in dangerous and exhausting jobs that paid meager wages and altered the very fabric of their bodies.

Irish immigrants in New York were well aware of this predicament and tried in a number of ways to improve their situations and those of their countrymen and women. Historical records tell us that those with means, including Dr. William MacNeven (1842a), formed emigrant aid societies. Those with fewer means worked hard to send their children to school, hoping that education would propel them away from the drudgery of manual labor. Some, including Frank Roney (1931), tried to improve laboring conditions through union organizing. Others became involved in politics and still others in small business ventures, such as saloons and groceries. Archaeology from the Five Points suggests that those with even fewer resources attempted informal business ventures, possibly selling homemade whiskey or home remedies. Archaeological remains from 472 and 474 Pearl Street also point to another important and previously overlooked strategy: using appearance-altering commodities to project identities distinct from the stereotypes of Pat and Bridget.

FASHIONING NEW IDENTITIES: COSMETICS AND OTHER SOCIAL "MEDICINES"

Writing from New York to his parents in Westmeath, Ireland, in 1849, Irishman Matthew Gaynor advised them about what to bring when they emigrated to New York. After suggestions about food, he warned that "it is foolishness to be bringing too much clothes that [are] friezes [a coarse woolen cloth] or corduroy for they are not the fashion. . . . I'd bring only as little as possible . . . only bring . . . money . . . for while you wear the friezes and corduroy you will be called a greenhorn." Gaynor was not alone in sharing sartorial advice or in quickly realizing that Americans reacted negatively to the appearances of newly arrived Irish immigrants (Chapter 2). Frank Roney (1931:182), the Belfast-born iron worker and labor organizer, also noted his poor clothing made it difficult for him to find good employment: "I bore the unmistakable marks of a recent arrival . . . the cut of my clothes marked me." Irish women shared similar concerns. Christine Stansell (1986:164) describes how "Irish girls, as soon as they could, shed their clogs and shifts—so different from New York styles that one guidebook warned they were apt to be 'laughed out of use'—for hoopskirts and flowered bonnets." Many Irish newcomers quickly grasped that among the myriad challenges they faced in New York City, they also had what today might be called an image problem. In order to control their own identities and destinies, they had to take control over how others saw them. Historical and archaeological records combined suggest that their attempts to alter their appearances extended beyond clothing, beyond assimilation, and beyond the body's surface.

Along with the plant remains and patent medicines they unearthed in the deposits associated with 472 and 474 Pearl Street, archaeologists also discovered several bottles of what could be categorized as cosmetics: one bottle each of Rowland's Macassar Oil (J+Z 1850), Lyon's Kathairon (O 1860), and Batchelor's Hair Dye (J 1870), and three bottles of Lubin Perfume (1 in O 1860 and 2 in J 1870).[65] These products were popular among native-born Americans to improve hygiene and appearance and were advertised in mainstream American and Irish American newspapers, where they were marketed as medicinal and magnificent.[66] Rowland's Macassar Oil was a British brand advertised as an exotic "purely vegetable" potion from Macassar in Indonesia that beautified hair, cured baldness, and rendered "use of the fine comb unnecessary," signaling that it killed headlice (*NYDT* 1854:7).[67] The makers of Lyon's Kathairon claimed their product was the finest *ever* made and cured hair loss, gray hair, and dandruff, in addition to making hair shiny and manageable (*NYDT* 1857b:5). The French company Parfums Lubin was one of the world's oldest perfume houses, at one time supplying French royalty, and their products were advertised as appropriate "for toilet use or the headache" (*New-York Daily Tribune* 1844:3). Although there is no direct evidence of precisely what effects individual Irish consumers desired when purchasing these products, applying the same principles used to assess patent medicines earlier in the chapter (considering Irish cultural perspectives and needs, product advertisements, and ingredients) suggests that Irish immigrants used these products not just to remedy dandruff, baldness, or lice, but ultimately to heal social problems related to Irish immigrant stereotypes. I suggest they were not simply concerned with assimilation, however, but with the opportunities these and other products noted in historical records afforded them to strategically present themselves to different audiences.

For women interested in finding employment as domestic servants, for example, Lyon's, Rowland's, and Lubin's products would have helped to make a good impression on potential middle-class native-born employers. Marie Haggerty, a domestic servant born in 1867, told a Works Progress Administration (WPA) oral history collector that appearance was a critical factor in attaining and maintaining a position, especially in "nicer" houses. "You got hired by your looks," she remarked (Banks 1980:171). Personal hygiene was a concern of many employers who worried that Irish help might contaminate their houses with typhus fever, cholera, or other diseases arising from their supposed poor hygiene and sanguine temperaments. Cleanliness and orderliness were the chief concerns of middle-class mistresses, and they themselves were judged by their ability to keep their household and servants in order (Stansell 1986:159–165). Neat and clean hair was a critical part of a respectable appearance, but washing hair in a tenement was a challenge, requiring either immersion in cold water in a rear yard, hauling buckets of water upstairs to heat on an apartment stove, or visiting a public bath. Scalp ailments, including dandruff and hair loss, that could have been a signal of poor health to employers, could have been more prevalent among Irish immigrants because such conditions are related to overall health and impacted by overwork, trauma, dietary deficiencies, and unsanitary living conditions, all problems that also affected the Irish in New York. Lyon's Kathairon and Rowland's Macassar Oil contained ingredients that discouraged lice and might have improved dandruff as well as pleasant-smelling aromatic oils—of rose in Rowland's and of bergamot, clove, rosemary, and lavender in Lyon's, "equalling Lubin's choicest extracts" (*NYDT* 1853:7).[68] Such products thus could have aided Irish women (and men) to style their hair neatly, extend time between laborious washings, and present a pleasant-smelling and clean appearance.

Potential employers also looked for workers who were young and strong. Such qualities were especially important for male manual laborers in competing for day-laboring jobs and skilled positions, as described previously. Men of more advanced ages might have sought cosmetics to present more youthful appearances. All three hair treatment brands found in Irish contexts at the Five Points—Rowland's, Lyon's, and Batchelor's Hair Dye—advertised they could restore color to gray hair and cure baldness, both usually interpreted as markers of age.[69] It is also possible that Irish residents looked to Batchelor's Hair Dye to enhance their job prospects in other ways. Advertisements often claimed that hair dyes changed "red hair to a beautiful brown or black," implying that red hair was neither beautiful nor desirable, likely because of its association with unfavorable stereotypes of the sanguine Irish temperament.[70] A Bellevue Hospital case record from 1874 of Kate, a 22-year-old Irish-born sewing machine operator admitted for lead poisoning from her use of "ball powder for her complexion," suggests some Irish immigrants also attempted to disguise a ruddy complexion associated with Irish stereotypes, to cover unsightly scars from injuries, and/or to lighten skin to conform to American and Irish aesthetic ideals (BHMCB 1874:389).[71] Although we cannot know exactly why Kate used ball powder, we can be sure that she applied it hoping it would make others see her the way she wanted to be seen.

Disguising Irish identity might have been attractive to youth who had immigrated as young children, sometimes referred to as the 1.5 generation, who often feel caught in between the culture of their parents and their host country and can be targets of harassment, especially if they stand out from native-born peers (Kasinitz et al. 2010). Some might not have sought to reject Irish identity but to participate in popular fashion to command respect and attention from other youth, including potential romantic partners. Dark and oiled locks were a critical element of American urban working-class masculine style in the middle of the 19th century, epitomized by the popular fictional stage character, the fireman and dandy, Mose the Bowery B'hoy. Mose dressed in a long tight jacket that accentuated his broad shoulders and narrowed at the waist. He was often accompanied by his fictional and flashy-dressing girlfriend, Lize the Bowery G'hal, who styled her hair in long "sausage" curls (Stansell 1986:90) (Figure 5.7). The complaints of middle-class American-born mistresses about the way their Irish female domestic servants outfitted themselves during their limited hours off suggest that they, too, often adjusted their images for their peers and potential partners. In contrast to mistresses' respectable middle-class attire in "muted colors that covered the flesh except for the face (including obligatory gloves and hat)," their servants adopted the styles of working-class American-born women who wore "startling combinations of colors," dresses that accentuated the hips and the thighs, and "ornate hats" that exposed their faces and gave them "full liberty to see what is going on in every direction" (Stansell 1986:93–94). Later combined advertisements for

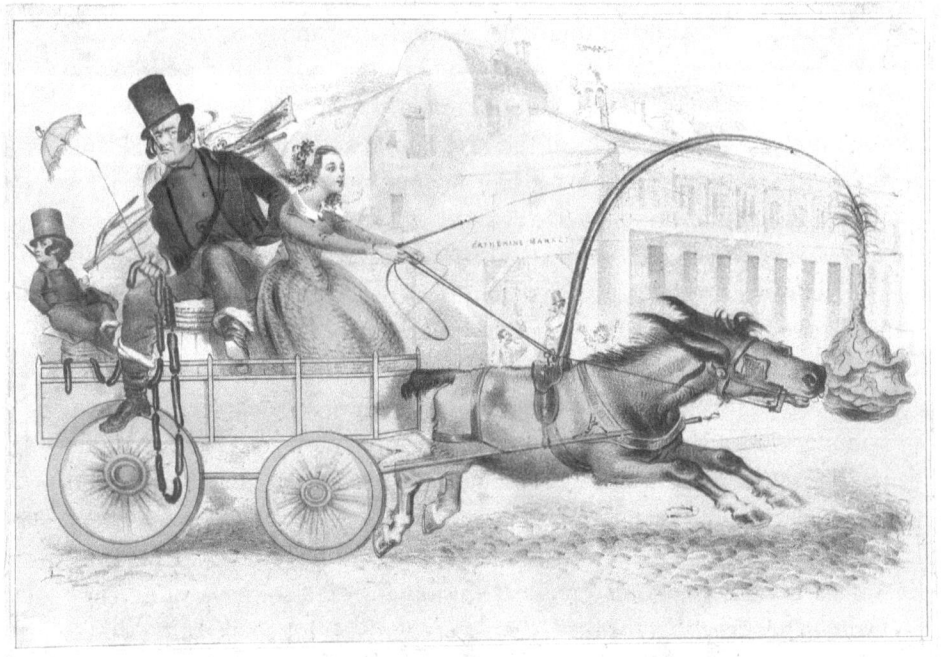

FIGURE 5.7. Lithograph titled "Mose, Lize & Little Mose Going to California" [during the Gold Rush] (Robinson ca. 1849). Courtesy of The Metropolitan Museum of Art.

Lyon's Kathairon and Hagan's Magnolia Balm for the complexion suggest these products increased customers' chances of finding partners: "Brothers will have no spinster sisters when these articles are around" (*NYT* 1870a:5). Census records indicate that there were, in fact, fewer spinsters and old bachelors among Irish immigrants in the Five Points than in Ireland. Men and women married earlier than their counterparts in Ireland (Griggs 2000:46). Most chose Irish spouses, cementing their place within the Irish American community, the support of which was critical for survival, as will be discussed further in Chapter 7.

Fair skin, dark and shiny hair, and a fashionable, clean, and healthy appearance were qualities appreciated by fellow Irish immigrants as well.[72] Shared preference for sleek hair was featured in the previously noted satirical report from a dispensary doctor in rural Ireland in *Harper's Weekly* (1879:806). The doctor was vexed by how youth used the castor oil he prescribed for them. At Sunday mass "there was an unmistakable odor in the air, and the unusually sleek hair of many of the boys and girls bore witness to the use the oil had been put to." This anecdote also points to the material similarity between the brands of hair products found in the Irish deposits at the Five Points and substances used similarly in Ireland, from oils for hair styling to extracts of rosemary for washing and darkening hair to counterirritants for hair growth (Purdon 1895a:217; NFCS 1938[364]:175; Logan 1994:115–117).[73]

Other evidence suggests that some Irish immigrants went to greater extremes to shape their appearances. Historian David Kunzle (1982:92) reports that corseting or "tight-lacing" was popular among not only middle-class women (and some men) to achieve an ideal form but also among working-class seamstresses for the same reason and to hide work-related back injuries, tuberculosis-related spinal deformities, and even pregnancy. Worn tightly, a corset would have restricted movement and oxygen intake, and thus seems like a counterproductive measure for Irish women who had to work for a living. Yet, some working-class women believed that the near-term costs of reshaping their bodies would be worthwhile in the end, while others, such as seamstresses, might have worn a looser fitting corset as a supportive garment to enable them to spend longer hours working and to counteract the negative effects of such work on their spines and posture. Similarly, Irish men, women, and children sought out orthopedic braces—which were often painful and debilitating—at the New York Orthopedic Dispensary (1870–1873) to remedy spinal deformities caused by injuries and tuberculosis and to cultivate a literally more upright appearance. Sculpting a respectable and attractive appearance increased their chances of finding better work or "marrying up" to escape hard labor altogether.

An example of how some Irish immigrants, especially younger men and women, might have utilized a variety of commodities to cultivate an appearance different from Irish stereotypes is suggested by a cartoon published in *Harper's Weekly* in 1867 (Figure 5.8). It depicts two Irish immigrant men in conversation. The "Ancient Hibernian" conforms to many aspects of the male Irish immigrant stereotype. He has the muscular hands and rounded posture of a manual labor, skin darkened and wrinkled from working outdoors, and the unfashionable but functional clothing of a laborer: an old overcoat, floppy hat, and shabby, baggy shirt and pants. He smokes a clay tobacco pipe and says, in accented speech, he prefers whiskey and wakes. He is a caricature—more sympathetic than some—of a backward laborer who clings irrationally to the past, a relic from an unfortunate and uncivilized place.

"Young Hibernia" presents a contrasting image. His upright posture and smaller hands suggest his body has not been sculpted by hard labor. His closer-fitting clothing approximates the fashionable style of a Bowery B'hoy dandy. He smokes a cigar, sports a walking stick, and speaks, without an Irish accent, of weddings and champagne. He is oriented toward the future and to new beginnings in this world, rather than toward the past and those moving on to the next. To complete his look, he has an oiled mustache and head of dark curly hair as well as an extraordinarily light and smooth complexion, suggesting use of cosmetics. Whereas the Ancient Hibernian's appearance suggests he would prefer to go unnoticed among strangers, Young Hibernia clearly wants to be seen and recognized as a legitimate player on the urban stage with opportunities for other roles besides "Pat," the Irish immigrant.

The cosmetic hair preparations and perfume bottles found at the Five Points contained substances that Irish immigrants used along with clothing and sometimes corsets or braces to refashion their bodies and their opportunities. Displaying good personal hygiene and style was important, but their goals were not always assimilationist, and they had a range of audiences in mind, from employers to peers to potential

230 Irish Remedies for Relief

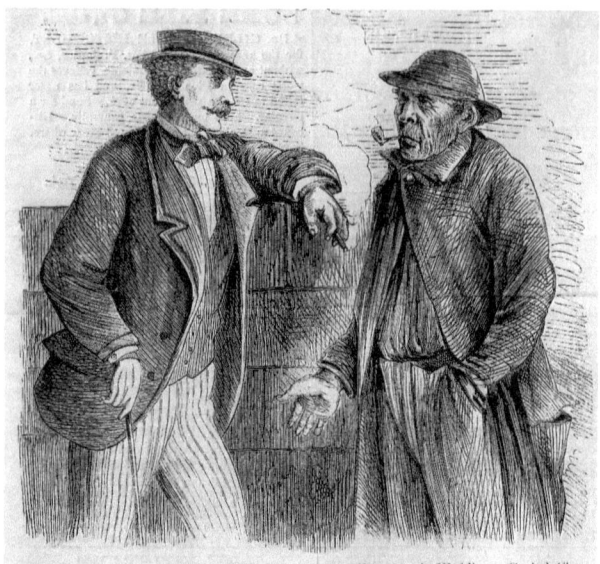

FIGURE 5.8. Cartoon of a young Irish immigrant conversing with an older Irish immigrant (*Harper's Weekly* 1867a:320).

YOUNG HIBERNIA. "Jolly day we had last week at O'Donohue's Wedding. Capital Champagne he gave us, and faith it was justice we did it, I can tell you."
ANCIENT HIBERNIAN (*who prefers a drop of Whisky*). "Widdings is well enough at yer time o' life, but give me a good Ould Wake."

spouses, native born and Irish born and more (see also Linn 2019). These appearance-altering commodities offered a chance to heal the underlying cause of myriad assaults to Irish bodies and minds in urban America: the endless cycle of work and injury. Over time, strategic use of such tools assisted Irish immigrants in discarding the stereotype of the sanguine Irish newcomer—the brutish, brawny, belligerent, bogtrotting, and whiskey-besotted Pat and Bridget—and embodying and expressing identities as complex and cosmopolitan Irish American individuals.

Conclusion

Many Irish immigrants in mid-19th-century New York City found work in jobs requiring physically demanding manual labor. Such work combined with an unfamiliar climate, dangerous conditions, and few workers' protections regularly resulted in bodily damage, ranging from everyday sore muscles to the more serious acute and chronic injuries detailed in the previous chapter. This chapter investigated the strategies that

Irish immigrants employed before seeking professional medical care in order to continue labor that was necessary to sustain their lives.

It suggested new interpretations for archaeological material uncovered from the deposits associated with Irish immigrant residences in the Five Points, viewing particular faunal and floral remains often interpreted as food remains or traces of the surrounding environment as well as household and personal items, such as teacups and tobacco pipes, as evidence of continued access to ingredients used in popular cures in Ireland and potential remains of continued use of such cures in New York City.

This chapter also suggested new interpretations of patent medicines at the same site as not necessarily the remains of low-cost self-medication resorted to out of desperation and alienation from professional medicine, but instead, as new healing options Irish immigrants incorporated into their popular ethnomedical system. Taking types, brands, advertisements, material qualities, and Irish immigrants' perspectives and needs into consideration, suggests that residents of 472 and 474 Pearl Street likely used most of the patent medicines discovered there to relieve pain and injury, either as convenient replacements for popular cures or as new resources to meet the increased physical demands of life and work in New York City.

Additionally recovered were a few bottles of cosmetics that this chapter has proposed were likely not simple reflections of residents' vanity but of attempts to strategically modify their appearances in order to be recognized as complex individuals different from the negative Irish stereotypes that restricted their opportunities. The next chapter will consider how tuberculosis, another affliction that disproportionately beset Irish immigrants, unexpectedly aided this effort.

CHAPTER 6

A Phthisical Paradox

Tuberculosis and the Beginnings of Irish Immigrant Incorporation

TUBERCULOSIS has often been called a "disease of civilization," a term that highlights its long-recognized prevalence in densely populated areas since ancient times (Jones 2001:34; Hayes 2009:156). By the early 19th century, deaths from tuberculosis had reached astonishing levels in industrializing Western cities including London, Paris, and New York; "it was the greatest epidemic killer in the nineteenth-century West," accounting for nearly one-quarter of all deaths (Barnes 1995:4; Hayes 2009:160).[1] Despite the disease's brutality, for much of the 19th century, pulmonary tuberculosis had a romantic reputation as a disease that most often afflicted and further refined sensitive, highly "civilized" individuals. Present-day studies have found that approximately 90% of healthy individuals exposed to tuberculosis will not develop symptoms or active disease, but those whose immune systems are compromised by internal or external factors are highly vulnerable. Thus today, the disease is regarded as a distinctly unromantic, painful, and debilitating infection that most often affects the poorest and most disadvantaged (Farmer 1999).

Suffering from tuberculosis can be a long, torturous battle that draws in family members and friends as caregivers, witnesses, and further casualties, as illustrated by the case of the McPeake family described in the obituary of James McPeake (Figure 6.1). The disease most often killed young adults between the ages of 25 and 40 years old who were in their peak productive years and often left behind vulnerable dependents (Barnes 1995:16; Board of Aldermen 1864:226). This chapter shows that the McPeake family catastrophe was not unique among the Irish in New York City. It was a tragedy that became increasingly prevalent in the

OBITUARY.

Died, on Thursday, the 27th. of August, in the 33d year of his age, after a lingering consumption, JAMES MCPEAKE, third son of John and Rachael McPeake, who emigrated to this country from the county Derry, Ireland, over thirty years ago. His father died in May, 1841, leaving a widow with four children, whom she succeeded in keeping together, until the fell destroyer —Consumption— snatched them from her one by one. Patrick Joseph McPeake, the eldest son, died on the 24th December, 1849, just as he had established a lucrative business in Broadway. Sarah A.C. McPeake, the only daughter, died on the 4th of November, 1854, after a long and painful illness, borne with Christian resignation. Thomas, the youngest, was one of those who sought fortune amidst the newly discovered gold regions of California; and as he has not been heard from for years, his friends have long given him up for dead.

The deceased—who leaves a devoted wife and infant child, in addition to his widowed mother, (who now parts with the last link that binds her to earth) to mourn his untimely loss—was brought up to the painting business, and was gifted in an eminent degree with that energy and tact for with Irish-Americans are remarkable. He was warm-hearted, generous and genial in his disposition, affable in manner, and kind, affectionate and dutiful in his relations of husband, father and son. His demise is deeply felt by his afflicted family, with whom we sincerely sympathise, and by a large circle of friends and acquaintances who universally loved and esteemed him. He was brother-in-law of Wm. L. Cole, of this journal.

His remains were deposited on Sunday last in the family vault, in the Roman Catholic Cemetery in 11th street. May he rest in peace. Amen.

FIGURE 6.1. Typographic Facsimile of James McPeake's Obituary (*Irish American Weekly* 1857:3).

1850s. With so much sickness and death among Irish immigrants in New York, tuberculosis threatened to destroy new Irish American communities and to further incite anti-Irish prejudice. Yet, neither happened. This chapter examines why and teases out the complicated causes and effects of Irish immigrant entanglement with this disease, beginning with an investigation of just how many Irish immigrants might have been afflicted. It suggests that while tuberculosis took a great toll on the Irish community, because of the way this disease was understood by White native-born Americans during the middle of the 19th century, it also helped native-born Americans to see beyond stereotypes and to recognize Irish immigrants as fellow human individuals.

"The Natural Death of the Irish Immigrant"

The diseases native-born Americans most associated with Irish newcomers in mid-19th-century New York City were feared epidemics, most notably typhus fever, a.k.a. the "Irish fever" (Chapter 2) and cholera (Rosenberg 1987a; Kraut 1994, 1995, 1996).[2] Outbreaks of these diseases caused by conditions of immigration claimed many Irish immigrant lives and fueled anti-Irish prejudice, especially in the late 1840s and early 1850s. Work-related injuries from dangerous and strenuous jobs were another major sources of Irish immigrant suffering and mortality from the 1840s through the 1860s (Chapter 4). In 1867, John Hughes, the Catholic Archbishop of New York, identified a new scourge, declaring that "between the ages of 25 and 40, tuberculosis was the natural death of the Irish immigrant" (Stuart 1938:13–14). This section investigates when tuberculosis rates began to increase among the Irish in New York and to what extent this disease afflicted this community. Results suggest that rates rose substantially in the early 1850s and quickly reached epidemic levels, peaking in the 1860s. This is significant because Americans did not seize upon the prevalence of tuberculosis among the Irish to further stigmatize this group. The timing of such high rates of infection also draws attention to living conditions in New York City.

Phthisis at New York City Healthcare Institutions: Rising Rates of Tuberculosis among the New York Irish

Precisely how many Irish immigrants were afflicted with and died from tuberculosis during this period is difficult to determine. In addition to the typical limitations and incompleteness of historical records, there are hurdles caused by how deaths were recorded and how tuberculosis was understood at the time. If a person suffering from consumption died from another cause, their tuberculosis infection was not indicated as the cause of death; conditions understood today to be tubercular were not always identified as such then. Tuberculosis is a complicated disease.

Today we know that *Mycobacterium tuberculosis* can attack almost any part of the body and manifest many different symptoms. It infects the lungs, producing the iconic pulmonary tuberculosis (then called phthisis or consumption), the bones and joints (e.g., Pott's Disease and *morbus coxarius*), eyes (*strumous ophthalmia*), brain (tubercular meningitis), lymph nodes (scrofula), peritoneum (peritonitis), skin (*lupus vulgaris*), small intestines, kidneys, bladder, fallopian tubes, adrenal glands, and more (Dormandy 1999:23–25).[3] Before the discovery of the germ theory, physicians did not understand the cause of tubercular illness or its complicated etiology. Additionally, they sometimes mistook tubercular diseases for other ailments, such as pneumonia, emphysema, lung cancer, pleuritis, or marasmus (Stillé 1994:113).

Tuberculosis also progresses differently depending on which body part and person it affects, adding to the challenge of diagnosis. Tubercular meningitis can cause death within 48 hours, while death from pulmonary tuberculosis can occur within a few weeks to a few decades, with initial infection ranging from asymptomatic to severe (Dormandy 1999:24). Healthy individuals are often successful at walling off the disease, but it can be reactivated by immune system weakening long after initial infection.[4] In its later stages, pulmonary tuberculosis is more distinctive and thus was more likely to have been correctly diagnosed. Symptoms include "obstinate cough, inclination to vomit, oppression of the chest, habitual fever which increases after eating, flushing of the cheeks, general paleness, high pulse, dryness and heat at night (night sweats), looseness of the bowels, loss of weight, loss of hair, swelling of the legs . . . exhaustion," pain, and coughing up of blood (hemoptysis) (Jones 2001:16).

Surviving records from New York Hospital, Bellevue Hospital, the New York Dispensary, and St. Vincent's Hospital together provide more details about tuberculosis among the New York Irish in the middle of the 19th century than offered by municipal or federal mortality records.[5] Case records from New York and Bellevue Hospital show how physicians diagnosed and treated tubercular patients, while annual reports from New York and St. Vincent's Hospitals and the New York Dispensary (Figure 6.2) help to identify when rates of tuberculosis began to rise significantly among the Irish and the extent of the outbreak. During the middle of the 19th century, the two most common diagnoses at New York and Bellevue Hospitals describing conditions we now understand to be caused by *Mycobacterium tuberculosis* were *phthisis* (pulmonary tuberculosis, also popularly called consumption) and *morbus coxarius* ("hip disease"), a tubercular infection of the hip. The number of patients admitted with these diagnoses was relatively low compared with those with some other ailments; it rarely approached even a quarter admitted for fractures at New York Hospital, for example. This is in part because consumptives avoided hospitals, then considered places of last resort, whenever they could and probably because of New York Hospital's policy discouraging admittance of terminally ill patients.[6]

Hospitals and professional physicians did not have much to offer tubercular patients in the mid-19th century. Physicians threw their full medical arsenal at patients to little avail, including bleeding (more rarely after midcentury); toxic purges of antimony or mercury; quinine; inhalations of iodine, creosote, turpentine, and coal gas; external application of iodine; massage with lard and other fats or oils; and surgery to remove necrotic bone for *morbus coxarius* (Dormandy 1999:44–48, 274; Jones 2001:18).[7] Case records from the 1840s and early 1850s show that physicians at New York Hospital typically prescribed purges, expectorants (particularly Stokes Expectorant, named after the famous Irish physician William Stokes), and opiates. By the 1860s, physicians there and at Bellevue Hospital favored a more nurturing approach, prescribing *oleum morrhuae* (cod liver oil), *cinchona* (Peruvian bark), iron, and nutritious diet, along with opiates (NYHMCB 1865; BHMCB 1866–1868, 1873–1875). This change in therapy, as I will show later in this chapter, appears to have been inspired by popular medicine. Despite some promising effects of cod liver oil on early-stage disease (Grad 2004), most 19th-century physicians felt that the "treatment indicated for tuberculosis, as an ancient adage put it, was opium and lies" (Rosenberg 1977:493–494).[8] Case records and annual reports show phthisis patients were almost never discharged as "cured." Some were "relieved," others discharged as incurable or "by request" of the patient. Between one-third and one-half of patients admitted to New York Hospital with tubercular diseases died there (NYHAR 1835–1866; NYHMCB 1847, 1852, 1865).

The number of Irish-born patients treated for phthisis alone each year at New York Hospital, as indicated by annual reports, suggest that tubercular illness began to affect Irish immigrants at rates disproportionate to those of non-Irish New Yorkers just before the Great Famine, and rates increased dramatically in the early 1850s. Figure 6.3 shows that from 1835 until 1843, U.S.-born phthisis patients were more numerous than Irish born (or German born). In 1844, the number of Irish-born

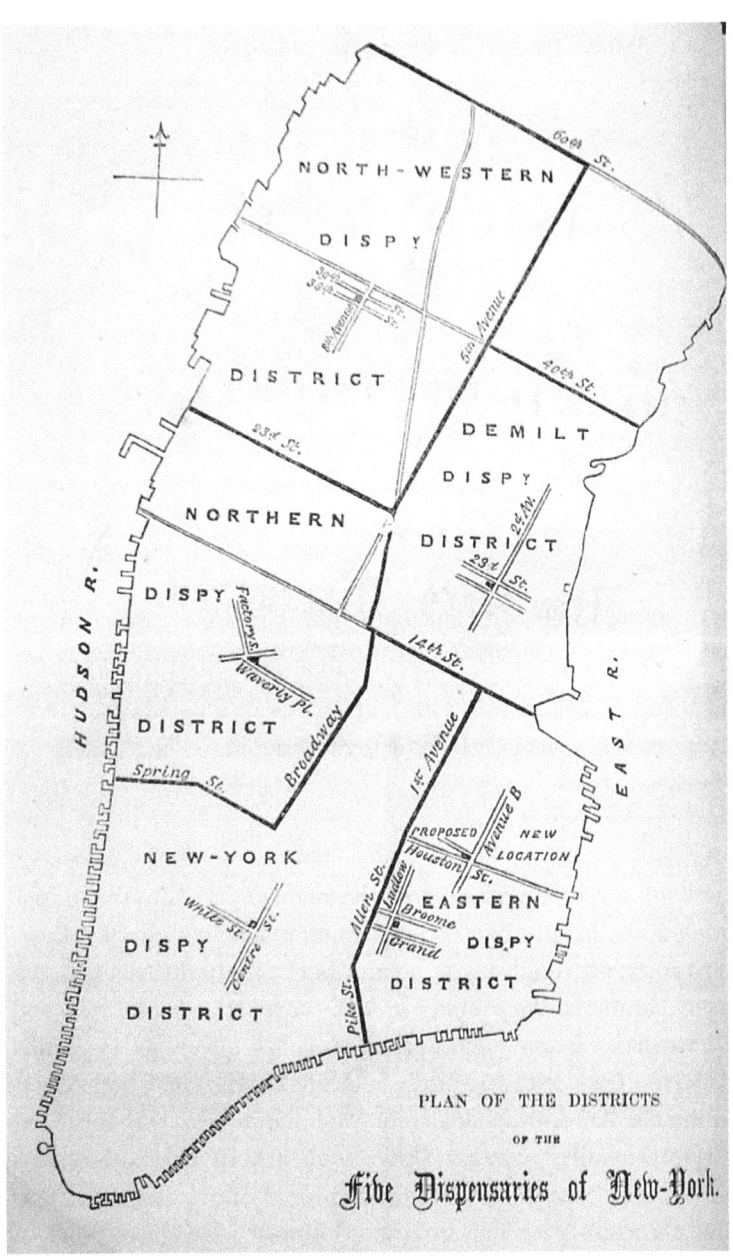

FIGURE 6.2. Plan of the dispensary districts of New York City in 1856 (NYDAR 1857). The New York Dispensary's district in the Sixth Ward was the closest to the Five Points neighborhood and to the McPeake family's residence at 28/30 Wooster Street.

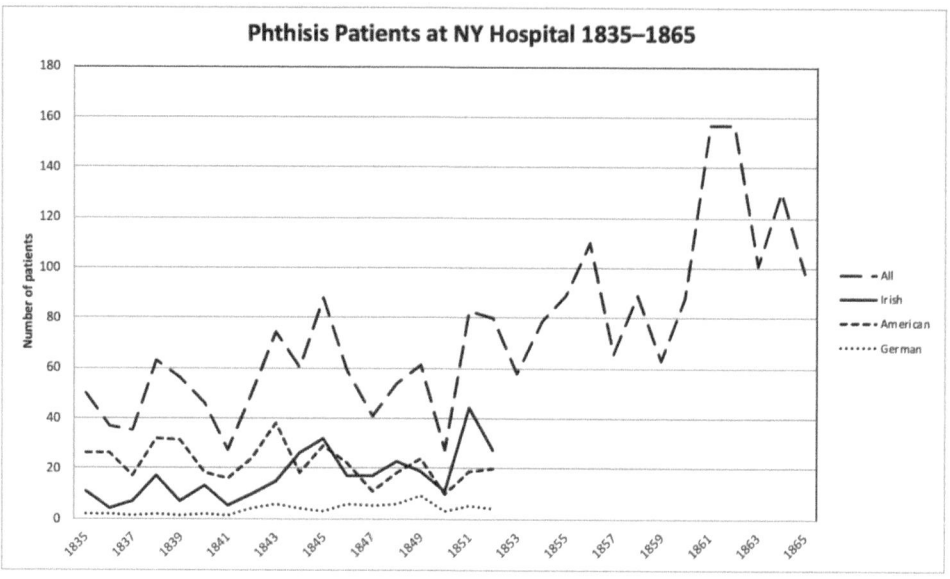

FIGURE 6.3. Graph showing the total number of patients admitted to New York Hospital and diagnosed with phthisis (pulmonary tuberculosis) annually from 1835 to 1865. Also included are numbers of Irish-, German-, and US-born phthisis patients admitted during those same years (Data from NYHAR 1836–1866). After 1852, the hospital's annual reports no longer tabulate diagnoses by patients' countries of origin.

phthisis patients increased, which also elevated the total number of patients treated at the hospital for this condition to a new high the following year. From 1844 through 1850, the number of Irish phthisis patients was relatively similar to the number of U.S.-born patients and followed the same pattern of increases and decreases. This is nevertheless significant, because the Irish made up only about 26% of the city's population in 1850, while the American-born composed about 54%, and Germans about 8% (Rosenwaike 1972:41; Diner 1996:91). In 1851, Irish-born phthisis patients at New York Hospital increased dramatically to more than double those of American origin and almost nine times those of German origin. Irish patients decreased slightly in 1852, but still outnumbered the others. This marked upsurge of Irish patients in the early 1850s compared with a trend of decreased American patients from 1844 on (and a relatively flat rate of Germans) suggests the Irish had embarked on a different tubercular trajectory.

The hospital stopped reporting diagnoses by patients' countries of origin after 1852, but we can assume that this different Irish path substantially contributed to the increase in phthisis admissions overall at New York Hospital between 1851 to 1865 and to the peak in the early 1860s (NYHAR 1836–1866).[9] The Irish also appear to have contributed to increased city-wide mortality from consumption, which crested to nearly 500 per 100,000 in 1854 and again in 1864, after hovering around 425 per 100,000 during the 1840s (Drolet and Lowell 1952:v).

Annual reports from the New York Dispensary (Figure 6.4) also suggest a substantial rise in tubercular illness in the city in the 1850s and 1860s, and similarly point to Irish immigrants as major contributors to this trend. The New York Dispensary treated 639 people (1.6% of all patients) for phthisis in 1856, 895 people (2.2%) the next year, and 1,235 people (3.0%) in 1858. By 1866, the dispensary treated a smaller number of individuals for phthisis (1,154), but they were a greater percentage of the total patient population (3.3%). The dispensary's annual reports do not record diagnoses by patients' countries of origin, but they do indicate the total number of patients treated by countries of birth. During the 1850s and 1860s, Irish-born individuals were the most numerous evaluated at this dispensary and outnumbered the American-born, the second most numerous group, by about 2 to 1 (NYDAR 1856, 1857, 1858, 1866). These figures underestimate the number of patients of Irish descent, because American-born children of Irish immigrants were recorded as U.S.-born. The dispensary was open for only a few hours during the middle of the workday and was frequented most by mothers and children with more flexible work schedules (Rosenberg 1974b:35). The dramatic increase in patients treated for phthisis at the dispensary, nearly doubling between 1856 and 1858, therefore, appears to have been generated by a great increase of this disease within the Irish immigrant community in the Lower Manhattan region served by this dispensary (see Figure 6.2).[10]

The annual reports of St. Vincent's Hospital also help to assess the extent of the outbreak, noting a large number of deaths of phthisis patients at this institution dedicated to serving the Roman Catholic community.

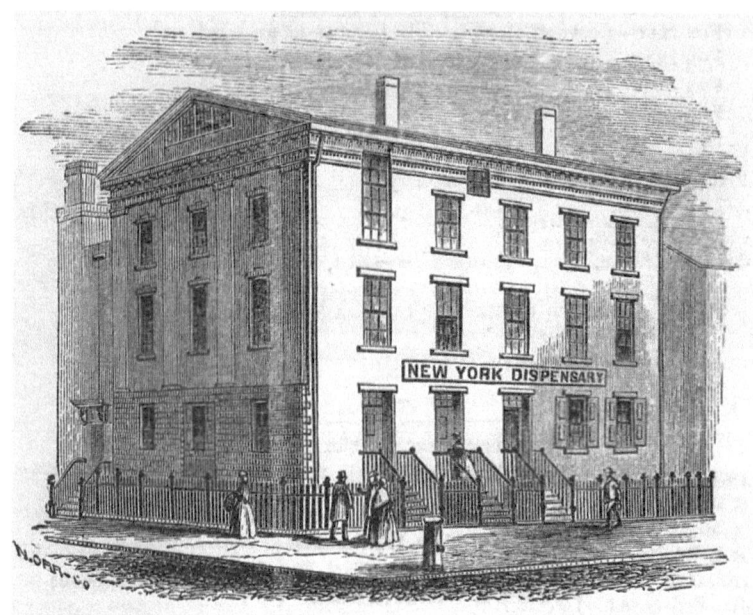

FIGURE 6.4. Illustration of the New York Dispensary on the corner of White and Centre Streets (Valentine 1860:358). Courtesy of Columbia University Libraries.

Dr. William O'Meagher, the editor of the Hospital's annual report for the years 1859 and 1860, explained that death rates were higher than the hospital administration would have liked because "many patients in the last stages of consumption, seek for admission in order to secure for themselves a home for the few remaining days of their lives—to have a place where they can make their peace with God, and quietly and peacefully glide down the stream of life" (SVHAR 1861:12). This statement that Irish Catholic phthisis patients sought out this institution over others is supported by other records. For example, a case record from Bellevue Hospital notes that the friends of Martha, a 19-year-old Irish-born domestic servant with "chronic pneumonic phthisis," asked that she be taken to St. Vincent's (BHMCB 1874:93). The familiar cultural atmosphere, access to priests and sacraments, and the care of the Sisters of Charity were no doubt appealing, although the hospital was small (Walsh 1965).[11] O'Meagher's use of the popular term consumption, instead of medical term phthisis, suggests that the staff at St. Vincent's might have avoided using specialized language that distanced patients, another aspect of the institution that probably appealed to Irish immigrants.

Annual reports from St. Vincent's also corroborate evidence from other institutions suggesting that tuberculosis had become a major affliction within the Irish community in the 1850s, and they additionally suggest rates declined beginning in the 1870s, when mortality from consumption began to decline citywide (Drolet and Lowell 1952:v). Unfortunately, reports from the early 1850s are not available, but phthisis was *the* leading condition for which patients were treated at St. Vincent's during each year available—1859 (107 patients or 22%), 1860 (172 or 29%), 1863 (162 or 22%), 1874 (142 or 16%)—except for 1881 (174 or 9%), when it ranked fourth (SVHAR 1861, 1864, 1875, 1882).[12]

The rarer forms of tuberculosis that appear in St. Vincent's annual reports help to assess the magnitude of the outbreak. Beginning in the early 1860s, more patients appear to have sought care at St. Vincent's than New York Hospital for rarer nonpulmonary forms of tuberculosis.[13] St. Vincent's staff diagnosed patients with tubercular meningitis and cephalalgia (tuberculosis of the brain/meninges), scrofula (of the lymph nodes), *morbus coxarius* (of the hip), *strumous ophthalmia* (of the eyes), and *strumous osteitis* (of the bones, especially the heads of long bones, vertebrae, wrist, and ankle) (SVHAR 1861, 1864).

Epidemiological studies today suggest that only about 10% of individuals with *active* tuberculosis develop tubercular meningitis, 3% to 6% develop tuberculosis of the lymph nodes, and only 1% to 3% develop tuberculosis of the bones or joints and that these nonpulmonary forms are most prevalent among young children and other individuals with weak immune systems (Daniel 1997:25; Malaviya and Kotwal 2003:319; Murthy 2010:716). St. Vincent's treated 10 patients with *morbus coxarius* and 6 with meningitis in 1863 alone (SVHAR 1864).

An even larger number of individuals were treated for *morbus coxarius* as outpatients at the New York Dispensary. The dispensary treated 28 patients in 1856, 25 in 1857, 26 in 1858, and 40 in 1866 (NYDAR 1856, 1857, 1858, 1866). If the present-day incidence of this nonpulmonary form of tuberculosis is projected into the past, it suggests that by 1856, anywhere from 2,800 to 8,400 people within the district served by the Dispensary had active tuberculosis, many more than the 639 seen for phthisis that year at this institution alone. Thus, even relatively small numbers of people infected with rarer nonpulmonary forms of tuberculosis indicate high levels of tuberculosis in the community and poor health among children, a topic that will be further explored in the following section.

These hospital and dispensary records together thus reveal a marked increase in tubercular illness among Irish immigrants, especially those residing near the New York Dispensary in Lower Manhattan, beginning in the 1850s and accelerating in the early 1860s, when admissions of American-born non-Irish patients appeared to have been decreasing. The Irish thus greatly contributed to keeping city-wide consumption mortality rates high, while rates were decreasing in London (Wilson 2005:522).[14] And yet, again, there is no evidence that Americans blamed the Irish for this or otherwise stigmatized them because of tuberculosis during this period. The timing of a city-wide mid-century consumption mortality peak in 1854 is also interesting in that it occurred slightly after the peak years of Irish immigration (1847–1853), as one might expect for newcomers who became consumptive in New York City, instead of arriving with the disease. These records thus suggest that living in New York City was an essential element in Irish immigrants' development of active disease. The next section examines the particular conditions that catalyzed high rates of tuberculosis among the New York Irish, using the McPeake family, whose tragic story was introduced in the obituary at the beginning of the chapter, as a primary example.

Consumptive Conditions

In 1830, the recently arrived McPeake family of eight lived together in a rented apartment in a brick building at 30 Wooster Street (Figure 6.5), on the southeast corner of Grand and Wooster Streets (USBC 1830).[15] By 1840, the family had lost two members, grandmother Allay McPeake and a male infant (*New-York Evening Post* 1830).[16] During the following year, John, the head of the McPeake family and a weaver-turned-grocer, perished from consumption (*Irish American Weekly* 1857:3). At least three of his four surviving children—James, Sarah, Patrick Joseph, and Thomas—succumbed to the same fate within the next 15 years. Where John McPeake was first exposed to tuberculosis is impossible to know. He could have been initially infected in Ireland or on the emigrant ship the *Robert Fulton*, which brought his family to New York City in 1827, and successfully "walled off" the infection for more than a decade in New York City (Passenger Lists 1827). Alternatively, he could have been infected in New York City, where tuberculosis rates were much higher than in Ireland (Jones 2001:36). Either way, it was in New York that John and his children became ill and died.[17] Conditions of life in New York City were an essential catalyst of the McPeake family tragedy and that of other families and individuals who similarly succumbed to tuberculosis.

Initially, the McPeake family had advantages over other Irish immigrants in the city, especially famine-era newcomers. The McPeakes arrived in 1827, when the city was more sparsely populated and there was less anti-Irish prejudice. Although James McPeake's obituary indicates they were Catholic, they were from County Derry in the north of Ireland. There they likely had more exposure to English language and urban life than Irish immigrants from more rural western and southern counties. John McPeake was skilled in weaving, literate in English, and started a grocery business within a few years of his family's arrival (New York Passenger Lists 1827; *Longworth's American Almanac* [*LAA*] 1830:412;

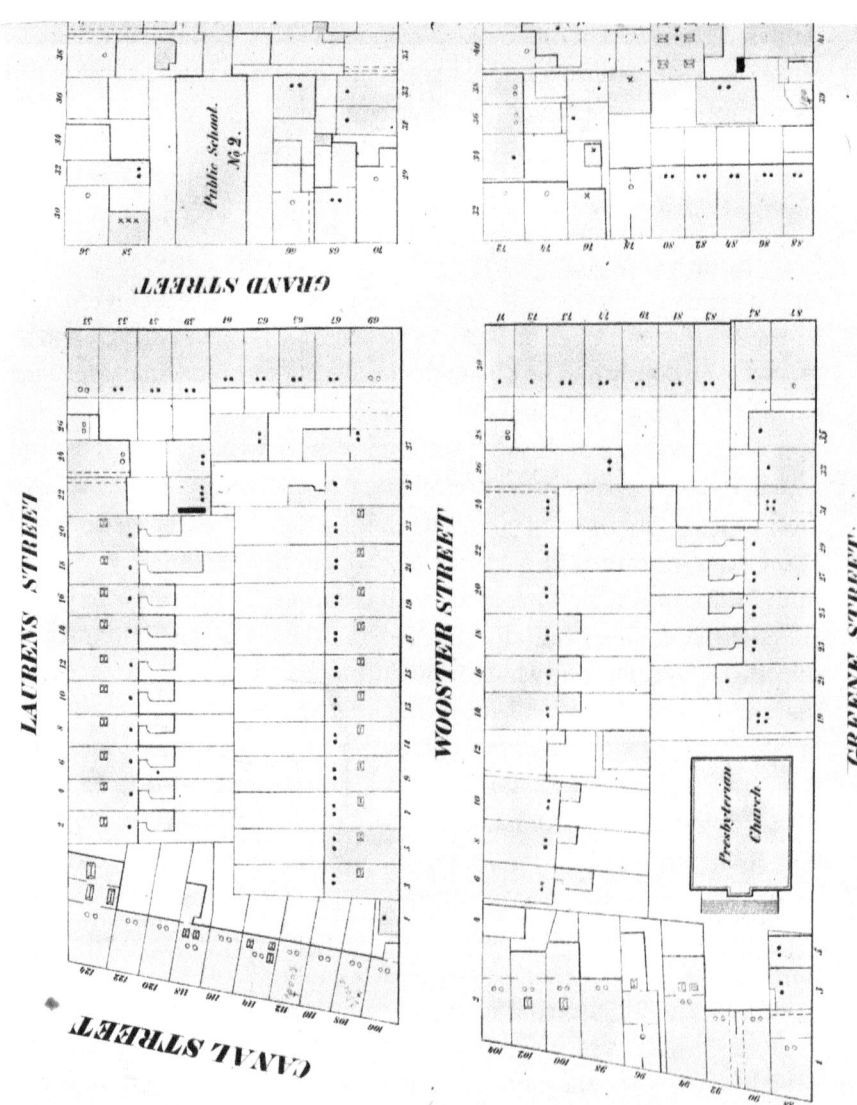

FIGURE 6.5. Section of the Perris Map of 1853. Courtesy of the New York Public Library Digital Collections. City directories indicate that the McPeake family lived at 30 Wooster from 1830 until sometime after John's death when Rachael and the children moved into his former shop next door at 28 Wooster. They lived there until about 1849, and then moved back into 30 Wooster, likely supported by brothers James and Thomas's painting business, then operated from 28 Wooster.

USBC 1840). Rachael, his wife, could not write in English, but she could read it, and might have helped John with the store (NYSC 1855). John's mother, Allay, likely aided in childcare and the healthcare of the family until her death in July of 1830 (*New-York Evening Post* 1830). The family settled in the Eighth Ward, a reasonably attractive part of the city, alongside other working- and middle-class immigrants from Ireland and Germany as well as native-born Americans (USBC 1830).[18] According to the Perris Map (1853:Plate 31), their apartment was in a building solidly constructed of brick with a slate or metal roof, instead of a timber-framed fire trap (see Figure 6.5). Nevertheless, a closer look at the family's living conditions reveals dangers that they shared with other newcomers from their native land, including the residents of 472 and 474 Pearl Street in the Five Points neighborhood. These conditions help to explain why tuberculosis plagued so many of the Irish in 19th-century New York.

HOUSING ENVIRONMENT

Like many other immigrant families, the McPeake household was large. It consisted of four to five children as well as extended family members and/or boarders. Sharing the same quarters with numerous family members was also common in Ireland, where much of the population resided in one- or two-room dwellings.[19] Apartment buildings in New York City were usually even more crowded and lacked the same access to fresh air, however. In 1850, for example, three other families shared 30 Wooster with the McPeakes, totaling 16 residents in the small three-story building (USBC 1850). As the city grew exponentially from migration and immigration in the 19th century, increased pressure was placed on the city's aging housing stock, and people packed more closely together, making it easier for tuberculosis to spread. More than 100 people lived in two brick tenements at 472 Pearl Street, after the rear building was added in the early 1860s (Fitts 2000a:69).

Scientists today believe that sleeping in the same room as a person with active tuberculosis is the most common way the disease spreads (Singh et al. 2005). The main vehicles of person-to-person infection are airborne droplets expelled through coughing, sneezing, speaking, and spitting. Momentary exposure usually does not lead to infection, but extended exposure does; and a single infected person can make many others ill

(Beggs et al. 2003). Sharing the same living, and especially sleeping, quarters was likely the means by which tuberculosis spread through the McPeake family. Dr. B. M. Keeney (1865), the Sanitary Inspector of the McPeakes' former neighborhood in 1864, shared this view of nearly all diseases. He felt that the high rates of illness largely resulted from people crowding into rooms with poor ventilation. The brick tenements were old, small, and crowded, with ventilation that was "entirely insufficient" (Keeney 1865:37). It was not until the Tenement Laws of 1867 and 1879 that much was done on a large scale to address housing ventilation.

Dr. Keeney (1865:41) found exceptionally high death rates from a number of diseases, including pulmonary afflictions, in the southern region of the Eighth Ward, where 28 and 30 Wooster Street were located. He noted the dampness and lack of drainage in this area built upon landfill deposited atop the former marshy Lispenard Meadow. While his particular explanations about the role of rotting organic matter in illness are no longer on the cutting edge of medical science, his observations that constant dampness and filth, including human excrement, clogging the streets and sewers were threats to health are still relevant. With regard to tuberculosis, darkness and dampness increases the lifespan of the bacillus, which can remain suspended in the air for hours (Beggs et al. 2003). Recent studies have also shown that exposure to mold increases rates of respiratory infection and asthma that, in turn, can weaken an individual's immune system and pave the way for tuberculosis (Dales et al. 1991). Similarly, although human waste is not directly involved in tubercular infection, it spreads other diseases, such as typhoid and cholera, that can make survivors more susceptible to opportunistic tuberculosis infection or reactivation.

The natural and built environment in which the McPeakes lived was thus hospitable to infectious disease as was the Five Points neighborhood in the nearby Sixth Ward. That neighborhood was built on the former area of the Collect Pond and its surrounding marsh; it was notorious for its dampness, exacerbated by improperly graded sewers, and privy waste that seeped into basement apartments, as well as high rates of illness. In 1863, the death rate in the Five Points was 1 in 24, three times greater than the city as a whole (Rosenberg 1987a:183). The Five Points was also infamous for its basement dwellings, used most often as lodging houses and apartments for the newly immigrated and the poor.

With few affordable alternatives and often used to semi-subterranean dwellings in Irish townlands—excellent structures for the Irish climate [Scally 1995]—formerly rural Irish might not have initially realized such apartments would be so dangerous.[20] Constant dampness, mold, seeping sewage, lack of disinfecting sunlight, and crowded conditions typical of such apartments—described by Sanitary Inspector of the 4th Ward, Dr. Ezra R. Pulling (1865:49)—made basement apartments veritable petri dishes for the hardy tuberculosis bacillus and a host of other pathogens. No amount of cleaning could make such a space safe. The only remedy was to move to a healthier environment.

INSUFFICIENT WARMTH AND INADEQUATE DIET

When John McPeake died in 1841, the family lost their major earner and likely experienced a period of hardship that contributed to the active tuberculosis infections of the McPeake children. A year after John's death, at least one creditor, a grocer named Stephen Wray, filed a complaint against John's wife Rachael, the executrix of John's will, for repayment of $100, a considerable sum. Rachael and her children did not lose their housing, but the absence of John's grocery business in city directories suggests they were not able to carry it on. The same directories indicate that the family moved from 30 Wooster into the smaller building at 28 Wooster that had housed the grocery, likely to trim their budget (*LAA* 1841; Doggett 1844, 1846, 1848).[21] To pay off debts and afford other necessities, the McPeakes might have used strategies employed by other Irish immigrant families: pawning possessions, including clothing and bedding, purchasing less fuel for heating and cooking, and skimping on food or purchasing discounted food, all of which would have made them more vulnerable to illness.

When Frank Roney, the Irish immigrant ironworker, was unemployed in San Francisco in 1876, his family adopted each of these strategies. He wrote, "While I regret my circumstances, I am aware others are a good deal worse off. I still keep house. Of course, in a poor fashion . . . my wife and children [are] pent up from week to week without a sufficiency of warmth or of warm clothing. They feel the effects of this mode of living, and it begins to tell upon them" (Shumsky 1976:257). Roney's wife was ill several times that year. Extended exposure to cold has been shown to reduce an individual's resistance to illness, giving some support for the Irish folk belief that catching a chill can lead to tuberculosis (Logan 1994:27). The surge of Irish immigrants admitted for phthisis at New York Hospital in 1851 might have been partially influenced by the unusually cold and long winter of 1851–1852. In addition to subjecting those without adequate shelter and clothing to physical hardship, the weather reduced many day-laboring opportunities, and thus wages, while increasing the price of goods and food.[22]

When given the choice between heating and food, available records imply most Irish immigrants chose food.[23] Reliance on sugar, tea, alcohol, and tobacco was a common economizing strategy in American and European cities that propelled work but did not provide adequate nutrition (Hayes 2009:163). There were a variety of foods available in New York City, and archaeological remains at the Five Points as well as immigrant letters and guidebooks indicate that Irish immigrants generally ate more meat and a greater variety of food than they had in Ireland (Stott 1990:139, 180; Milne and Crabtree 2000). Some of what was on offer was not fit for consumption, however. Studies of the city's food markets suggest that some foodstuffs, especially the most affordable provisions, were unsafe and spread illness (Pulling 1865; Baldwin 2012; Lobel 2014; Baics 2016). Swill milk (see Chapter 1), for example, was a major contributor to scrofula—caused by both human and bovine forms of tuberculosis—and other diseases among children (McNeur 2014). Meat from infected cows can also transmit tuberculosis. Gastrointestinal diseases caused by spoiled foods of many kinds produced sickness and death on their own, especially in children, and also contributed to susceptibility to tuberculosis (City Inspector's Department 1855, 1858; Board of Aldermen 1864, 1866).[24]

Sanitary Inspector Dr. Pulling (1865:59) investigated the city's markets and found plenty of causes for concern: "Unwholesome meat, particularly slunk veal [meat from miscarried calf fetuses or sickly newborn calves], is constantly vended and consumed. Piles of pickled herring are exposed to the air till the mass approaches a condition of putridity; and this slimy food, with wilted and decayed vegetables, sausages not above suspicion, horrible pies, composed of stale and unripe fruits, whose digestion no stomach can accomplish, all find ready purchasers." While the doctor's vivid description is not without class bias, the questionable quality of meat and dairy products and the poor condition of unrefrigerated perishable foodstuffs in the city combined with an alarming lack of government regulations cannot be doubted. On Saturday evenings after it sat out all day, marketers discounted food, since the markets were closed on Sunday and it would no longer be sellable on Monday (Figure 6.6). Some peddlers specialized in purchasing less-than-fresh produce from wholesalers to market to the poor for days afterward (Baldwin 2012:113).

Even if consumers did not contract an illness directly from the food they ate, malnutrition from poor or insufficient diet has been identified in recent studies as a tuberculosis risk factor; individuals who are 10% underweight are more than three times more likely to develop tuberculosis as those who are similarly overweight (Daniel 1997:38).[25] Many refugees from the Irish famine arrived underweight and malnourished.

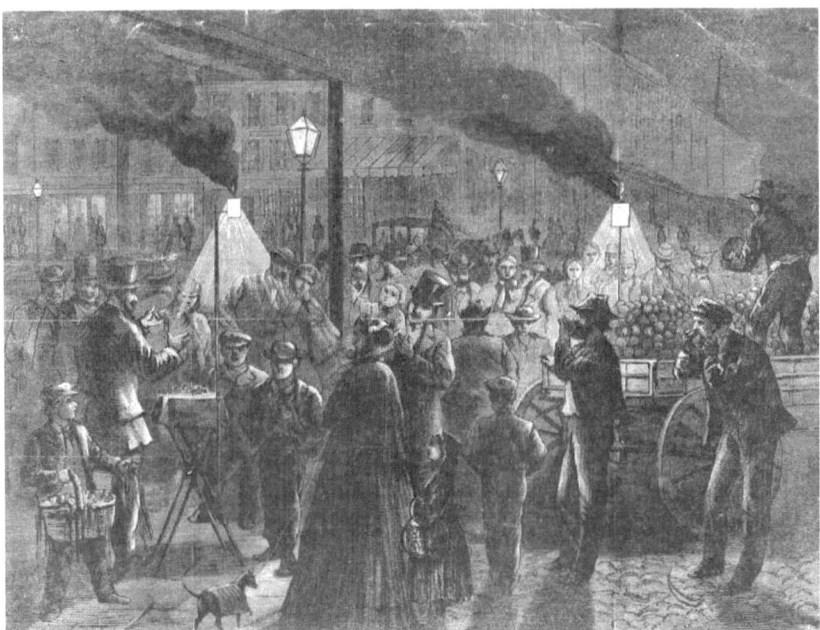

FIGURE 6.6. Illustration of "A Saturday Night Scene in the Bowery, New York," showing hawkers and vendors selling food late into the night at discounted prices (*Harper's Weekly* 1871:469). Courtesy of the New York Public Library Digital Collections.

Living and working conditions in New York City might have kept some from being able to achieve a healthy weight, despite the imagined sturdy build of Pat and Bridget. The case of Ann, an Irish-born 41-year-old dressmaker admitted to Bellevue Hospital in 1874 with phthisis, is an example of how malnourishment can play a significant role in tubercular infection. Upon admission, the doctor found her to be "weak, anemic, and poorly nourished." Ann explained that she "was a strong healthy woman up to seven years [prior]. Since then she has been obliged to work very hard and live poorly and she has not had sufficient food and has gradually lost flesh strength and appetite" (BHMCB 1874:265). Similarly, Philip, a 27-year-old laborer admitted to the same hospital during the same year had recovered from a cough that began the previous fall but fell ill again because he was "out of employment and lived very poorly . . . sleeping in an unoccupied house" (BHMCB 1874:268). As these cases illustrate, poor living conditions, insufficient food, and loss of income made many Irish immigrants more susceptible to tuberculosis. Ann's case additionally highlights tuberculosis-related risks of strenuous, low-paying jobs.

OVERWORK AND DANGEROUS WORK

The period of adversity the McPeake family appears to have endured after John's death in 1841 likely also necessitated more work from each of the surviving family members. The eldest son, Patrick Joseph, was about 19 years old and the only male child of legal age at the time. He is absent from city directories until shortly before his own death from "consumption" in 1849, just after he had established a business selling "looking glasses" [mirrors] on Broadway and two years after his younger brothers James and Thomas established a painting business (Doggett 1849; *Irish American Weekly* 1857:3). It is possible that after his father's death much of the responsibility of supporting the family fell on Patrick Joseph, initially forcing him to take a variety of day-laboring jobs that wore him down—as it wore down other Irish men (see Chapter 4)—and contributed to active tuberculosis infection.

Among male patients treated for phthisis at New York and Bellevue Hospitals, the most common occupation was that of laborer or longshoreman (NYHMCB 1847, 1852, and 1865; BHMCB 1866–1868; 1873–1875).

Other well-represented occupations were painters, printers, and metalworkers (including blacksmiths and refiners), jobs that were dubbed the "dusty trades," because of the lung-irritating airborne particulates to which workers were regularly exposed. Stonecutting, carpentry, masonry, lens grinding, engraving, and linen manufacturing (in which John McPeake had been engaged in Ireland) are other occupations that are also considered dusty trades. Such trades are known today to have high rates of respiratory diseases among workers that, in turn, raise risks of developing active pulmonary tuberculosis and increase the severity of the infection (Cohen 1989:167; Jones 2001:17, 42, 70). Lead poisoning, common among painters (like James and Thomas McPeake) in the 19th century, also could increase susceptibility to tuberculosis, because lead negatively interferes with the immune system (Dietert and Piepenbrink 2006). Data compiled by the Workers Health Bureau in the early 1920s found that painters died from lead poisoning more often than other workers and that their rate of death from tuberculosis was double that of carpenters (Zausner 1941:135). John and Rachael McPeake's sons were only three of thousands of Irish immigrant men employed in types of work that put them at greater risk of active tubercular infection. Census records show that between 1850 and 1870 about 30% of the adult male residents of tenements at 472 and 474 Pearl Street were engaged in the strenuous positions of laborers or porters, and many others were involved in dusty trades, including seven carpenters and one carpenter's apprentice, three coopers, three tinsmiths, and one coachmaker, marble cutter, mason, printer, blacksmith, brass turner, cutler, and glasscutter (USBC 1850, 1860, 1870).

Pulmonary tuberculosis was also observed to be prevalent among seamstresses, tailors, shoemakers, and those in other trades involving indoor work in factories, sweatshops, or apartments. An anonymous contributor to the *Boston Medical and Surgical Journal* proposed in the 1830s that the "sedentary, bent position, and great exercise of the upper extremities" was the cause, but it is more likely that a germ-laden, poorly ventilated environment combined with insufficient diet and rest were the real catalysts (Feldberg 1995:30). Next to laborer, tailor was the most common occupation of Irish-born men treated for phthisis in the records surveyed from New York and Bellevue Hospitals; several seamstresses were treated as well (NYHMCB 1847–1853, and 1865; BHMCB

1866–1868;1873–1875).[26] Between 1850 and 1870, a number of Irish-born residents of 472 and 474 Pearl Street were occupied in this constellation of trades. There were at least eight tailors, nine seamstresses/tailoresses, one dressmaker, one artificial flower maker, three sailmakers, two capmakers, two milliners, and five shoemakers (USBC 1850, 1860, 1870). A close examination of census records shows that, along with washing laundry and taking in boarders, sewing was among the most common occupations recorded for widowed women and half-orphaned daughters residing in these buildings.

Domestic service was another occupation well represented among Irish immigrant women in New York, as discussed in previous chapters. Phthisis rates among domestic servants in the late 19th and early 20th centuries in Dublin, Ireland, were lower than among other working-class women. Historian Greta Jones (2001:77) explains this trend as a result of superior wages and living environment. Domestic servants who boarded in their employers' houses tended to have better quality housing, food, and clothing than other working-class women, as these resources were supplied or gifted by their comparatively wealthy employers. They might also have had less exposure to tuberculosis because of lower rates of tuberculosis among the wealthy (Dubos and Dubos 1952:98). In New York City, wages of domestic servants were also significantly higher than those of most other female workers, and some enjoyed the other benefits Jones describes (Stansell 1987:157; Stott 1990:62–63; Ó Gráda 2005:8). Hospital records from New York and Bellevue Hospitals, nevertheless, show that Irish domestic servants in New York City frequently fell ill with phthisis, particularly those who were under the age of 25 or over the age of 40 (NYHMCB 1847, 1852, 1865; BHMCB 1866–1868, 1873–1875). Most gave case histories of continuing to work until they were so ill that they were no longer able. Performing the strenuous labor required of domestic servants might have hastened the progression of the disease. Aimee, a 21-year-old Irish-born domestic, for example, had a cough for three years before it became so severe that she had to stop working. Aimee's condition was so advanced that she passed away only seventeen days after she was admitted to Bellevue (BHMCB 1867:145). Had she been able to afford to take a break from her job earlier in her illness, she might have been able to keep tuberculosis at bay for several more years or even decades.

DEMOGRAPHICS: AGE AND GENDER

One of the many tragic aspects of the McPeake family's history is the young ages at which John and Rachael's children perished, in the prime years of their lives. Pulmonary tuberculosis was a leading killer of young adults, not just the very young and the very old, the age groups typically most vulnerable to disease (*Science* 1885:35; Barnes 1995:9; Jones 2001:16). Sickness and death of young adults puts great strain upon communities, since they are often the most energetic contributors and the caretakers of parents, siblings, and children, putting all at greater risk with their loss. The demographic trends of mid-century Irish immigration, with family members of various ages (including children and older adults) emigrating together during the famine and mostly young adults (and slightly more women than men) just after the famine, meant that by the late 1850s and early 1860s, the Irish community in New York City was largely composed of young adults, a sizable number of very young children, and a smaller but significant number of adults of advanced age. The demographics of the tenements at 472 and 474 Pearl Street are consistent with this description (USBC 1850, 1860, 1870).

Consumption mortality rates in the U.S. during the 19th century were generally higher for young women than for young men until the 1880s, when the situation reversed and young men perished at higher rates. Both of these trends have puzzled historians. Some now believe that the high female tuberculosis mortality rates do not necessarily mean that women were more susceptible than men, but that men were more likely to die from other causes, such as the work-related accidents described in Chapter 4 (Barnes 1995:9; Smith 2008:31). Whether or not they were more susceptible, there were a number of tuberculosis-related health risks more common among or particular to women. These include the additional domestic labor that traditional roles demanded of women, even if they also worked for wages outside of the home (Stansell 1986; Foner 1999). This "second shift" (Hochschild and Machung 1989) made it—and still makes it—difficult for many working-class women to attain adequate rest and nutrition. In the 19th century, this labor included cooking over stoves or fires and tending them for heating, subjecting women more often to this lung-irritating smoke. Women were also expected to take lead roles in caring for the sick, increasing their exposure to contagious disease. In addition, in households without enough food, studies suggest that women more often than men sacrificed their own portions for their children or other family members (Hayes 2009:163). It is possible that some of these factors contributed to Sarah McPeake's demise.

Other stressors on women's bodies were pregnancy and infant nursing (Jones 2001:68; Smith 2008:44). The needs of growing fetuses and infants require a mother to consume more calories to maintain health, which was not always possible for poor women. Tuberculosis also caused miscarriages and stillbirths, which put both physical and emotional strain on mothers, additionally reducing the efficacy of their immune systems. Immigrant women on average bore more children and lost more children to disease than White native-born women in the 19th century.[27]

By the early 1860s, children of immigrants were 10 times more likely to die by the age of 20 than children of native-born parents (Blackmar 1995:57). A census taker in the Five Points in 1860 remarked that the vast majority of the 414 childless families he visited had not chosen to be so; their children had died, sometimes two or three children in the same family (Groneman Pernicone 1973:60). In the Sixth Ward in 1864, Sanitary Inspector William F. Thoms M.D. (1865:82) also found "fearfully high" child mortality. "Many families have lost all of their children, others four out of five or six. The proportion of still-births, also, is almost unparalleled."

Case records from New York City hospitals provide examples of individual women who endured multiple childbirths and child deaths. Margaret, a 50-year-old Irish widow and domestic servant who succumbed to phthisis at Bellevue Hospital, told her physician that she had borne nine children, and all were dead but one (BHMCB 1874:635). Another woman of the same age who also died of phthisis was the "mother of four children, three alive and healthy and one died of whooping cough," and she had had five miscarriages (BHMCB 1874:254). Losing adult children might have been as or even more traumatic than younger ones, whose lives were understood to be more fragile. James McPeake's obituary hints at the suffering of "his widowed mother," who "now parts with the last link that binds her to earth" (*Irish American Weekly* 1857:3). Rachael's death less than four years later might have been hastened by heartbreak.

The large numbers of American-born children in the Irish community in New York, as well as the continual stream of new immigrants with little prior exposure to the disease, were new hosts for tuberculosis, enabling it to remain at epidemic levels in the community for many years. Children have weaker immune systems than adults and are more likely to develop extrapulmonary forms of tuberculosis. Case records from New York Hospital show the majority of patients admitted for *morbus coxarius* were Irish-born children, such as 12-year-old Peter. Peter had previously suffered from pain in his hip, but it had improved until he contracted a case of measles. The hip pain then returned and was so severe that he could not straighten his leg. He was treated with counter-irritation, cathartics, and rest, and he became well enough to go home (NYHSCB 1852:C539). Other children were not as lucky. Tubercular infection of the joint can destroy the femoral head and hip socket, a horribly painful problem with a terrible prognosis in the 19th century.[28]

Individuals of more advanced age within the Irish community in New York, including Rachael McPeake, as well as several residents of 472 and 474 Pearl Street (Chapter 3), were also vulnerable to tuberculosis. Weakening of the immune system is part of the aging process, and each year brings increased risk. Mortality rates among older men were higher than among older women in the U.S. and Europe, as well as in New York City specifically.[29] Historian Greta Jones (2001:78) suggests that men had more repeated exposure because they remained longer in the labor market. This trend was thus also entwined with class. Those who could not afford to retire or shift to less demanding or hazardous jobs were more likely to become ill.

In the sample of phthisis patient records surveyed from New York and Bellevue Hospitals, nearly twice as many Irish women than men over 50 were admitted, but approximately 80% of male patients died in the hospital versus 50% of female patients. The occupations of these men fit the profile of strenuous and/or dangerous labor, including laborers, longshoremen, and tailors. The women were predominantly widows and unmarried domestic servants (NYHMCB 1848, 1852, 1865; BHMCB 1866–1868;1873–1875). High rates of death from tuberculosis and work-related accidents (see Chapter 4) among older men help explain the preponderance of older Irish women in the Irish community, a pattern also observed in the demographics of 472 and 474 Pearl Street. Census records show Irish female residents of 472 and 474 Pearl Street in the Five Points aged 50 and over outnumbered men of the same age group 23 to 12 between 1850 and 1870. Only 4 of those 23 women were living with husbands, 7 headed households with children, 4 were grandmothers living with family, and the rest were boarders (NYSC 1855; USBC 1850, 1860, 1870). Rachael McPeake also outlived her husband and all her children, dying at the age of 68 on June 1, 1861 (New York City Municipal Death Records 1861).

In addition to age- and gender-related demographics, the regions in Ireland from which the majority of famine-era Irish immigrants who settled in Lower Manhattan wards originated contributed to their susceptibility to tuberculosis. As will be further explained later in the chapter, these regions had low rates of tubercular infection, meaning residents had little exposure or immunity (Breathnach and Moynihan 2003:151; Hayes 2009:164). In summary, the age- and gender-related demographics of the Irish community in New York City are another set of factors that contributed to high rates of tuberculosis among Irish immigrants from the 1850s through the 1860s. Reasons do not end there, however. There are also cultural factors that increased their risk, factors that Americans could have used to stigmatize the Irish as tubercular, had they understood the disease differently.

CULTURAL PRACTICES: SOCIALITY AND SOCIAL DRUGS

The cultural practices that the Irish had long used to sustain individuals and communities—smoking, drinking, and offering hospitality—likely contributed to the high incidence of tuberculosis among immigrants to New York City. While none of these practices are unique to the Irish, they were of particular importance to them and were at times more prevalent among them than among native-born Americans.

In the 19th century, smoking was a popular practice among working-class people for socializing and to stave off fatigue and hunger, and they projected identities and loyalties through pipe decoration (see Chapter 5). Irish men and women smoked pipes in New York and in Ireland. In Ireland, pipe smoking among elders was also seen as an honor they had earned. It was also an important substance at Irish wakes (Figure 6.7), where mourners smoked and drank whiskey to honor the dead and console themselves and one another (Ó Crualaoich 1998:184). An informant explained to folklore collector S. P. Ó Piotáin (NFC 1935[227]:92–93): "It was the blessed Virgin that was the first

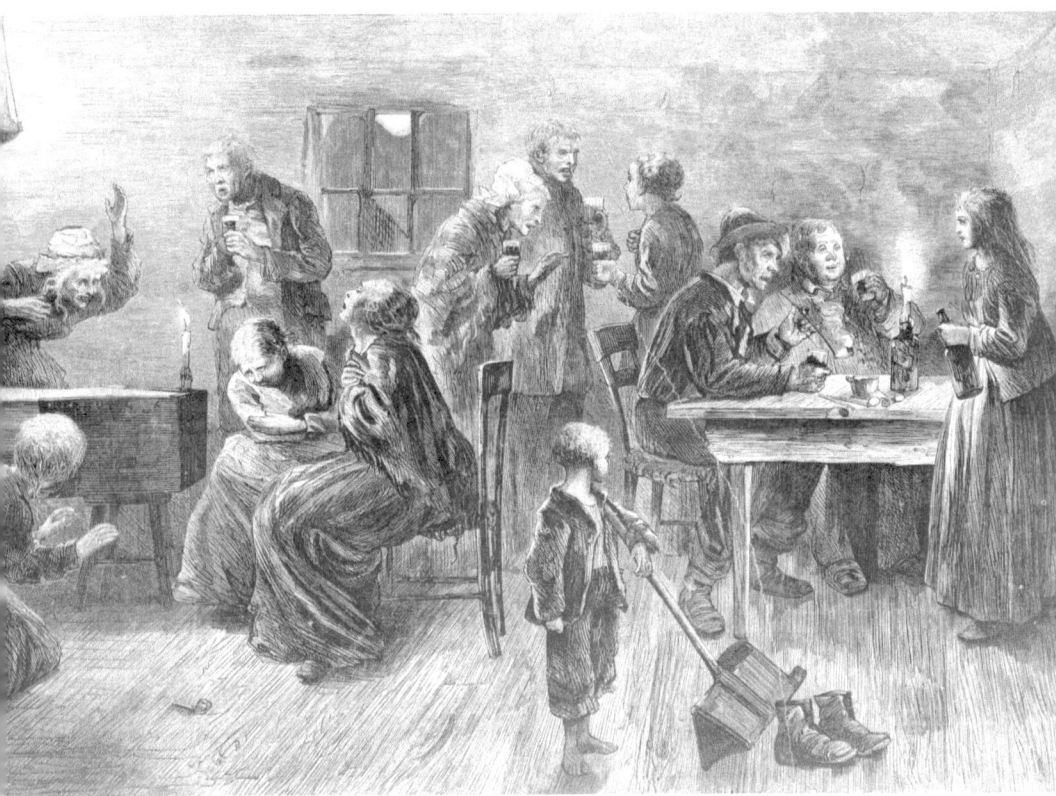

FIGURE 6.7. Illustration titled "An Irish Wake—From a sketch by M. Woolf" (*Harper's Weekly* 1873a:204). Courtesy of the Library of Congress.

to have tobacco at a wake and for that reason people has it ever since. She was terrible sorry and broken hearted the day her son was crucified and for comfort she got a pipe and 'tobaccy' and took the first few draws herself." Ó Piotáin further noted, "Whether you are a smoker or a non-smoker, it is right, according to custom to take a few 'draws' out of a pipe you get at a wake house; and say in an undertone 'The Lord have mercy on the dead.' On several occasions I have seen young ladies light their pipes and just take three draws." As mentioned in the previous chapter, the Irish also used tobacco to alleviate headaches and toothaches and to poultice wounds.[30] Irish immigrants brought these traditions to New York City. Despite these positive cultural meanings and uses, smoking tobacco also likely contributed to tuberculosis infection in the Irish community, jeopardizing the health of smokers as well as those subjected to secondhand smoke. Contemporary studies have shown that pulmonary tuberculosis is among the many respiratory problems that tobacco smoking exacerbates. It is also thought to induce reactivation of prior infection (Davies et al. 2006; Yen et al. 2014).

Alcoholic beverages played even more important roles in Irish social and economic life in Ireland and in New York City, and were used as medicines, as described in previous chapters.[31] They were also substances that some imbibed in excess to manage or escape difficult and/or heartbreaking conditions. A sanitary officer recorded one Irish-born mother's explanation for immoderate drinking, for example. He encountered her living in a dismal rear tenement, and she explained, "If you lived in this place, you would ask for whiskey instead of milk" (Maguire 1868:228). Like smoking, habitual alcohol consumption is also understood today to contribute to active tubercular disease and it too was probably a factor in the high levels of tuberculosis among the Irish (Lönnroth et al. 2008). The heavy involvement of many Irish men, such as John McPeake, in liquor businesses gave them even easier access to alcohol for personal and social use. Additionally, in positions such as grocers and saloon-keepers, these men would have come into regular contact indoors with many Irish immigrants daily, some of whom were most certainly in poor health, exposing them and their families to illness.

Sharing tobacco and alcohol—as well as other objects and favors—, nevertheless, was an essential aspect of the Irish social and moral code that required collectivity and reciprocity. This code was shaped by rural conditions and valuable in urban areas as well. Proper hosting required presenting tobacco, whiskey or beer, tea, or food to guests, while proper guest behavior required accepting what was offered. Refusal to offer or accept signaled lack of desire to enter into or continue a social relationship; this would have jeopardized subsequent requests for aid and perhaps suggested an embrace of English-influenced Protestant, capitalist individualism and a rejection of Irish Catholic collective values and identity. Some Irish immigrants recoiled at American notions of individuality. Maryann Tetherston (1864) wrote home to Ireland, for example, "I cannot remain in afford [*sic*] (foreign) country like this where people can make themselves comparatively independent of everyone." Collective values, along with the pressures of anti-Irish prejudice, contributed to a desire to interact mainly with likeminded countrymen and women, partially explaining so-called Irish "clannishness." These Irish social values would have obligated John McPeake to extend to Irish neighbors goods from his grocery store on credit, or risk being ostracized. Such favors ideally would have earned him friends who he could call upon in times of need. Nevertheless, because poor health and misfortune were so common within the Irish community, especially by the 1840s, it is possible that the inability of some friends to repay their debts contributed to John's own financial debts at the time of his death. These debts put more strain on his widow and their children, but it is likely they, in turn, got by with the help of others.[32] Similarly, James McPeake's own widow and infant daughter were helped by the "large circle of friends and acquaintances who universally loved and esteemed" this "generous... and kind" man, including William L. Cole, his brother-in-law and author of his obituary (Figure 6.1).

Some Irish immigrants were attracted to temperance, advocated by both middle-class White native-born American reformers and some Catholic leaders—most notably the Irish priest Father Theobald Mathew—, but whiskey drinking and tobacco smoking and sharing these substances with a large circle of friends and acquaintances remained important within the Irish community in New York. Such practices created vital networks of assistance and belonging among Irish immigrants in New York City, but present-day understanding of tuberculosis suggests such practices also helped to spread the disease along these networks. These practices likely caused or hastened the deaths of *individuals* and even families, but they, nevertheless, appear to have enabled the long-term survival of the Irish American *community* in New York City, as will be discussed further in the next chapter.

RIPE FOR STIGMATIZATION

In summary, given what we now know about tubercular disease today, it is not surprising that it afflicted Irish immigrant families like the McPeakes in 19th-century New York City. The living conditions that the majority of immigrants could afford were extremely hospitable to *Mycobacterium tuberculosis*. The necessity to labor incessantly for wages, and the strenuousness or outright dangerousness of most available jobs, made workers less likely to be able to fend off the bacteria that was nearly everywhere in the city. Milk and meat from sick cows was another source of infection, and the spoiled and inferior foods most accessible to the laboring poor led to food poisoning and malnourishment that can catalyze and exacerbate active tuberculosis infection. The age and gender-related demographics of the Irish immigrant population, especially when combined with the working-class status of the majority, made them a population ripe for this infection. Finally, whiskey drinking, tobacco smoking, and offering hospitality to guests, some of the very cultural practices that the Irish relied on to build vital social ties, provide economic support, and offer comfort for the sick and the traumatized, contributed to tubercular illness as well.[33]

High rates of tubercular illness among the Irish could not have escaped the notice of their American-born neighbors or the physicians who treated them at city hospitals and dispensaries. *Yearly* deaths from consumption in New York City between 1850 and 1870 outnumbered total deaths from the infamous 1832 cholera epidemic and were two to three times more than the yearly deaths from typhus fever during the epidemic years of 1847 and 1851. Given how Americans responded to typhus epidemics in the late 1840s and early 1850s, blaming Irish immigrants for the disease and using typhus to support ideas about essential Irish difference and inferiority, one might think that Americans would have responded similarly to the disproportionate suffering of Irish immigrants from tuberculosis. If typhus fever was the "Irish fever" in the eyes of Americans, caused by inferior Irish constitution and character and irresponsible Irish practices (such as drinking and smoking and living in "dirty hovels"), Americans could have regarded tuberculosis as a "Paddy phthisis" with similar roots. Tuberculosis could have further destroyed the reputation as well as the health of the Irish in New York City. Remarkably, however, it elicited a different reaction from Americans, one that can only be understood by examining Americans' incompatible conceptions of tubercular illness and Irishness in the 1850s and 1860s.

The Unnatural Death of Irish Immigrants: The Incompatibility of Irishness and Consumption

In the late 1840s when Irish immigrants began to arrive in large numbers, those among them suffering from fever elicited strong negative reactions from native-born New Yorkers. New Yorkers avoided contact with them in public places, refused them lodging, detained them on ships in the harbor, ordered them to hospitals, and even burned down the Quarantine Hospital on Staten Island. This physical and social distance, combined with typhus's symptoms, contributed to Americans' essentialization of the Irish as a naturally different and lesser group of people (see Chapter 2). In contrast, when Irish immigrants fell ill with tubercular disease, New Yorkers did none of these things. The absence of such actions suggests that New Yorkers did not see the increasing number of Irish consumptives as cause for alarm or proof of Irish difference. Instead, in this section, I propose that, to New Yorkers, the death of Irish immigrants from consumption was *unnatural*, or at least unexpected. To them, consumption was an urban disease that targeted individuals with qualities that were the exact opposite of those they believed the Irish possessed. The incongruity between New Yorkers' ideas about the typical consumptive and the typical Irish immigrant caused them to question their views about the latter.

Consumption as a Part of Urban Life

Although deeply destructive, dreaded, and long misunderstood, tubercular disease was unlike cholera or typhus fever in that it was neither new nor rare among the native-born population of 19th-century New York City. Tuberculosis had been the leading cause of death in New York City since at least 1804, before the McPeakes immigrated and well before famine-era Irish arrived.[34] Consumption was not only a leading cause of death in the 19th century, but also a "formative influence" on life that could not be reasonably attributed to the Irish (Dormandy 1999:12).

Tubercular disease was so prevalent in 19th-century cities that nearly every urban resident would have been exposed to the disease and would have known someone who suffered from it (Barnes 1995:4). Although it was long recognized to claim the most lives among the poor, tuberculosis cut across age, class, gender, religion, and ethnicity. A popular saying in the late 19th century was that "everyone is some time or another a little bit consumptive" (Ott 1996:1). Because of this, it did not incite the same kind of fear as typhus fever, with which New Yorkers had had little experience until the 1840s. Consumption was feared, but it was familiar, and seen as an almost inevitable aspect of urban life.

Another factor that distinguished pulmonary tuberculosis (the most common form) from typhus fever and many other epidemic diseases was its relatively slow progression. This feature of the disease informed the names most often used to describe it: phthisis (from the Greek "to waste away") and consumption. The prolonged time span aided some patients, and their families and friends, to come to terms with mortality. After suffering from "long and painful illness[es]," that could last years or decades, some consumptives, like Sarah McPeake, were able to bear the disease "with Christian resignation" (*Irish American Weekly* 1857:3). Sudden epidemic diseases, such as typhus fever, conversely, caused death within hours or days, leaving little time for contemplation, and left survivors in shock. Because of their suddenness and deadliness, epidemic diseases tend to elicit greater social and psychological responses than their overall death rates would suggest (Condran 1995).

Tubercular disease elicited social responses, but ones that were less reactionary and more independent of Irish immigrants. It was such a regular part of 19th-century urban life that it informed broader cultural attitudes toward both life and death (Sontag 2001). As pathologist and medical historian Thomas Dormandy (1999:12) writes, "For a century and a half it became a formative influence in art, music, and literature ... it compelled doctors to question the very purpose of their calling—or its lack of purpose. It mocked statesmen and social reformers. It challenged the churches and the agnostic scientific establishment equally." From our perspective today, much of how tuberculosis was understood in the 19th century was incorrect, but it nevertheless had significant social and cultural implications that ultimately helped to change Americans' views of Irish immigrants.

Misunderstanding Consumption's Contagion

In 1882, the German scientist Robert Koch identified *Mycobacterium tuberculosis* to be the source of pulmonary tuberculosis. This was a landmark discovery that, over the following three decades, helped to convince physicians of the germ theory of disease. In the decades before Koch's breakthrough, as well as the one immediately after, however, most physicians' conceptions of consumption did not differ much from those of physicians for the two millennia prior. Most then believed that consumption was not a contagious disease but instead resulted from the conjunction of two elements, "exciting causes" and a heritable condition. Given the complicated nature of tubercular infection and the demise of entire families, such as the McPeakes, the noninfectious thesis was not as unreasonable as it might sound today. It also had the result of reducing fear and stigmatization of consumptives.

As related previously, tuberculosis's most common manifestation is pulmonary, but it can affect nearly every organ. Tuberculosis was often mistaken for other diseases and vice versa, making the etiology of the disease difficult to discover. It was widely observed that individuals who nursed consumptive relatives often later suffered from the affliction themselves, but some, such as Rachael, the matriarch of the McPeake family, appeared to escape unscathed (Bowditch 1994b:52). Doctors and nurses attending to patients with phthisis also frequently remained healthy, whereas many perished attending typhus and cholera patients in New York City alone (Commissioners of Emigration 1861:83, 111). Thus, even attentive observation suggested a predisposition was especially significant in tubercular illness.

Most physicians in Northern Europe and the U.S. throughout the 19th century vigorously insisted that tuberculosis was not contagious (Rosenberg 1974a:163; Barnes 1995:42-46).[35] Health inspectors did not reject immigrants at landing depots in the U.S. for being consumptive, even later at Ellis Island (est. 1892), where evidence of contagious disease was a leading reason for nonadmittance (Kraut 1996:156). The New York City Health Department did not add tuberculosis to the list of communicable diseases until 1897 (Fee and Hammonds 1995:177). Instead, most physicians during the middle and late 19th century believed, like their ancient Greek and Roman predecessors, that only people with a particular heritable constitutional predisposition to the disease, a "consumptive diathesis," fell ill from tuberculosis.

Although there were different hypotheses about the particular mechanisms of the disease, belief in a required heritable predisposition held sway throughout the 19th century (Rosenberg 1974a:167; Grad

2004:106–107). Virtually every tubercular patient had a consumptive relative, making heredity impossible to rule out (Bowditch 1994b). Medical case records from Bellevue Hospital (1866–1867;1873–1874) and the New York Orthopaedic Hospital and Dispensary (1870–1873) regularly solicited information about a patient's family history of consumption.[36] The idea of a heritable consumptive constitution hung on even after scientific experiments suggested contagion, because it satisfied people on both sides of the political spectrum. For those who retained conservative Puritanical beliefs in sickness as a divine punishment, heredity helped to explain why so many innocent children were afflicted; they suffered because of the mistakes of their parents or other ancestors. As medical historian Charles Rosenberg (1974a:167) writes, "In the post-Darwinian years especially, a surprising variety of articulate Americans found in heredity a plausible mechanism with which to restate in appropriately secular form a lingering commitment to 'original sin.'" For those who were more liberal, the heritable diathesis thesis protected the afflicted. There were some physicians who refused to entertain in public the idea that consumption was contagious, for fear that it would lead to social unrest, turning family members against one another and inciting prejudice against the vast number of tuberculosis sufferers (Hayes 2009:171).

Most physicians thus were committed to the idea that a heritable diathesis, catalyzed by "exciting causes" including bad air, dirt, dust, irritation of lung, lack of exercise, and poor diet, led individuals to develop consumption. Some even initially insisted that the bacillus Koch discovered was merely a more specific "exciting cause." Thus, Irish immigrants suffering from this disease were not considered to be contagious threats to public health, but individuals who, like many native-born New Yorkers, fell ill because of a predisposition that was a tragic cost of urban life, and one that conflicted with Irish stereotypes.

The Consumptive Diathesis

The idea that the Irish were predisposed to consumption appeared occasionally in Britain and America, where they were noticeably afflicted by the disease, but according to historian Greta Jones (2001), it did not have influence until the 20th century. Jones (2001:36) argues that the low rates of consumption mortality in Ireland until the 1880s easily refuted this idea. Throughout the 19th century, rates were lowest in the mostly rural counties of the island's north and west, where Irish rural culture dominated. The northern county of Derry, where the McPeake family originated, for example, had a consumption mortality rate of 122 per 100,000 in 1840, while rates in the west southwestern counties of Kerry, Cork, Clare, and Sligo, from where many Irish in the Sixth Ward originated, ranged from 128 to 148 (Figure 6.8). Rates in the country's east were the highest, over 290 in and around Dublin, but even these were still much lower than the rate in New York City of over 400 (Drolet and Lowell 1952:v; Breathnach and Moynihan 2003:151). Outbreaks in mid-century Ireland have been attributed to individuals who had spent time in England: laboring men who contracted the "English cold" in inexpensive lodgings known as "Paddy Houses" and poor women who had spent time in English workhouses (Jones 2001:2, 36–39; Farmar 2004:103).

Physicians and scientists were aware of this lower incidence of tuberculosis in Ireland; they keenly observed the frequency of illnesses in many different places and populations, hoping to find cures or methods of prevention for a variety of ailments. Edward Jenner famously developed the

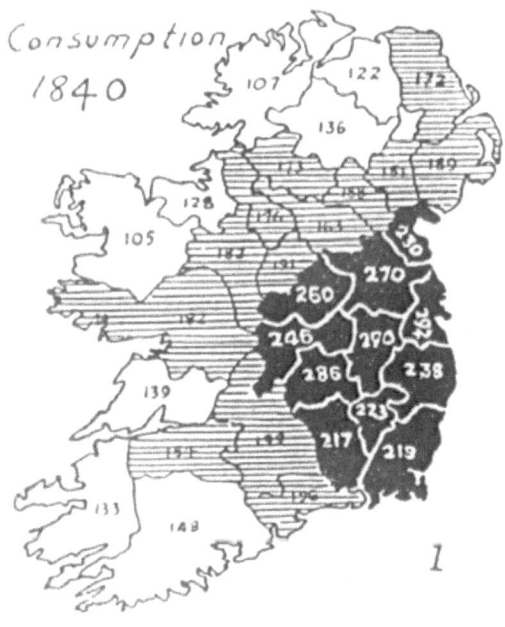

FIGURE 6.8. Map showing consumption mortality by county in Ireland in 1840, as determined by Irish statistician Robert Charles Geary's analysis of data collected in the 1841 Census (Breathnach and Moynihan 2003:151). The shaded areas indicate higher prevalence of tuberculosis in eastern Ireland, while the unshaded areas show the lowest rates in the west and north. The numbers indicate rates of death per 100,000 people in each county.

smallpox vaccine in 1796 from observations that cowpox offered dairy farmers and milkmaids protection from smallpox in England, for example.[37] Also in the late 1790s, the Quaker physician John Coakley Lettsom opened a facility for scrofula sufferers on the coast of Kent, England, based on his observation that fishermen, who were regularly exposed to sea air, rarely contracted scrofula (Hayes 2009:169). Similar perceptions about the good health of Northern European, including Irish, coastal dwellers led other English and German physicians to experiment with cod liver oil, a substance used in popular medicine in these areas. German physicians in the 1820s and 1830s reported good results for treatment of scrofula, rickets, and rheumatism and, later, consumption. In 1847, John Hughes Bennett published results of successful treatment of early-stage consumption in Edinburgh, and cod liver oil became a standard treatment for pulmonary tuberculosis (Grad 2004:106–110). Physicians continued to prescribe it into the 20th century. It helped some patients, but it was not the magic bullet.

Lower rates of tubercular mortality in mid-19th-century Ireland help to explain why tuberculosis was so deadly for Irish immigrants in New York City—they had little prior exposure and thus little immunity—but they do not fully explain why Americans did not view the Irish as predisposed to this disease.[38] Stigma and incidence are often not directly related. Later in the century, for example, scientists showed that mortality from pulmonary tuberculosis was considerably lower among Jewish immigrants in the U.S. than among the American-born, but that did not stop Americans from stigmatizing Jews as tubercular (Kraut 1995:75). A more significant reason the Irish escaped this stigma is that the stereotypes of the Irish were incompatible with Americans' image of the "consumptive diathesis," the heritable predisposition to consumption.

As mentioned previously, the idea of a consumptive diathesis was ancient. Hippocrates believed this inherited phthisical *habitus* was evident in an individual's pale coloring and slender and delicate frame with wing-like shoulder blades (Daniel 1997:18, Ott 1996:11). This image persisted into the 19th century (Dormandy 1999:41–43). For example, 19th-century physician Frederick Roberts (1884:21) described the physical signs of the consumptive diathesis, which coincided with greater physical and emotional sensitivity, as "tall, slim, erect delicate looking, having scarcely any fat . . . pretty oval face, a clear complexion, bright eyes and large pupils, the skin is very thin, soft, and delicate, and through it bluish veins are visible. The hair is fine and silky, often light, the eyelashes being long."

The consumptive diathesis was believed to be inherited from a parent, or earlier ancestor, who was naturally weak in constitution or who had been weakened by their lifestyle (Hamlin 1992:55).[39] Wealthy individuals were thought to be enfeebled by overindulgence in luxuries, food, drink, sex, anxiety, "sorrowful passions," and lack of physical exercise, while these same factors and/or deprivations, overwork, and unhealthy environments debilitated the poor. Urban life was thought to foster lifestyles on both ends of this spectrum, which popularly explained why consumption was so prevalent in cities. Weakness in body was thought to be a cost of modern civilization. Simple heredity alone did not explain all cases of consumption, however, particularly why some offspring of the same parents fell ill and others did not. So, physicians explained that an "exciting cause" (a deleterious activity, environment, or state of mind) was sometimes necessary to activate consumption. They believed these exciting causes were more prevalent in cities and could affect the outcome of the illness.[40] "Without predisposition," however, "no amount of exposure to an exciting cause would lead to the disease" (Hamlin 1992:55).

Nineteenth-century conceptions of the consumptive predisposition are closely connected to long-held ideas about the humoral temperaments. The humoral types physicians most associated with it in the 19th century were the phlegmatic (later called lymphatic) and the melancholic (later called nervous) temperaments, which both supposedly weakened the body in different ways (Murray 1870:23–24; Sontag 2001:32). The phlegmatic/lymphatic temperament was thought to produce positive attributes, such as mental acuity, reason, and civility but to make some people "languid and sluggish" (Barnes 1995:40). The melancholic/nervous temperament was thought to produce the positive qualities of creativity and sensitivity but to provoke anxiety and mental anguish that consumed vital energies (Barnes 1995:49; Ott 1996:11). Just as it contributed to the consumptive diathesis, civilized urban living was believed also to have cultivated phlegmatic and melancholic temperaments. Urban living, at least the lifestyle of the middle and upper urban classes, was thought to produce rational and refined temperaments, capable of complex intellectual tasks and possessing genteel tastes and manners but lacking the bodily vigor necessary to fend off consumption or other illnesses (Pernick 1985:151–154). Physical weakness and related high rates of tubercular infection were the costs of these otherwise "superior" temperaments. Again, as explained in previous chapters, in the 19th century, these humoral temperaments were understood as evidence of natural, essential difference; Americans believed that the "civilized" English and German "races" were phlegmatic in temperament while the "uncivilized" Irish "race" was sanguine in temperament.

There were gendered aspects to this discourse as well. Physicians explained higher consumption mortality rates among women than men to greater prevalence of the consumptive diathesis among women, aided by the belief that the phlegmatic temperament was "incontestably more frequent among women than men" (Barnes 1995:40). In fact, they gendered consumption itself, and understood it to be the result of the feminization of modern American urban society. Some physicians even spoke of hemoptysis (coughing up blood) among consumptive men as vicarious menstruation (Ott 1996:6). Historian Georgina Feldberg (1995) argues that through consumption Americans expressed concerns about industrial capitalism, the increased participation of women in work outside the home, and the greater number of men who labored in city offices instead of fields. Consumption "seemed just punishment for deviation from the habits of rugged masculinity that mid-nineteenth-century Americans equated with health, strength, and virtue" (Feldberg 1995:31).

Given these conceptions of the consumptive diathesis, it is not surprising that Americans did not imagine the Irish to be naturally predisposed to consumption. Descriptions of the consumptive diathesis profoundly clashed with the stereotypes of Irish immigrants detailed in Chapters 2 and 4.[41] In fact, they were polar opposites. Americans imagined Irish immigrants as ruddy and muscular, not pale and thin; red or dark haired, not fair haired; rugged and coarse, not delicate and fine; having veins filled with hot red, not cold blue blood; well adapted to strenuous labor and primitive living conditions, not comfortable with intellectual labor or luxuries; and freely expressive and carefree, not mannered and anxious. Even Irish women were stereotyped as unfeminine. The sanguine (Irish) temperament was thought to be prone to fevers (including typhus fever) and to alcoholism, but to be relatively immune to consumption, unlike the genteel phlegmatic Anglo and German temperament. Alfred Stillé (1861:149) a leading 19th-century American physician and professor of medicine at the University of Pennsylvania Medical School explained, "The temperament and constitution which lead to abuse of alcoholic drinks are antagonistic . . . to those which belong to the phthisical diathesis. The sanguine are fond of excitement and of the association which lead to convivial excess, but the nervolymphatic of small appetite and feeble digestion, and who court quiet and loneliness rather than scenes of boisterous mirth, are the predestined victims of consumption."

Americans believed the sanguine temperament was less than ideal in many ways, but producing overly civilized and physically weak individuals was not one of them. Paddy and Bridget might have been weak of mind in Americans' estimation, but Americans credited them with strength of body, cultivated in the rugged Irish rural environment and demonstrated in the hard labor that so many Irish performed in the U.S. This perceived physical prowess was one advantage that Americans believed the Irish possessed, and it offered the Irish protection from being seen as prone to consumption. In contrast, the Anglo and German "races," with which Americans identified, were weaker in body and predisposed to consumption; this was the cost of being "civilized." Within this context, unlike typhus fever, tubercular disease was not a social liability for an Irish immigrant. Instead, consumption was a condition that made those who suffered from it seem more genteel, more interesting, and more like White native-born Americans.

Meaningful Suffering

On an evening in 1842, the American writer Edgar Allen Poe and his ailing young wife, Virginia Eliza Clemm Poe, were entertaining guests at their home in Fordham in the Bronx. Virginia, dressed in white, was singing and playing the harp. According to her husband, she appeared "delicately, morbidly angelic," and "suddenly she stopped, clutched her throat and a wave of crimson blood ran down her breast. . . . It rendered her even more ethereal" (Dormandy 1999:94). Edgar Allen Poe was not alone in having this bizarre reaction to hemoptysis from pulmonary tuberculosis. As numerous medical historians have noted, many 19th-century Europeans and Americans romanticized a consumptive death as a good death. Many believed—and arguably needed to believe in order to cope with so many deaths—that the disease refined the spirit and intellect, enhanced physical beauty, and articulated individuality (Dubos and Dubos 1952; Sontag 2001; Ott 1996; Dormandy 1999).

This view is evident in 19th-century novels, stories, poems and plays. Louisa May Alcott's account of the death of Beth March, the saintly sister in *Little Women* (1868 and 1869), is an iconic example. Alcott wrote that the illness acted upon Beth "as if the mortal was being slowly refined away, and the immortal shining through the frail flesh with an indescribably pathetic beauty" (Krieg 1992:90). This image obscures the terrible pain caused by the disease. Alcott's own real-life sister, Elizabeth, died like so many others in agony and exhaustion, possibly eased somewhat by liberal use of opiates (Krieg 1992:90–91). Romanticizing Beth March's death as meaningful was a way for Alcott to make sense of her own sister's anguish.

A diagnosis of consumption in the middle of the 19th century was a death sentence that conveyed a limited but unknown amount of time to live. It encouraged sufferers to make the most of their remaining time. Consumptives who could afford it traveled the world—to locations including the Kent coast of England, the French Riviera, North Africa, the Alps, and later the Adirondacks and the Rocky Mountains—in search of clean air and a cure. Sanatoria in seaside and mountain towns became the recommended antidotes for this disease of urban life (Hayes 2009:169–170). Travel to beautiful places and exposure to different cultures added to the romantic image of the wealthy consumptive. Poorer consumptives were directed to more mundane locales. A doctor at St. Vincent's Hospital, for example, advised his patient to buy herself a "peanut stand on the windiest corner of Brooklyn" (Walsh 1965:69).

The romantic image of consumption expressed the "value of being more conscious, more complex psychologically;" it was the mark of poets, artists, and intellectuals (Sontag 2001:26). Physicians wrote that they observed consumptives to be more brilliant and creative, to have increased sex drives, and to experience moments of euphoria (Ott 1996:27). In contrast, "health [was] banal, even vulgar" (Sontag 2001:26). The English poet Lord Byron remarked to a friend, for example, "I should like to die of a consumption . . . because the ladies would say, 'look at that poor Byron. How interesting he looks in dying'" (Daniel 1997:32). Similarly, Henry David Thoreau's friends described the wondrous effect consumption had upon him: "A flush had come to his cheeks and an ominous brightness and beauty to his eyes, painful to behold. His conversation was unusually brilliant, and we listened with a charmed attention." (Krieg 1992:92).

The physical changes brought upon by the disease were also considered to be aesthetically pleasing. The characteristic pallor, emaciation, and sunken eyes made Virginia Poe "more ethereal," Beth March "pathetic[ally] beaut[iful]," and Thoreau "bright." Such attributes were the antithesis of the stereotypical Irish appearance, and were fashionable for both men and women throughout much of the 19th century. The paintings of the Pre-Raphaelite artists Dante Gabriel Rossetti and Sir John Everett Millais, for example, depicted women with the feminine consumptive phenotype that was the standard of beauty in the West for decades: "The fragile silhouette, with long limbs, long throat, the tired head leaning on a pillow, the prominent eyes and twisted sensual mouth, became the unhealthy, perverted symbol of Romanticism" (Dubos and Dubos 1952:57).

The consumptive appearance was fashionable at least in part because of the intellectual and spiritual virtues associated with it (Hayes 2009:158–160). The emaciated figure of the consumptive contributed to the already popular practices of corseting, which some physicians argued exacerbated consumption (Kunzle 1982:92). "Whitening powders replaced rouge," and pale clothing colors and ethereal fabrics became popular among the genteel (Dormandy 1999:12; Hayes 2009:158). Irish working-class women, in contrast, paraded around the Bowery in "startling combinations of colors" that were tight around the hips and low cut at the breast, emphasizing voluptuous portions of the female form (Stansell 1986:94). The differences between these two styles of dress were stark and could accentuate the perceived differences between these two groups of women, both in their physiques and their tastes. But, as noted in the previous chapter, there is evidence that Irish immigrant women and men skillfully manipulated their appearances, sometimes adopting clothing, corsets, face powders, and more, to make a more genteel impression. Pulmonary tuberculosis arguably had similar effects, thus making Irish consumptives appear as natural equals.

When Americans encountered Irish consumptives, there is no indication that it caused the kind of alarm incited by typhus fever. Instead, Irish immigrants with the delicate appearances of consumptives, seem to have taken some Americans by surprise, because the stereotypes of the brutish Bridget and Pat were so pervasive. A physician at New York Hospital, for example, took the time to note that an 18-year-old Irish patient, named Maria, had "a rather handsome countenance, black hair, hazel eyes, and fair skin" (NYHSCB 1848:C1632). None of the doctor's notes about his other patients included remarks about their aesthetic appearances, implying Maria was not what he expected of an Irish woman, and he did not know quite how to categorize her. Over time, more encounters like this slowly shifted what Americans identified as the attributes of Irishness.

Consumptive Irish immigrants were thus a challenge to American stereotypes of the Irish and conceptions of Irishness for two reasons. The first was conceptual; the consumptive diathesis and the constitution of the Irish, both as imagined by Americans, were incompatible. The second was aesthetic; the disease caused physical transformations that Americans considered to be beautiful. The existence of Irish men and women, in particular, who were equal in beauty and individuality to Americans, challenged Irish stereotypes, and ultimately, ideas of essential Irish difference.

Consumption Humanized the Irish

In 1868, *Harper's Weekly* published a melodramatic moralizing tale titled "Eva Eve" that illustrates how consumption had begun to complicate and soften Americans' views of Irish immigrants. The story's protagonist is Eva Eve, the eldest child and "the pride and the pet" of an Irish immigrant family in the Five Points neighborhood. Eva's parents had been a respectable chamber maid and porter in a dry goods store upon their marriage, but over time they fell into poverty and succumbed to drunkenness—in that order. Eva's mother occasionally brought Eva to the Five Points House of Industry, a Methodist mission in the Five Points, for meals. Eva also attended Sunday School on her own there and absorbed the catechism lessons. Eva's intellect, beauty, and sensitivity attracted the attention of a genteel middle-class American couple,

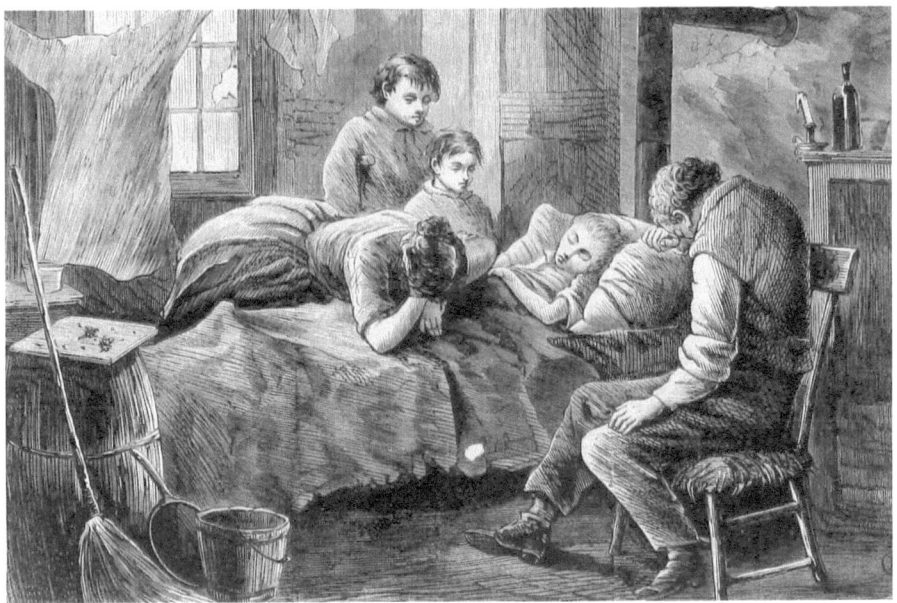

FIGURE 6.9: Illustration titled "He Giveth His Beloved Sleep," depicting the death of Eva Eve at the conclusion of the short story "Eva Eve" (*Harper's Weekly* 1868:725).

who tried to persuade her parents to allow them to adopt Eva. Eva's parents, who are portrayed somewhat sympathetically as proud and loving, but made unfit by their life circumstances, refused. Months went by. During this time, Eva's parents continued to drink away their meager earnings which deprived their children of regular food, heat, and adequate clothing. The fair-skinned, chestnut-haired, and blue-eyed Eva secretly wished she could have gone to live with the American couple, but dutifully remained with her parents, earning money for them by selling flowers on the street. Nevertheless, she became paler and thinner, developed a cough, and had fever-induced dreams about being a sheep watched over by the Good Shepherd. The story ends with Eva's peaceful death in her sleep on Christmas morning—illustrated in the accompanying drawing (Figure 6.9)—after dreaming Jesus led her to a green, sunlit pasture (*HW* 1868:725–726).[42]

The purpose of this story was ostensibly to highlight the negative effects of poverty, especially when combined with Irish proclivity toward drink, to illustrate the positive effects of the House of Industry's civilizing efforts upon poor Irish American children, and to make a case for adoptions.[43] Eva's death from consumption is not an incidental element in the story. It would have impacted the middle-class American-born readership of this newspaper as an indication that through some combination of innate gifts and the mission's instruction, Eva did not inherit the Irish temperament. Eva's death from consumption argued that she and, by extension, other Irish American children like her, were not so different from the readers' own children, who also fell victim to tubercular disease. In the wake of the Second Great Awakening, many Americans—and reformers, in particular—began to view their own children as innocents in need of protection and instruction in order to become responsible citizens in a dangerous world (Fitts 2000b:423–424). Through Eva's character and her manner of death, the author made a case that even the children of Irish immigrants were capable of being civilized and worthy of adoption into the American "family."

The persuasive impact of this story was heightened by another association readers would have made between Eva Eve and the character Eva in Harriet Beecher Stowe's *Uncle Tom's Cabin* (1852). Eva, a slave owner's daughter who befriends the protagonist, Tom, was the prototype for the Irish American Eva; she was sensitive and innocent, despite the evil context in which she was raised. Stowe's Eva also dies from consumption, and her death from this condition confirms her moral goodness and refined sensibility (Krieg 1992:91). "*Uncle Tom's Cabin* became the nation's most popular stage presentation; the death of little Eva was considered to be the height of pathos" (Krieg 1992:91). The connection between these two Evas intensified readers' feelings for the fictional Irish American girl and drew their attention to the plight of real-life Irish American children, who were served by the nonfictional Five Points House of Industry, the Five Points Mission, and other city institutions (Fitts 2000b).

Eva Eve tragically wasted away from consumption, but her story has a bittersweet ending; her suffering further refined her spirit and enabled her to enter into eternal bliss. Her suffering, like that of real girls, boys, men, and women, was meaningful and redemptive. Recall the description of Sarah McPeake's death in her brother's obituary: "After a long and painful illness, borne with Christian resignation" (*Irish American Weekly* 1857:3). Because of this conception of consumptive suffering, real Irish immigrants could similarly appear refined by the disease and, in turn, be socially redefined. In this context, consumption humanized the Irish. It drained Irish consumptives of their supposed brutish sanguine temperament, both literally—through illness-induced pallor, emaciation of muscles, and hemoptysis—and metaphorically—by showing White native-born Americans that the Irish were not so different from themselves. As more Irish immigrants and their Irish American children suffered from consumption in the 1850s and 1860s, more stood out as different from the stereotypes of Pat and Bridget. This realization helped to reframe how Americans saw the Irish.

The stereotypes of Pat and Bridget that had been centuries in the making were not immediately dispelled, of course, and they were a convenient font of vivid imagery from which native-born Americans drew whenever they wished to disparage someone of Irish descent. Some of the most insulting and dehumanizing written descriptions and cartoons of the Irish (such as Figure 2.4), for example, were published between the late 1860s and the 1880s. These depictions of the Irish as apish brutes have garnered much attention, but scholars have argued that Irish men, and especially women, were more often depicted as normal humans during this period, albeit sometimes with mild facial prognathism indexing lower class status that was not necessarily essentializing. Extremely simianized representations were created by a few particular artists and were reserved for depicting political activists, rioters, and members of gangs or secret societies; these depictions responded to specific violent events, such as the New York City Draft Riots (1863), the Fenian Rising in Ireland and the St. Patrick's Day Riot in New York (1867), and the Orange Riot in New York (1871) (Curtis 1997; de Nie 2004:34; Kenny 2006; Garner 2015).[44] During this time, Irish nationalists themselves mobilized the ideas of race scientists that the Irish were descended from a distinct "Celtic" race to galvanize an Irish diasporic community no longer united by shared presence on Ireland's soil (McMahon 2015a). Such rhetoric also drew upon humoral theory to vividly describe the merits of the Irish "race." In praising Irish Civil War soldiers, for example, the *Sydney Freeman's Journal* (1863) noted their "recklessness in danger and death": "The wide world knows how Irishmen fight, 'fast, fiery, and true' for there is scarce a battlefield from the North Pole to the South that Irish blood has not crimsoned" (quoted in McMahon 2015a:12, 24, 139).

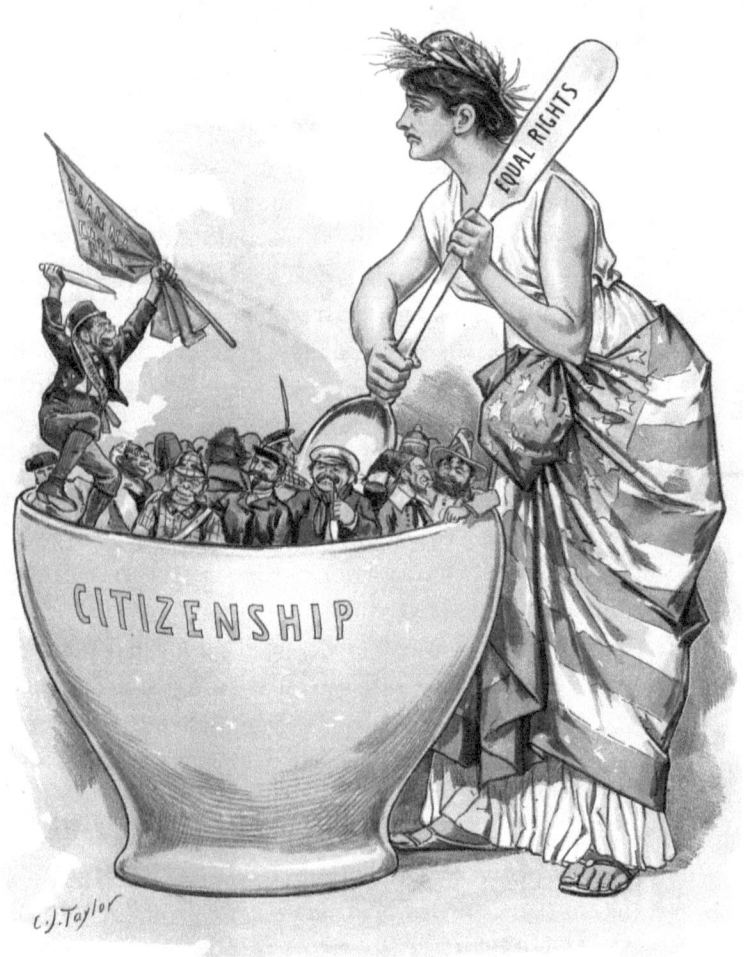

FIGURE 6.10. "The Mortar of Assimilation—and the One Element That Won't Mix" by Charles Jay Taylor (*Puck* 1889). Courtesy of the Smithsonian National Museum of American History. This cartoon shows Lady Liberty mixing the immigrants from many nations into the American melting pot, but an Irish nationalist resists, holding a bloody knife and a flag emblazoned with the name of the Irish republican organization Clan Na Gael.

The extreme cartoons were thus published during a time when Irish nationalists asserted natural Irish difference that was becoming less and less apparent or meaningful to native-born Americans who were increasingly willing to believe the Irish could be integrated along with newcomers from many other nations, as long as the Irish themselves were willing (Figure 6.10).[45] This chapter proposes that both the high rates of tubercular infection in the Irish community in New York and individual cases of suffering Irish-born or Irish American individuals, especially young people, contributed to this shift in Americans' perspective.[46]

Conclusion

Beginning in the 1850s, there was a major outbreak of tubercular illness among the Irish in New York City. Hospital and dispensary records provide a sense of its magnitude. Over the next two decades these institutions would treat far more Irish immigrants for tubercular illness than they ever had for typhus fever. The causes of tuberculosis, as we understand them today, shed light on the living and working conditions the Irish endured in the city. Tuberculosis was not a disease that was prevalent in Ireland, but one that the Irish succumbed to in New York. Overwork, undernourishment, poor living conditions, other illnesses and injuries, and lack of previous exposure made Irish bodies particularly vulnerable, while crowded quarters and even Irish traditional forms of comfort and community building—such as drinking, smoking, and sharing food and lodging with guests—spread the bacteria and lowered immune resistance.

That the Irish suffered heavily from this disease was recognized outside of their communities as well, by physicians and hospital staff, druggists, neighbors, employers, and the broader American public. Nativists could have interpreted consumption in ways that stigmatized the Irish and supported preexisting stereotypes, as they interpreted typhus fever, but they did not. This curious inconsistency is important, and it can only be explained through an appreciation of how tubercular illness was understood differently in the middle of the 19th century, as a "natural" and all-too-familiar part of urban life, a cost of civilization that affected those with a hereditary predisposition. Thus, there was no need to ostracize or quarantine Irish immigrants suffering from consumption; it was not contagious or a foreign or Irish disease. Moreover the appearance and character of the consumptive diathesis—pale, thin, sensitive, refined, phlegmatic—was the polar opposite of Irish stereotypes. Resistant to the idea that consumption was contagious or that the terrible suffering of their own friends and relatives who were not spared by tuberculosis might be meaningless, most Americans did not question their views of consumption when large numbers of Irish immigrants began to suffer from it. Instead, this trend seems to have prompted many to question the Irish stereotype.

The physical changes tuberculosis wrought, emaciation and pallor, created a more naturally genteel appearance than even the best combination of face-whitening powders, red-hair-obscuring dyes, and fashionable clothing (Chapter 5). The disease metaphorically and visibly—and literally in the form of hemoptysis—drained the sanguinity from Irish immigrants afflicted with it. In individual Irish consumptives, Americans came to recognize individuals not so different from themselves. As the American writer O. Henry, who had lost his mother and first wife to the disease, described, there was a "freemasonry among consumptives: 'A cough is your [calling] card; a hemorrhage a letter of credit'" (Ott 1996:24).

Consumption thus fostered a counternarrative to prejudiced views of essential Irish difference by prompting Americans to see Irish individuals beyond the stereotypes, perhaps beginning first with Irish American children, like the fictional Eva Eve, and more assimilated Irish immigrant men and women who had grown up in New York City, such as James and Sarah McPeake. In a sense, consumption brought to fruition American nativists' desires that exposure to the American environment would transform rural Irish aliens into civilized Irish American citizens. The next chapter investigates Irish immigrants' perspectives and how their own efforts to contend with consumption in New York City also contributed to their acceptance as Irish Americans .

CHAPTER 7

Consumption and Community among the New York Irish

ALTHOUGH TUBERCULOSIS was comparatively rare in Ireland until the late 19th century, the Irish had long recognized illnesses that cause progressive wasting. The ancient Brehon Laws, dating to the 5th century A.D., for example, decreed that if a mother developed *anbobracht,* a terminal condition in which she became "devoid of juice or strength," the father would be responsible for raising their child(ren) (Kelly 2001:76). By the middle of the 19th century, *anbobracht* popularly denoted tuberculosis (Blake 1918:220), as did the terms *seirglighe* (decay), *seirgean as* (shrinking of oneself), *cnaoid* (wasting), *etige* (decline, pulmonary consumption; used in the West of Ireland), and *Creacht na Sgamhain* (ulcer of the lung) (Wilde, W. 1856:447; Purdon 1904:41; Breathnach and Moynihan 2003:44). Like the English term "consumption," these Irish terms focus upon tuberculosis's debilitating effects.[1] The popular Irish perspective differed not in appreciation of symptoms but in how to explain consumption and how to treat it.

This chapter investigates 19th-century popular Irish views of tubercular illness and shows that it was understood to be caused primarily by external factors. Irish informants reported to folklore collectors that individuals living in poverty, those who had been blessed by good fortune, and those who had accumulated wealth without sharing were particularly at risk. Thus, in contrast to the American perspective that acknowledged the role of "exciting causes" but saw an individual's internal constitution as the necessary ingredient, the popular Irish perspective viewed socioeconomic conditions and/or social relationships as critical. Each group's conception of the causes of consumption reflected their differing perspectives of both illness and personhood. Americans emphasized the internal qualities of individuals, while the Irish focused upon individuals in relation to their community. The American ideal was self-reliance, while the Irish valued mutual aid. The differing perspectives that these ideas about consumption underscore contributed to some of the misunderstanding between Irish immigrants and Americans in New York City.

What follows will first describe 19th-century popular Irish understandings of consumption and forms of treatment for this illness. It will then interpret traces in archaeological and historical records of how Irish immigrants treated tuberculosis in New York City, where the previous chapter established this disease afflicted so many Irish individuals and families, including the McPeakes, with a vehemence and ubiquity previously unknown to the Irish. These records reveal that in New York City Irish immigrants responded to the "disease of civilization" with popular Irish strategies and new American resources. In the process of struggling against tuberculosis, they increased their own participation in the American marketplace as avid consumers of patent medicines, cod liver oil, and soda water. They also strengthened social connections within Irish communities and expanded contact with non-Irish neighbors. Consumption was not simply the "natural death of Irish immigrants," as Archbishop John Hughes opined; it also prompted creative responses from Irish immigrants that further integrated them as a group into American life. Both American and Irish reactions to this terrible affliction ultimately assisted the development of Irish American identity in New York City.

Irish Popular Causes and Cures of Consumption in Ireland and New York I: Fairy Capture and Bewitching

In 19th-century Ireland, as in the U.S., it was recognized that consumption often attacked the young, innocent, beautiful, and talented, and Irish people also searched for meaningful explanations for such terrible suffering. Irish informants reported to folklore collectors that some cases resulted from poor material conditions, which will be discussed in the next section, and others from fairy or human interference. These ideas provided means for the afflicted and their families to cope as well as reinforced rural Irish social norms.

Fairies are supernatural creatures in Irish folklore, sometimes said to be fallen angels, guardians of the dead, or deities of pre-Christian

Ireland (Wilde, W. 1852:124–125; Wilde, L. 1887a:169–170; Mac Cárthaigh 1988:90). They were said to have great power as well as humanlike personalities and foibles. If treated respectfully, they could help humans, but they caused illness and misfortune if disrespected, jealous, or they simply felt mischievous. Humans who entered fairy territory, logged fairy trees, or ploughed fairy fields unannounced and without offering anything in return, for example, could receive a fairy "blast"—described as a sudden chill, painful sensation, or even being knocked off one's feet—in retribution that caused sudden paralysis (NFC 1935[54]:204; NFC 1937[463]:44–45; Glassie 1985). In contrast, "many a [*poitín*] still-owner was warned of coming of the police by the fairies; if he was prone to giving the fairies a sample or first shot" (Dorian 2000:270). One of the most prominent legends about fairies was that they kidnapped children, especially extraordinarily beautiful ones, and occasionally adults, particularly pregnant women, replacing the stolen human with a fairy changeling, who was cross and sickly and soon wasted away (NFC 1941[782]:258; Gregory 1920:104–147).[2] There are a variety of conditions that might cause a young child to fail to thrive, but in the opinion of the 19th-century folklorist and physician William Wilde (1856:455), tubercular and scrofulous infection "gave rise to the popular ideas respecting the 'changeling' and to the many superstitious notions entertained by the peasantry respecting their supposed 'fairy-stricken' children."[3]

Humans were also said to cause illness in one another through conscious or unconscious bewitching, also sometimes called the "evil eye" or "overlooking." Around 1950, Peig Minihane, an elderly woman from the isolated Beara Peninsula in County Clare, explained,

> If you had any complaint then [when she was young] ... the mother or the woman of the house, she would say: "You didn't have any complaint until that man came in a while ago, maybe he's bewitched you." Bewitching comes from begrudgery.... When a person with the evil eye commented on the beauty of a child, the fineness of someone's cow, the excellence of someone's work, etc., without saying "God bless it" afterwards, it could cause that thing or person to become bewitched. (Verling 2003:86)

This explanation that "bewitching comes from begrudgery" adds insight into an account of a woman who was said to have perished from consumption because she did not give charity to a person who asked for it, recorded by Lady Gregory (1920). Fairy capture and bewitching, from an outsider's perspective, functioned to explain emotionally traumatic and otherwise unexplainable illnesses and deaths in the 19th century, when deaths of young children and of women in childbirth were frequent (Mac Cárthaigh 1988:29). These ideas also encouraged resource sharing and conservation of the environment and discouraged the accumulation of wealth or showing off special gifts or accomplishments that might spur jealousy and conflict.[4]

When an affliction was perceived to have been caused by bewitching or fairy capture, the Irish generally chose a remedy that was also considered to be in the realm of supernatural or personalistic power. Examples to counter consumption resulting from fairies include making the sign of the cross, invoking the Holy Trinity, imbibing or applying holy water, visiting holy wells, and seeking a cure from a baptismal sponsor.[5] Peig Minihane completed her remarks stating that to break an enchantment, a family member would be sent to retrieve the bewitcher. The bewitcher "would have to spit on that [sick] person three times . . . 'in the name of the Father and of the Son and of the Holy Spirit'" (Verling 2003:86). To recover a baby who was "away" with the fairies, a farmer in Kerry recommended giving the changeling a cup of holy well water or "spring water to drink . . . [with] the sign of the cross . . . made over it" (NFC 1941[782]:255).

Wisewomen and fairy doctors were sought to resolve fairy capture (Figure 7.1). Lady Wilde (1890:41) recorded one remedy: make a "good fire" and throw a "handful or more of certain herbs ordered by the fairywomen." Then carry the changeling three times around the fire and "recite an incantation against evil and sprinkle holy water all around." One of the plants used in this remedy was likely foxglove (*lus mór*, also called "fairy fingers" and "fairy thimble"), noted in many sources as a cure for witchcraft and fairy capture (Wilde, L. 1887b:18, 101; Allen and Hatfield 2004:254). One of Lady Gregory's (1920:150) informants, Mrs. Quaid, told her that "the *lus mór* is the only one [herb] that's good to bring back children that are away [with the fairies]." Similarly, Tom Kearns, an informant in Kerry, reported that giving a changeling an infusion of foxglove leaves was said to bring the real child back (NFC 1941[782]:192). This potion could have caused the child acute distress, because foxglove has heart-stimulating properties and effects upon the central nervous

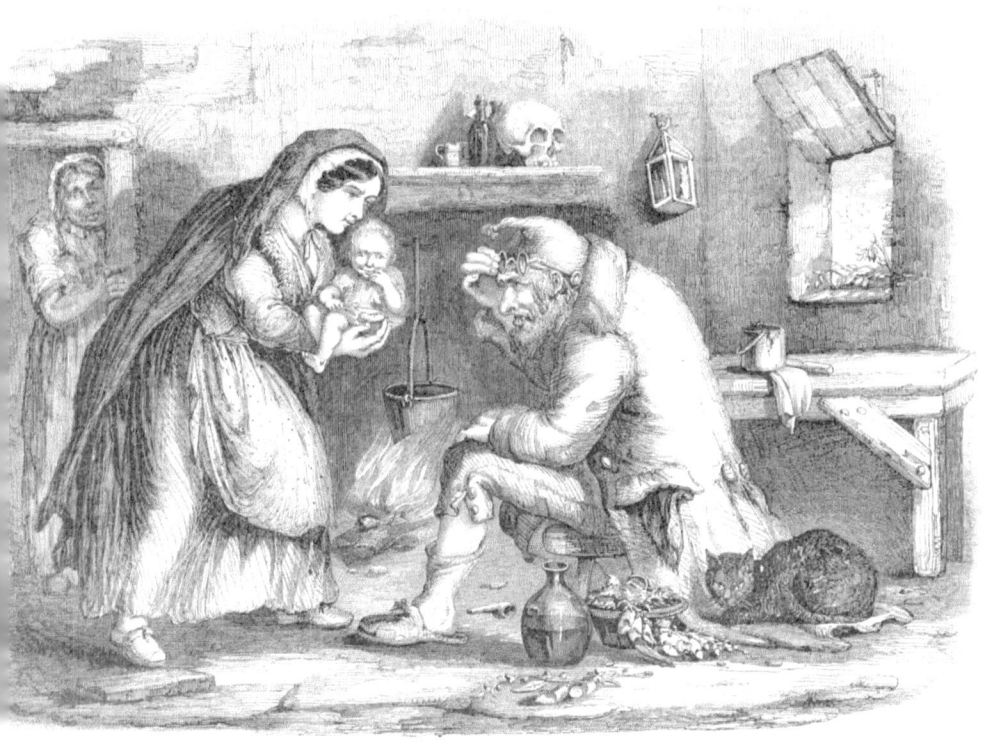

FIGURE 7.1. "Manners and Customs of the Irish Peasantry: The Fairy Doctor—From a Drawing by E. Fitzpatrick" (*Illustrated London News* 1859:635). This illustration depicts an outsider's view of an Irish mother's visit to a fairy doctor with a suspected changeling. The accompanying text describes the doctor as a charlatan, but the illustration contains objects reported to folklore collectors as having been used by fairy doctors and wisewomen in healing—*lus mór* (foxglove), a liquid-filled glass bottle, and a clay smoking pipe in the foreground and additional dark bottles and a human skull on the mantle and a pot over the hearth fire. The black cat resting on the doctor's coattails suggests his connection to supernatural power.

system; the drug digitalis was originally derived from it, and older legal records in Scotland note "numerous cases of children's deaths" from drinking infusions of foxglove (Allen and Hatfield 2004:254–257).[6] The idea behind these cures was to make the changeling so uncomfortable that the fairy would leave and return the child.[7]

There were also measures taken to prevent enchantment and fairy capture; many drew upon Christian symbols. Making the sign of the cross or putting one's thumb in between one's middle finger and forefinger when passing fairy-inhabited areas was recommended (Wilde, W. 1852:16, 128). To protect babies and young children from accidental bewitching, any adult who picked them up should say "God bless it" (NFC 1941[782]:191). It was advised to be extra cautious around red-haired women who were thought to often have the evil eye, although they might not know it themselves (Wilde, L. 1887a:43, 1890:64; Doherty 1897:16). It was also recommended never to leave babies, young children, or pregnant mothers alone and to have babies receive the sacrament of baptism as early as possible (NFC 1941[782]:191; Mac Cárthaigh 1988:29, 35; Gillespie 1998; Dorian 2000; Verling 2003:41). Iron was used as protection from fairies, reportedly because of its connection with the iron nails of the crucifixion. Popular preventives included placing iron tongs over a baby's crib (NFC 1941[782]:192; NFC 1974[1837]:42, 59), putting an iron horseshoe over the door of the house (Dorian 2000:267), or sewing a bit of iron into a child's clothes (NFC 1941[782]:192).

Other preventive actions included sewing a bit of burnt sod from St. John's Eve into the child's clothes; having the child wear a "gospel" (a small rolled or folded piece of paper with gospel verses written upon it) around his/her neck (Wilde, W. 1852:130); making the sign of the cross over a child and giving him/her a cup of spring water to drink; putting a few drops of the water in which the baby was first washed in his/her mouth; sprinkling holy well water around the house; and burning candles, especially around Whitsuntide, to protect a sick person in the house (NFC 1941[782]:191, 192, 248, 255). Additionally, young boys were dressed in skirts to disguise them from fairies, who were said to prefer male children (see Chapter 1 and Figure 1.2) (Evans 1957:289).

The degree to which Irish people in the middle of the 19th century believed in fairy capture and/or bewitching versus used it as a metaphor cannot really be known. There is plenty of evidence, however, that many people spoke about enchantments and employed measures against them. There is also evidence that they did not leave these ideas or practices in Ireland but brought them wherever they migrated.

Preventing Enchantment Beyond Ireland

Fairy lore was not limited to Ireland. The Irish used it to make sense of misfortune wherever they migrated. Irish residents of New York declared that banshees (fairies who mourned deaths in certain families) were present in the city, for example, and that fairies wore red clothes and caps there, the dominant color also associated with them in Ireland (Lees 1979:188; Hand 1981:142; Hutchings 1997:59). The Irish in Paterson, New Jersey, said that there fairies disguised themselves as old women, walked down the street using canes, and begged for money (Lees 1979:188 citing the *Paterson Evening News*, 1900). Fairy capture was thus a threat on this side of the Atlantic too. The *Boston Pilot* (1863:5) reported that a woman in New York inadvertently killed her three-year-old child, a suspected changeling, by placing the child on a red-hot shovel, a "cure" for fairy capture later reported to Lady Wilde in Ireland (1890:49). In the 20th century, American folklorists recorded measures Irish Americans took to prevent fairy malevolence and bewitching. Masons in California embedded horseshoes and other iron items in building walls, while residents of Illinois and New Jersey hung horseshoes "with the points down" over the door (Hyatt 1935:527; Hand 1981:145; Francis L. Boyle 1988, pers. comm.). Similar practices to protect 19th-century households have been discovered by archaeologists within the walls and foundations of houses in other parts of the U.S., as well as in the British Isles and Australia (Manning 2014).[8]

Some practices that had been used in Ireland were difficult to replicate away from Ireland's social and physical environment. As will be suggested later in this chapter, Irish immigrants might have looked to commodities, including soda water and patent medicines as substitutes. Additionally, many Irish sought out formal organizations for protection, such as churches and charitable organizations. Many measures to prevent and cure enchantment in Ireland drew on symbols and rituals of the Roman Catholic Church, but informally, usually requiring neither a priest nor church, likely a response to reduced access to both because of the Penal Laws' suppression of Catholicism. In cities abroad where clergy were accessible, such as London, Irish immigrants were eager to have their children formally baptized, even though they did not show enthusiasm for regularly attending Sunday mass (Lees 1979:180). The priests at the Transfiguration Church, located only two blocks from the Five Points in New York City, similarly performed many baptisms, marriages, and last rites for Irish immigrants, but regular mass attendees and pew subscribers were few (Dolan 1975:51; Griggs 2000:47). In these cities, Irish immigrants focused upon sacraments they deemed essential for protecting their children (baptism), dying good deaths (last rites), and building strong community ties (marriage).

Irish immigrants in New York City also participated in variety of religious, benevolent, political, and nationalist organizations that provided support to their communities (Miller 1985:328, 533; Brighton 2005:126–129). Given the idea that "begrudgery" could make a person susceptible to bewitching, involvement in these organizations could be viewed as a protective strategy. Financially successful Irish immigrants sat on the boards of hospitals, orphanages, and benevolent societies, but immigrants of more modest means participated in these kinds of institutions as well. For example, according to the records of the Emigrant Industrial Savings Bank, Robert Hamilton, a Sixth Ward Mott Street resident and painter by trade, was the Treasurer of the charitable Catholic St. Vincent de Paul Society in 1860 (Yamin 2000 [3]:25–28). Eliza Garrick, who also lived nearby at 25 Church Street, was the Directress of the St. Theresa Society of St. James Church in 1860 (Yamin 2000 [3]:25–28). Peter McLoughlin, who was able to purchase the tenement at 472 Pearl Street by running a successful liquor store, served on the executive committee of the Irish Emigrant Society, was Controller of the Citizens Savings Bank, and Treasurer of the Roman Catholic Orphan Asylum (Yamin 1998:78).

In their private lives, many Irish immigrants also continued to mind social conventions that encouraged mutual aid and discouraged inciting envy and ill will. After his purchase of 472 Pearl Street, for example, Peter McLoughlin built an improved five-story brick tenement on the property and upgraded the sanitary facilities in the yard. These were unnecessary measures had he been primarily interested in profit, since many absentee landlords had become wealthy by renting substandard housing in the neighborhood at exorbitant prices (Yamin 2000[1]:98).

Some of the Irish residents of Peter's building and the neighboring 474 Pearl Street took in friends during times of need and/or pulled resources together for mutual survival. Listed among members of the undertaker John Ward's household at 474 Pearl Street in the 1855 New York State Census was an eight-year-old girl named Ellen Flyn, who had been adopted by the family, for example.

Documents including diaries and letters attest to how important the help of fellow Irishmen and women was in obtaining a place to stay, food to eat, clothes to wear, jobs to earn money, etc. (Maguire 1868; O'Connell 1980; Roney 1931; Anbinder et al. 2019a; McMahon 2021). The desire to remain in a community kept Irish immigrants in cities, a fact that dismayed advocates who felt that rural immigrants would be better suited to rural America (Maguire 1868). Irish immigrants feared the isolation of dispersed American farms (O'Donnell 1997:7). A lonely newcomer in Missouri lamented, for example, that he missed Ireland, where "I could then go to a fair, or a wake, or a dance, or I could spend the winter nights in a neighbor's house cracking jokes by the turf fire. If I had there but a sore head I would have a neighbor within every hundred yards of me that would run to see me" (Miller 1985:270).

Rural Irish values emphasized that the world was a difficult place in which to live and that cooperation with neighbors, human and fairy, and sharing of resources was required for the mutual benefit of everyone (Glassie 1982:143). Those who did not play by the rules and those who did not have others to help protect them were in danger of fairy capture, fairy blasts, bewitching, and more. Each of these consequences could manifest in the form of consumption or other tubercular illness. For the Irish, there was an important relationship between consumption and community and between the individual and the larger social group. These links are also prominent in other explanations the Irish offered for tubercular illness, those centering on natural causes.

Irish Popular Causes and Cures of Consumption in Ireland and New York II: Difficult Life Conditions

When three-year old Huxley McGuire (Chapter 1) fell ill in the late fall of 1847, it is possible that his grandmother feared consumption. Huxley had a fever, cough, and congestion. These are symptoms that his grandmother, and most of her neighbors in New York, Irish and American, thought could develop into pulmonary consumption (Logan 1994:27; Jones 2012:39). Mrs. Huxley sought the knowledge and assistance of a number of people in her community to restore the boy's health. She used popular Irish remedies of warming and strengthening care that she had learned from her own relatives or friends, relied on her niece and boarders to provide Huxley with constant attention and to help administer nourishment, and sought a specialized healer with a good reputation in her community, Dr. Townsend (1847:1–17, 42–51). It is also possible that Mrs. Huxley employed some of the preventive measures or cures described in the previous section, depending on what she thought was the cause of Huxley's illness. Mrs. Huxley's multipronged healing strategy involving a number of community members and substances was not unusual in 19th-century Ireland or New York, just as it is not unusual today to use home remedies and consult professional physicians and alternative medical practitioners simultaneously. Consumption was a condition that encouraged multiple approaches, because its symptoms were variable, and in the later stages severe, and it was incurable, so no single approach could bring complete relief. In 19th-century Ireland, remedies for tubercular illnesses included recipes to attend to perceived causes as well as symptoms. This section outlines additional remedies and healers the Irish drew upon to cure consumption in Ireland and then considers evidence of continuity and change in New York City.

Many remedies for consumption preserved in Irish folklore records focused on strengthening the body. These include eating particular plants or drinking infusions made from their leaves or roots. The most frequently mentioned include dandelion, chamomile, carrageen, garlic, mint, myrtle, watercress and chickweed, and nettles.[9] These plants might have had some beneficial effects. For example, dandelion is high in vitamins A, B complex, C, and D, as well as iron, potassium, and zinc; these are vitamins and minerals we now recognize as necessary for a well-functioning immune system. Dandelions were a mainstay in the Irish popular medical kit, and consumption was only one of many ailments that the Irish used dandelions to cure.[10] Bridget Ruane, a renowned Irish wisewoman, said that the dandelion and plantain plant could "bring back the dead" (Gregory 1920:148).[11] Stinging nettles, another plant that was frequently used, is rich in vitamin A and a good source of iron, calcium, and protein (Rutto et al. 2013). Some informants told folklore collectors that eating boiled nettles could cure cancer (NFCS 1938[35]:237). In 19th-century rural Ireland, where diets were based largely on potatoes and meat was scarce, wild and cultivated plants were important sources of nutrition, especially for the sick. The Irish also recommended the following high-protein animal foods to strengthen the sick: milk, eggs, snails, fish, and fish oil.[12] The milk of goats, donkeys, and Kerry cows, in particular, was prescribed for consumptives. These animals were believed to be immune to the disease.[13] Other informants told folklore collectors that inhaling the breath of a goat or sleeping next to a goat could cure consumption (NFCS 1938[624]:77; Logan 1994:23). Similarly, sleeping next to a stronger person was said to cure a person in "decline" by absorbing some of the stronger person's strength or by passing the disease to them (NFC 1930[80]:19; Ní Bhrádaigh 1936:267). This might have been among the reasons Mrs. Huxley shared her bed with her sick grandson, to share some of her strength and the burden of the illness with him.

Other Irish popular cures for pulmonary consumption were plant-based mixtures thought to expel sickness-causing "poisons" from the body through purging and/or by increasing urine production. Infusions were made from bogbane, burdock, dandelion, dock, flaxseed, furze, knapweed, garlic, nasturtium, and sorrel.[14] In addition to the benefits of dandelion mentioned above, it was well known for its diuretic effects (Schütz et al. 2006). Spring water and whiskey, which also act as diuretics, were common ingredients in these mixtures, or recommended on their own as cures. A mixture of knapweed (*Centurea nigra*), purging flax (*Linum catharticum*), and maidenhair was a favorite purging remedy in Donegal for "the decline" (Allen and Hatfield 2004:284). Nettles were also thought to have blood purifying properties. It was widely reported that eating three meals of boiled stinging nettle leaves in May was a "spring tonic" that prevented sickness for the whole year.[15]

There are suggestions in the folklore records that the Irish understood worms to be the cause of scrofula and sometimes attributed pulmonary tuberculosis to them. For example, a girl dying of consumption was convinced by her friends to see a woman who administered the same cure described in Chapter 5 for "heart fever" and "heartache," filling a cup with oatmeal and applying it to her chest. In the process, some of the oatmeal disappeared. The old woman explained that the cure would work because she gave the meal to the worms that were eating the girl's heart (Mooney 1887:159). Given that worms can cause weight loss, fatigue, pain, and nausea, symptoms that can also be present during the early stages of pulmonary consumption, it is not unreasonable to associate worms with that disease. Dock and nettle roots that were used to treat consumption and scrofula were strong purgatives also used to expel intestinal worms (NFC 1930[80]:20; Logan 1994:35). The use of the same cure for consumption and "heartache" also suggests the Irish viewed a connection between depression or grief and consumption. Annie McCrea, an informant in County Tyrone, told a folklore collector in 1951 that "heart fever is what they call consumption today" (NFC 1951[1220]:45). Irish healers, like many folk healers everywhere, were attentive to patients' psychological states and physical symptoms (NFC 1974[1838]:161; Buckley 1980).

The positive psychological effects of being treated by a trusted healer helps to explain another Irish popular cure for consumption and scrofula, seeking a touch from a "seventh son." The seventh-born son, and sometimes daughter, in a family was believed to be able to cure all types of illnesses, especially worms and ailments then popularly thought to be caused by worms, including ringworm, now known to be caused by a fungus, and scrofula.[16,17] Other cures for scrofula included poultices of buttercup, burdock, walnut leaves or watercress; applying the blood of a wren; and drinking holy well water or decoctions of meadowsweet (*Filipendula ulmaria*), which might have had an analgesic effect from the salicylate it contains.[18] Poultices were also the favored remedy for a variety of skin and joint complaints and would likely have been used to treat tubercular infections of these parts of the body.

The Irish also had a number of remedies to relieve cough and chest pain, symptoms of pulmonary tuberculosis. For example, smoking rosemary leaves was said to improve asthma and the cough of phthisis (Purdon 1895a:217). Cough syrups traditionally made yearly by women in the family to have on hand would have been soothing. Typical ingredients included wild mint (horehound), liquorice, cherry, and carrageen, often mixed with whiskey.[19] Other cough remedies included: drinking infusions of mugwort (*Artemesia vulgaris*), mullein (*Verbascum thapsus*), ox-eye daisy (*Leucanthemum vulgare*), self-heal (*Prunella vulgaris*), elderberry, thyme, or, more rarely, foxglove (*Digitalis purpurea*).[20]

Of these, mullein was the "favorite remedy for pulmonary tuberculosis in Ireland throughout recorded history" (Allen and Hatfield 2004:250).[21] An informant in County Galway recommended to boil "the big blankety leaves," then "strain and sweeten" them, and "add whiskey for bottling and preserving" (NFCS 1938[45]:201). Recent studies have found mullein to have emollient and expectorant properties effective for relieving cough, as well as compounds that can kill bacteria (Turker and Camper 2002). Mullein was so valuable in 19th-century Ireland that people grew it in their gardens and advertised its sale in newspapers, including at some of the best chemist shops (Allen and Hatfield 2004:250). A Dublin hospital physician experimented with the plant in the early 1880s and published a note in the *British Medical Journal* reporting its positive effects upon his consumptive patients (Quinlan 1883:149–150).

Other cough remedies that crosscut Irish popular and mainstream medicine include applying warming and/or strong-smelling substances to the chest, such as mustard, camphorated oil, or goose grease, which Mrs. Huxley used on her grandson.[22] Restoring warmth was deemed to be a critical step in restoring health, because exposure to cold and wet was thought to trigger illness, and it was a popular belief that "neglected colds" could lead to tuberculosis (Jones 2012:39).

In summary, popular remedies for tubercular illness in Ireland drew upon a variety of resources in Irish communities and local environments. In order to remain healthy or to regain health, the Irish saw the assistance of others, and of the natural and sometimes supernatural world, as essential. The next section probes how Irish immigrants in New York attempted to remedy unprecedented levels of tubercular illness in their families and communities.

Cures for Consumption in New York City, Old and New

Medical case records from New York and Bellevue Hospitals show that Irish immigrants carried Irish popular views about consumption with them to New York City. Irish phthisis patients usually told the physicians taking their case histories that they had fallen ill because of some combination of poor living, previous illness, and exposure to cold (NYHMCB 1848:C59; NYHMCB 1852:C768; BHMCB 1867:48, 74, 97; BHMCB 1874:265, 268). For example, Ann, a 19-year-old single woman, described that she began to cough after "exposure to wet and cold" during the winter of 1852 (NYHMCB 1852:C768). Another Ann, a 41-year-old dressmaker, and Philip, a 28-year-old coachman, both mentioned in Chapter 6, explained that hard work, insufficient food, and "living poorly" caused them to fall ill (BHMCB 1874:265, 268). These case histories attest that in New York City the Irish continued to see difficult material conditions of life as primary causes of consumption.

Hospital case records also offer a few glimpses into the ways in which Irish consumptives treated their illnesses before arriving at the hospital, including self-medicating with whiskey. Case records state that Ann the dressmaker had been a "steady drinker," and Elizabeth, an emaciated 27-year-old Irish-born woman, "had been taking" a "large amount of whiskey" (BHMCB 1867:67; 1874:265). Similarly, James, a 24-year-old painter, had been "drinking freely and suffering the effects of it" (NYHMCB 1865:C116). These patients might have been mixing whiskey with herbs about which physicians did not know to inquire. Hospital patients with nonpulmonary tuberculosis reported other strategies. Michael, a 41-year-old laborer with a tubercular infection of his femur, treated it intermittently for seven years with poultices. The infection worsened, and Michael consulted a physician outside the hospital who made an incision to drain the infection. This did not bring relief, so he sought treatment at New York Hospital (NYHSCB 1852:C183). Michael, like Mrs. Huxley, first tried traditional home remedies and then supplemented them with attention from the specialized healers in the city.[23]

Another patient, 19-year-old Mary, had taken medicine before admission to New York Hospital that caused her breath to have "a mercurial odor." Mary was diagnosed with a tubercular infection of the peritoneum, the membrane that lines the inside of the abdomen and contains the internal organs. This is a rarer form of tuberculosis, which, again, points to the great extent of tubercular infection within the Irish community in New York. Mercury was not part of the Irish popular pharmacopeia, but was regularly used by physicians, available at drugstores, and contained in some patent medicines. Mary fell ill just after she gave birth to a child, a month before her admission to New York Hospital (NYHMCB 1848:C622).[24]

While these case records provide some insight into Irish immigrant approaches to tubercular illness, all were written by American physicians, not Irish patients themselves, and only a small percentage supply such details. Archaeology can help to corroborate these written records and shed light on practices omitted from them. It is not known for certain whether any residents of 472 and 474 Pearl Streets suffered from consumption during the years with which the archaeological deposits correspond (late 1840s through the early 1870s). The likelihood is great, however, given the high rates of infection within the Irish community in Lower Manhattan, as evidenced by the records of the New York Dispensary and the generally high rates of illness in the Five Points neighborhood. All three archaeological deposits of most interest for this study, two associated with 472 Pearl Street (one with a TPQ of 1850 and the other 1870) and one associated with 474 Pearl Street (with a TPQ of 1860), were built up gradually over several years. They resulted from residents depositing waste in a backyard privy, cesspool, and an old cistern. The materials within these deposits are thus more likely to reflect activities over time, such as medication of work-related chronic pain, as described in the previous chapter. Consumption is also a condition suffered over a period of time, and thus treatments for it are likely to be discernible in the deposits.

The archaeological deposits at 472 and 474 Pearl Street, in fact, did contain a variety of substances used in Ireland to treat tubercular illness and that residents of these tenements could have similarly employed. They include strengthening foods, such as meat and fish; plants also used for strengthening and others for purifying the blood and/or in cough medicines; and liquor bottles, which could have been taken alone or as part of plant-based medicinal mixtures. The archaeological remains also contain indigenous American plants and patent and prescription medicines advertised for treatment of consumption, suggesting that Irish residents also looked to new healing substances to remedy tubercular illness as they had to remedy pain and injury, and were similarly advised by neighbors, friends, druggists, and others (Chapter 5). These medicinal substances and the methods by which residents probably acquired them will be examined here in more detail.

Food, Drink, and Friends

The liquor and wine bottles found in these deposits are likely to be traces of continued use of whiskey or whiskey-based remedies for a number of ailments, including tuberculosis, and that could have also been part of a "hidden industry" and used in important social rituals such as hosting and wakes to build crucial social bonds. (See Chapters 3 and 5 for more discussion of these bottles.) Numerous bones of fish and mammals found in these deposits suggest that even in this poor neighborhood, Irish residents were able to consume foods valued in Ireland for strengthening the body (Milne and Crabtree 2000). Meat was a coveted resource rarely available to people of modest means in Ireland. Irish immigrants' letters home suggest they were astounded by the abundance of animal foods accessible to them for a low cost in New York City. Not all of this meat was of the best quality, however, and as mentioned previously, some could have contributed to tubercular illness. Archaeological remains, nevertheless, show that residents took advantage of high-protein food sources. The particular bones found by archaeologists indicate that residents occasionally ate leg of mutton, beef shank steaks, and local fish (especially porgies), and that they more frequently ate ham steaks and roasts, pigs' feet, and bacon. They probably used bones in soups and stews, could have added small pieces of bacon to a quick "Irish fry," which also included potatoes and eggs, and might have simmered the pigs' feet in wine and spices, a traditional Irish dish (Milne and Crabtree 2000:181–185).

In times of need, those who could not afford meat or fish sometimes drew upon Irish social rules of sharing and acquired it through the help of friends. American mistresses complained that their Irish servants shared food from the household with the servants' own friends and family (Stansell 1986; Diner 2001). A cartoon (Figure 7.2) from *Harper's Weekly* (1874:112) presents mistresses' view that Irish friends demanded too much and their employees too often gave it to them. The cartoon suggests that meat, spirits, and tea were most in demand, substances perceived by the Irish to be important for strengthening bodies and for providing good hospitality. Written accounts from Irish individuals, themselves, corroborate this form of resource sharing. For example, James Michael Curley, a mayor of Boston, recounted how his mother nearly lost her job because she gave a leg of Thanksgiving turkey to a policeman (Curley 1957:9–10 cited in Diner 2001:119). Sharing was important; it enabled the possibility of calling upon a favor in return.

Consumption and Community among the New York Irish 295

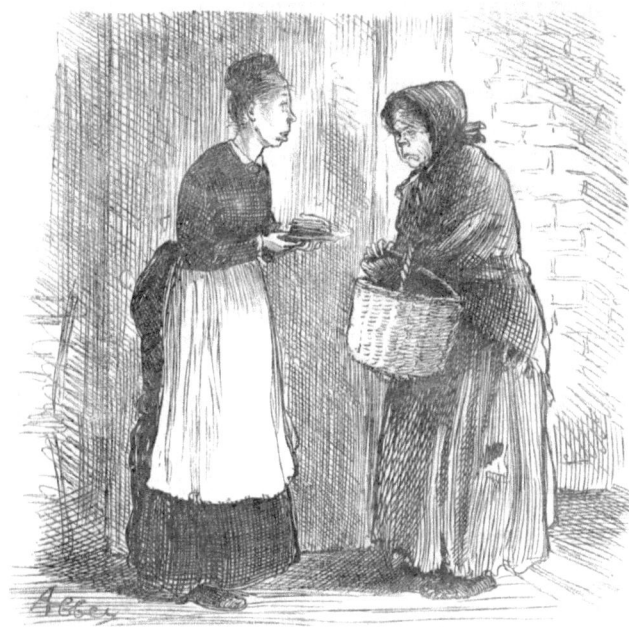

WHAT NEXT?
OLD SALLY. "I can't be a'tin' Bread all the while, along av the Dyspepsy. 'Avent yez a dit av Mate, or a sup av Tay—or just a wee dhrop av Sperrits to give a pore Crather?"

FIGURE 7.2. Cartoon titled "What Next?"; "Old Sally," an Irish woman, asks for more than the bread the domestic servant offers to her (*Harper's Weekly* 1874b:112).

Herbal Remedies from Neighbors

Of the types of plants the Irish used to treat consumption, remains of only a handful were present in the archaeological deposits at 472 and 474 Pearl Street. They include blackberry, dock, cherry, elderberry, and mint. But, as noted in Chapter 5, the city's markets, home cultivation, and gathering in less populated parts of the city could have provided access to other plant ingredients used in home remedies for consumption. Mullein, so revered as a consumption cure, had been introduced to the Americas but was so widespread on the East Coast that it was thought to be native by 1818 (Mahr 2022). Additionally, archaeologists found traces of jimsonweed (*Datura stramonium*) and wormseed (*Chenopodium ambrosoides*) (Raymer et al. 2000). Native Americans and African Americans used both of these plants to treat worms, and they also smoked jimsonweed for relief of asthma and coughs and in poultices for wounds (Covey 2007:100–101). Given the interest that the Irish had in the plants that grew around their homes and villages in Ireland, it would not be surprising if they asked neighbors about new weeds they encountered in American cities. Folklore records indicate that the Irish shared a widespread popular European belief that "for each disease God inflicted upon people He supplied a cure" (Farmar 2004:64; MacNamara 1963:120). Some Irish immigrants in New York might have thus felt that a cure for the consumptive diseases that plagued them in America could also be found in the American environment through the help of the American people. Archaeological and documentary records suggest that in New York City some Irish immigrants also looked to other new resources: patent medicines, alternative physicians, druggists, and soda water.

Patent Medicines

Despite the romantic image of consumption, historical accounts of individuals' experience of the disease remind us that pain was a major symptom, and one that many sought to remedy. The obituary of James McPeake, for example, notes that his sister, Sarah, died after "a long and painful illness" (*Irish American Weekly* 1857:3). Philip, the 28-year-old coachman mentioned earlier in the chapter, told physicians that what finally brought him to the hospital was "severe pain in [the] chest . . . [and] the sensation of suffocation and impending death if he stooped or rose or suddenly took a deep breath" (BHMCB 1874:268). Even those who survived hospital stays were almost never discharged "cured" and would have had to continue to manage the disease and its painful symptoms after discharge. It is thus likely that many of the patent medicines found within the archaeological deposits at 472 and 474 Pearl Street (see Tables 5.1 and 5.2) and discussed at length in Chapter 5 as remedies for injuries from labor, had been used also or alternatively by consumptive residents.

A laborer laid low by pulmonary tuberculosis, for example, might have tried one of the liniments, such as Radway's Ready Relief, that he originally bought upon recommendation from fellow laborers to ease sore muscles. Rubbing the product on his torso might have brought some relief from the pains caused by coughing, while the pungent odors of the turpentine and camphor the product contained might have cleared congestion, or at least provided a momentary distraction (Hiss

1900:183–185). A mother might have purchased Hunt's Ointment to try to heal her child's scrofulous wound that was not responding to her own ointment, or because she was unable to make a traditional preparation due to lack of knowledge, funds, or time. A concerned father could have administered the opium-based Godfrey's Cordial to a child suffering from painful *morbus coxarius*, because the product's advertisements claimed it was safe for children. Alternatively, a seamstress with advanced phthisis might have acquired this same product because a hospital stay had introduced her to opium, the only painkiller she had found that could enable her to rest without pain. Purchasing a bottle of Godfrey's Cordial would have drawn less attention at the drugstore than asking for morphine or laudanum.[25] Someone at 474 Pearl Street had used morphine, as attested by several glass and metal hypodermic syringes found by archaeologists (Yamin 1998:80). The hypodermic syringe was a new technology, used primarily for injecting morphine (Haller 1981b). It is quite possible that unrelenting tuberculosis was the reason one or more residents filled their veins with this powerful painkiller.

Still other residents might have looked to other types of patent medicines uncovered in their backyard for the near-miraculous cures they promised: balsams, bitters,[26] sarsaparillas,[27] and cough medicines. In the case of a sick child, especially, desperate parents might have spared no expense nor left any stones unturned. And, as discussed in Chapter 5, these substances were materially familiar. They were mixtures of plants and liquor that resonated with Irish popular whiskey and plant-based cures. Additionally, the advertisements of the specific brands found at the site suggest that they presented themselves in ways that were compatible with Irish popular understandings of illness causation and curing. Many advertised that they were excellent and safe "blood purifiers." An 1857 Hyatt's Life Balsam advertisement, for example, claimed it was a "potent, yet purely vegetable purifier ... the only reliable curative for all diseases flowing from great impurity of the blood," among which Irish immigrants would have included consumption. In addition, the advertisement claimed the balsam was "powerful yet mild" (*NYT* 1857:5). This notice, and others like it, aimed to convince undecided consumers that the product was worth trying; the risks were small and potential grains great.

Several of the brands represented in the archaeological deposits claimed specifically to cure consumption and/or scrofula, a tempting message, especially for those who had not found relief from other remedies. J. R. Stafford's Olive Tar, the only brand of cough medicine that was found in both tenements' deposits, for example, advertised in *Harper's Weekly* (1867b:479) that it could cure "all diseases of the throat and lungs," including "consumption" and "bleeding of the lungs" (Figure 7.3). The presence of this over-the-counter product suggests that residents of 472 Pearl Street sought a cough medicine that could do more than homemade cough syrups. Perhaps the statement in the advertisement that "thousands are saved annually from an untimely grave" caught the eye of someone desperate to save a family member, friend, or beloved. They might have hoped the image of a dove within the advertisement was a sign the medicine contained extraordinary power, and that it could be suitable for treating illnesses caused by supernatural forces, such as enchantment from a jealous neighbor or insulted fairy. The dove, the traditional symbol of the Holy Spirit, one of the three persons of the Holy Trinity, was at minimum compatible with Irish popular cures that evoked the Trinity.

Returning to Hyatt's Life Balsam, advertisements for this product also made grand claims about its ability to cure tubercular illnesses: "Diseases flowing from great impurity of the blood," including "rheumatism, *scrofula*, old ulcers, fevers, sores, mercurial, eruptive diseases, disease of the kidney, liver, and spleen, *debility*, and *incipient consumption* [emphases added]" (*NYT* 1857:5). Hyatt's Life Balsam was one of the two most represented brands of patent medicine in the Irish tenement deposits at the Five Points, found in the 1850 and 1870 layers of Feature J, and archaeologists also found two bottles associated with Irish households in Paterson, New Jersey. In contrast, archaeologists did not find any Hyatt's bottles in non-Irish contexts at the Five Points or at two comparative non-Irish sites in Greenwich Village (see Tables 5.1 and 5.2). Irish immigrants seem to have preferred this product.

Hyatt's Life Balsam was one of several balsam brands. As described in Chapter 3, an ingredient in balsams was an aromatic resinous sap with which most Irish immigrants would have been familiar prior to emigration in a mixture called friar's balsam, which was also the name of an English patent medicine. One of the purposes it was used for in Ireland was to create aromatic steam for relief of sore throats and congestion (Logan 1994:56, 74, 104). Additionally, balsams were a main ingredient

Consumption and Community among the New York Irish   299

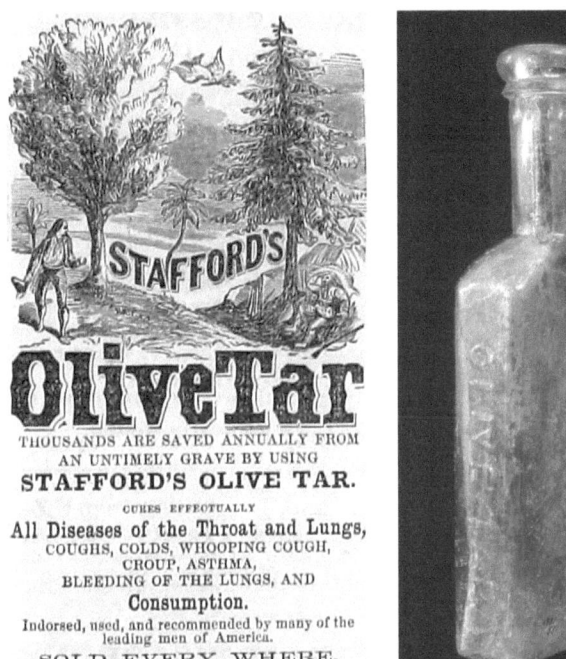

FIGURE 7.3. Left—Advertisement for J. R. Stafford's Olive Tar featuring a dove (*Harper's Weekly* 1867b:479). Right—Photograph of J. R. Stafford's Olive Tar bottle recovered from Feature J. Image courtesy of Rebecca Yamin and the New York City Archaeological Repository: The Nan A. Rothschild Research Center.

in the incense burned in Roman Catholic churches and in consecrated oil used in important rituals, including baptism, which, as mentioned, the Irish believed could offer protection from bewitching and fairy capture (Meehan 1907).[28] To Irish immigrants, Hyatt's Balsam would have appeared materially familiar, and the distinct odor could have signaled familiar, strong, and even divine, healing power.

Hyatt's Balsam also stood apart from other balsams because of the color of its bottles. Of 39 brands of balsams that Richard Fike (1987:22–29) describes as having been available in the U.S. between 1840 and 1870, only Hyatt's Infallible Life Balsam was sold in a green bottle. Folklore records indicate the Irish believed in the healing strength of certain colors by virtue of association with powerful people or things.[29] Although green was and still is sometimes considered unlucky in Ireland, it became a preeminent symbol of Irish nationalism by the 1840s; in the U.S., the color green was inseparable from the concept of the Irish homeland (Hutchings 1997:55; Owens 1998:252–253). In Ireland, green threads, ribbons, and stones were also occasionally used in healing and had positive connotations of growth and fertility (M'Clintock 1912:474; Hutchings 1997:57). At least one famous Irish wisewoman, Biddy Early, dispensed medicines in "dark" bottles, which were likely dark green, based on the types of dark glass readily available in the 19th century (NFC 1938[560]:464–466; NFCS 1938[596]:126; Brew 1990; O'Regan 1997:6).[30] Green things thus likely signaled to Irish immigrants not only nationalism, but also the healing potency of the natural world and of people, places, and things left behind in Ireland. In the absence of these powerful Irish sources of healing, the promises made by patent medicine producers and others who recommended them proved irresistible to at least some Irish immigrants in New York City who were desperate for a cure for consumption.

Hyatt's Life Balsam advertisements likely appeared trustworthy because they were published in mainstream American publications, including the *New York (Daily) Times* and *Harper's Weekly*. Inclusion in these newspapers might have seemed to vouch for the product's credibility among Americans, who Irish immigrants knew had more experience with consumption. Many ads even included testimonials with the names and addresses of individuals supposedly cured of incurable conditions. For example, one in 1855 included, "A lady in the family of F. W. Gilley, Esq., of the well-known Bowery dry-goods store (No 126) has just been cured of a case of scrofula of nine years standing. . . . Many of the most scientific of the medical profession had failed to cure . . . it. Mr. Gilley will cheerfully give any information . . . to any person who may desire it" (*NYDT* 1855:5). To Irish immigrants who were used to obtaining information about the quality of healers from neighbors and who were naïve about marketing techniques, testimonials like these were probably quite convincing, as they were for many Americans as well.[31]

Advertisements for the previously mentioned J. R. Stafford's Olive Tar also used testimonials. An 1860 ad in *Harper's Weekly* (1860:318), for example, stated that among several healed was "O. Charlick, Esq.,

President of the Eighth Avenue Railroad;" he "considers Olive Tar the best external remedy he has ever seen used . . . whether inhaled or applied, [it] is very beneficial for the diseases of the throat or lungs." The idea that these medicines had been used by "important" people, such as railroad presidents and successful dry goods store owners further increased the product's cachet, like celebrity endorsements today. Even readers who were more sophisticated might have been willing to suspend their disbelief in the veracity of the testimonials because they had already tried everything recommended by family members, friends, and neighbors, and they were willing to take a chance even on the advice of strangers.[32]

Alternative Physicians

Two medicine bottles embossed with "Dr. S. S. Fitch" were discovered in the cesspool associated with 472 Pearl Street, one in each layer. Dr. Samuel Sheldon Fitch was a self-proclaimed third-generation physician who professed to have had a uniquely successful method of treating consumption. It involved separate medicines for each symptom and a "pure silver inhaling tube" to inflate the lungs. Fitch (1854) published an "Almanac for 1855" containing his "Guide to Invalids," which explained his background and methods, listed the medicines and services he offered, and included testimonial letters. Consultations were free of charge, and interested parties could write to him to receive his medicines; but he preferred to assess patients in person. His guide was thus well crafted to appeal to people suffering from this then incurable and complicated disease.

Several aspects of his approach likely appealed to Irish immigrants, including the idea that he inherited cures passed down from his father and grandfather, his confidence in his curing abilities, his offer of free consultations, and his use of multiple medicines for different symptoms, all designed to build up the body instead of depleting it: "Nothing to break you down, or take away your strength, or appetite, or pleasures, or occupation, but all to cure and build up the health and strength" (Fitch 1854:6). In addition to his medicines, Fitch recommended good food, including meat, and frequent meals as well as a lot of sleep and moderate exercise (Fitch 1854:11–12). Fitch's background and approach was thus consistent with traditional Irish expectations of healers and traditional methods of healing via strengthening (Buckley 1980—also see Chapter 1). Fitch also advertised his services and products in the *New York Times* (1858c:5). He noted that he had given a series of public lectures and published them in book form. All these activities probably made him seem like a healer who had stood up to public scrutiny. Thus, although Fitch's shameless self-promotion diverged from Irish norms, a consumptive resident of the Five Points was willing to try his product.

Druggists

The presence of two bottles embossed with the names of nearby drugstores, Hegeman & Co. and M. E. Halsey & Co., within the Irish deposits at the Five Points are evidence that Irish residents also sought local pharmacists for healing. Pharmacists worked in drugstores that stocked myriad ingredients that they transformed into medicines. They also often dispensed advice and prescriptions of their own, filled prescriptions, sometimes performed minor surgical procedures, and sold soda water and patent medicines. Irish immigrants who had come from rural areas probably did not have much experience with druggists, but those who had spent time in cities might have been used to relying upon them.[33] In both New York and Dublin, druggists dispensed more affordable advice than physicians and developed relationships with their customers (Kearns 1994:103–105; also see Chapter 5). Customers did not just seek druggists' advice, they also obtained from them ingredients for home remedies; in Ireland this included mullein, the preeminent popular remedy for consumption (Allen and Hatfield 2004:250; Farmar 2004:34). In Ireland, druggists thus occupied an important position in between folk healers and professional physicians, and they helped bridge popular and professional medicine.

Druggists seemed to have occupied a similarly important role in Irish American communities and to have been similarly well regarded. The Irish writer Jeremiah O'Donovan (1969:292), for example, noted in his 1864 book that in New York City "druggists generally speaking, are a class of men of fine taste, solid education, refined manners, and invariably democratic, who would relieve, if possible, the woes and afflictions of an oppressed nation." In New York, druggists were also willing to supply ingredients for popular cures. R. Dillon, for example, advertised that "physicians' and *family* recipes [were] carefully dispensed [emphasis added]" at his shop (*NYFJ* 1854c:6). Dillon's shop was located within the Five Points at 421 Pearl Street, and it had been previously known as M. E. Halsey & Co.—the name embossed on one of the excavated bottles (Bonasera 2000a:379). Dillon might have been an Irish immigrant himself; there were Irish druggists in the neighborhood (see Chapter 5). His advertisement in the *New York Freeman's Journal and Catholic Register* was aimed at the paper's Irish Catholic readership. Some of his competition also seemed eager for Irish customers and advertised in the same newspaper, including Hegeman & Co.—the name embossed on the excavated cod liver oil bottle—, which was one of the first chain drugstores with branches at 161, 399, 511, and 756 Broadway by 1862 (*NYFJ* 1860b:5; *HW* 1862:175). The two bottles excavated from 472 and 474 Pearl Street and embossed with the names of these two nearby drugstores certainly underrepresent the amount of medicine residents obtained from druggists and only hint at their importance in residents' lives.

Cod Liver Oil

The bottle embossed with "Hegeman & Co. Cod Liver Oil" (Bonasera 2000a:379) contained a substance that bridged professional and popular medicine, Ireland and New York City. Fish oil was used as a popular medicine in Ireland, was adopted by physicians in New York, and probably extended the lives of many consumptives. This one bottle helps to further illuminate the relationship between Irish immigrants, consumption, and native-born Americans.

Folklore records indicate that the Irish had long used (cod)fish as a food to strengthen the sick, as Mrs. Huxley and her boarders attempted with her grandson. Pregnant women in Ireland had also been advised to eat fish brains during their pregnancy to ensure an easy delivery (Logan 1994:15). As mentioned in Chapter 6, fishermen in northern Europe, including Ireland, had long consumed fish oil to keep themselves and their families healthy. A few NFC Schools Manuscripts recommend cod liver oil for consumption specifically (NFCS 1938[268]:117; NFCS 1938[532]:193) or for "delicate people" (NFCS 1938[775]:245).[34] Present day studies have shown that the omega fatty acids in fish oil and the additional vitamins A and D in cod liver oil have many health benefits (Mayo Clinic 2023).

Low rates of consumption among fishermen attracted the attention of physicians, encouraging them to employ cod liver oil for phthisis in the mid-19th century. By the early 1860s, cod liver oil had become the most successful professional and popular medical treatment for consumption in the U.S., accepted by physicians and patients alike, despite, or partially because, of its revolting taste.[35] By the 1860s, many physicians believed this folk remedy saved the lives of phthisis patients, and its success changed their approach to disease. They used fewer purgatives and emetics and instead employed this oil, iron supplements, a hearty diet, and even whiskey. Demand for cod liver oil was so great that it helped to revive the then-ailing New England fishing industry (Grad 2004).

It is likely that the thousands of Irish immigrants afflicted with consumption and the increasing numbers of Irish immigrants employed as druggists, nurses, and physicians played a part in this shift in treatment in New York City. A variety of historical sources show Irish patients complained to physicians about harsh treatments, convinced nurses to provide them with more nutrition than physicians prescribed, and disobeyed physicians' orders outright, while archaeological remains from the Five Points show that they avidly self-medicated (Townsend 1847; Duffe 1853; MacLean 1886–1900; Bonasera 2000a; Brighton 2008). Physicians, meanwhile, read medical journals that published the latest good results of cod liver oil experiments and saw some of their patients improve with rest and good diets, supporting their patients' demands. The number of Irish-born nurses in New York City hospitals increased over time, infusing these institutions with Irish Catholic ideas and practices of care. Sister Claudia, an Irish-born nurse in the order of the Sisters of Charity interviewed for a history of St. Vincent's Hospital who began her seven decades of work there in 1889, remarked, for example, "Two things I never measured, cod-liver oil and whiskey. Cod-liver oil was best mixed with grape juice and a bit of egg white on top. The whiskey mixed well with anything, of course, and the patients never seem to tire of it. There's nothing to compare with it, therapeutically" (Walsh 1965:72). These Irish popular medicinal practices left a mark upon American medicine.

In ingesting cod liver oil, Irish immigrants suffering from tubercular illness strengthened themselves in a manner both recognizable to them and acceptable to native-born Americans. They participated in, and likely contributed to, making this familiar medicine the standard of care. The Hegeman & Co. Cod Liver Oil bottle found at the Five Points also indexes the variety of people Irish immigrants drew upon for healing, because fish oil could have been something recommended by any one of them: a family member in Ireland who had long ago shared a recipe, a neighbor from an Irish coastal village who had taken fish oil as a child, an American physician who had read of John Hughes Bennett's research, a druggist trained in Germany (where physicians had also experimented with this substance), an American employer whose own private physician had recommended it to him, etc. Cod liver oil was a substance upon which Irish immigrants, non-Irish immigrants, and Americans could agree. The experience of acquiring it from a drugstore or physician and taking it to manage consumption was something they shared, and something through which they could forge mutual understanding and compassion. The next section focuses on another commodity of interest to all three groups, soda water.

Soda Water: Elixir of Emigration

One of the surprises in the archaeological deposits associated with the Irish tenements in the Five Points was the number of soda and mineral water bottles: a total of 40, which significantly exceeded those found in association with the neighborhood's non-Irish residents (Figure 7.4).[36] Archaeologist Michael Bonasera (2000a:387) suggested Irish residents acquired them as alternative, low-cost medical treatments. This section digs deeper into a previously unappreciated relationship between Irish immigrants and bottled water in 19th-century New York City and beyond. Comparisons with contemporaneous sites in the New York area—Greenwich Village and the Dublin neighborhood of Paterson, New Jersey—also show more soda water bottles in Irish contexts than in non-Irish contexts (Geismar 1989; Salwen and Yamin 1990; Bodie 1992; Bartlett 1999; Yamin 1999).[37] In San Francisco, California, archaeologists found a cache of 127 soda water bottles related to an 1870s dwelling of an Irish laborer and his wife (Jack McIlroy 2006, pers. comm.; Praetzellis and Praetzellis 2009). Historical documents show Irish immigrant involvement in soda water production and sales. This section

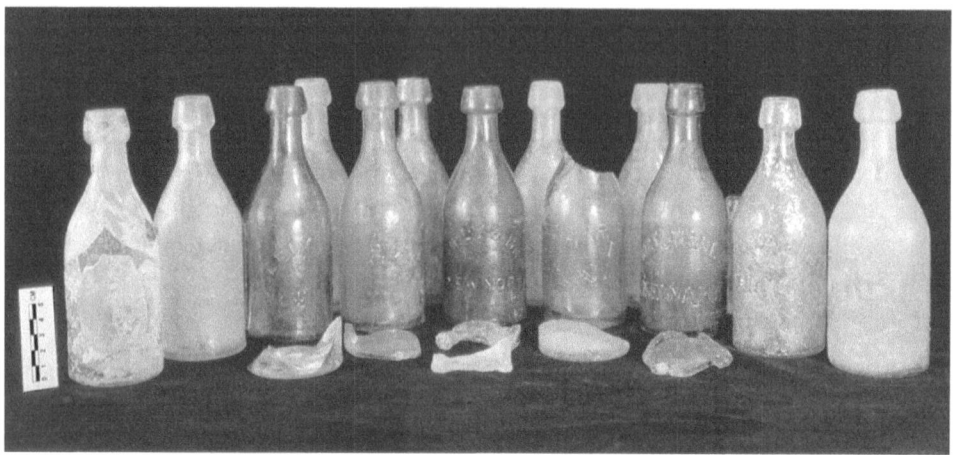

FIGURE 7.4. Photograph of soda water bottles found in Feature J, associated with 472 Pearl Street. Brands include Seely & Bros., Morton & Bros. Newark, and T&W (Bonasera 2000a:382). Courtesy of John Milner Associates, Inc., and the New York City Archaeological Repository: The Nan A. Rothschild Research Center.

proposes that like cod liver oil and certain patent medicines, soda water was a familiar substance in commodified form that appealed to Irish immigrants to treat illnesses, including consumption. Involvement with soda water also expanded their social and economic networks, vital for their long-term survival in a new land.

Before Soda Pop

In the U.S. and Europe in the 19th century there was a surge in interest in using water for healing, personal hygiene, and as an alternative to alcoholic beverages that was supported by the convergence of a variety of religious, social, and scientific ideas from Methodism to middle-class domesticity to sanitarianism and the rejection of heroic medicine (Numbers 1977; Porter 1990; Croutier 1992; Brown 2009; Linn 2010). The wealthy flocked to natural springs/spas, such as Bath, Evian, San Pellegrino, Poland Spring, and Saratoga Springs, for "water cures" and continued treatment at home with bottled water from those springs (Coley 1990:64). Many experienced relief largely from rest and imbibing cleaner water, but the natural mineral content of some springs might have had beneficial effects.[38] Spas were the precedents of tuberculosis sanatoriums.

Scientists eagerly isolated the constituents of spa waters, making them available to druggists for reconstituting in ordinary water; Epsom salt is an early (17th-century) example (Coley 1990:66). By the 19th century, druggists added carbonation. Technically, soda water is any type of water that is artificially carbonated, while mineral water contains minerals and might or might not be carbonated, naturally or artificially.[39] Because both of these products were commonly called soda water, that is the term I will use here, unless distinction is important. They were available for purchase in bottles or from fountains at drugstores, and peddlers sold cups of fountain soda from carts. True spring water from places such as Saratoga Springs cost nearly $2 per pint (Chapelle 2005:110), but fabricated bottled soda water was less expensive, and still cheaper was soda from fountains that chilled and carbonated the water (Figure 7.5): a cup cost between 2¢ and 10¢ (Funderburg 2003:20).

Until at least the early 1860s, the primary advertised uses of mineral and soda water were medicinal. Proprietors claimed their water could cure gout, rheumatism, kidney trouble, debility, catarrh, and consumption, for example (*HW* 1857:483; *NYT* 1866a:1). Physicians experimented with different mixtures of minerals and water to treat consumption. American Dr. J. F. Churchill claimed to cure 41 people of consumption with a mixture of hypophosphates of lime and soda in sweetened water (*Chicago Press and Tribune* 1858a:3). A man in Wisconsin said he cured scrofula and consumption with a mixture of baking soda and water. To mothers he advised, "If your nursing babies be sick, drink soda freely yourselves, and let your babe nurse, and your babe will soon get well" (*Chicago Press and Tribune* 1858b:2). Physicians, scientists, and the public were all anxious to find cures for many then-incurable ailments, especially consumption.

By the 1850s, flavored sodas had become popular as refreshing treats, especially during the summer months when sunstroke/heat stroke was a concern (Funderburg 2003:42).[40] Temperance reformers bolstered sales by advocating soda water as a refreshing alternative to alcohol. Enterprising individuals created soda-fountain shops separate from drugstores; by 1870 some offered more than 30 different flavored syrups (*NYT* 1870b:6). As a result of these businesses and changing attitudes

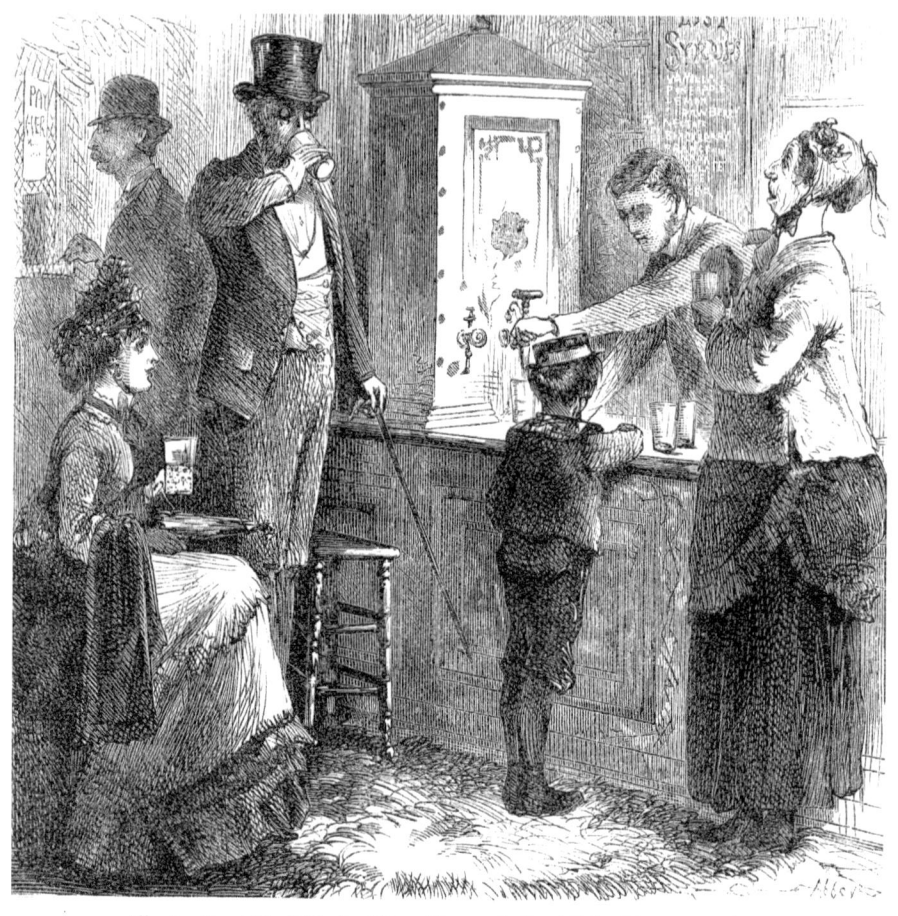

FIGURE 7.5. Illustration titled "Soda-Water Fountain," published in *Harper's New Monthly Magazine* (Snively 1872:341).

about medicine, most sodas consumed in the U.S. today are sweetened, and they are a major contributor to poor health. In the middle of the 19th century, however, soda water was a substance with perceived and real ability to improve health. The soda water bottles at 472 and 474 Pearl Street probably grossly underestimate what residents consumed, given the number of nearby drugstores and the abundance of peddlers in the neighborhood.

Interpreting Soda Water: Materiality in the Context of Diaspora

Because of these known meanings and uses of soda water among native-born Americans, archaeologists have often interpreted soda water bottles as objects that signal middle-class values and temperance or low-cost healthcare. Such interpretations importantly establish both social norms and disadvantages wrought by poverty, but they can underemphasize agency and inaccurately assume consumers understood and used these items as producers intended. As argued in Chapter 5 with respect to patent medicines, this premise is particularly suspect when the consumers come from different cultural backgrounds than the producers. Many scholars have long noted that people rarely adopt unfamiliar commodities wholesale, but instead employ them in creative and sometimes surprising ways, influenced by their own cultural worldviews and the material qualities of things. Certain textures, colors, and scents, for example, can trigger memories of (or resonate with) previously known items and inspire particular responses (or reverberate) (Thomas 1991; White 1991; Burke 1996; Howes 1996; Wilkie 1996; Linn 2010:71). Objects are not merely static markers of class status or ethnic affiliation. Instead, they participate in identity creation and social life; attention to "materiality" recognizes this recursive relationship between people and things (Latour 1992; Miller 1998; Buchli 2002; Rothschild 2003; Meskell 2005; Linn 2010:70–72).

In the context of immigration, particularly diaspora, material objects that resonate with people or places left behind can take on particular significance. Diasporic populations are especially resourceful and skilled in combining elements from their new and old homes. Attachments to the homeland and premigration worldviews are reservoirs from which migrants draw in practices ranging from artistic endeavors to religion to healing to community-building (Hall 1990; Boyarin and Boyarin 1993; Gilroy 1993; McCarthy Brown 1999). The next section considers Irish immigrants' premigration experiences with and ideas about healing water to enhance interpretation of the soda bottles found in Irish immigrant archaeological contexts.

Water in 19th-Century Rural Ireland

It is unlikely that most Irish immigrants would have had much premigration exposure to bottled or fountain soda water, especially those from rural areas.[41] Irish reactions to soda water in New York City were shaped by water from natural sources, particularly springs and holy wells. In Ireland, certain springs were said to have healing power through connection with particular saints or holy figures and were called "holy wells." Reverence for springs probably predates Christianity in Ireland, however, and is related to the reflective, hypnotic, life-giving, and shape-shifting properties of water (Strang 2005). Springs had prominent roles in Irish mythology. The Well of Segais was the source of all knowledge in the Celtic Otherworld (Bord and Bord 1985:4); in the Fenian Cycle the hero Fionn mac Cumhaill gains wisdom from drinking from it and eating the salmon that swam within it and the hazelnuts that grew above it (Brenneman and Brenneman 1995:27).

Holy wells could be visited by any individual on any day, and they were the sites of important religious and social events in Ireland: patterns and fairs. These events usually took place on holy days, such as the feast day of a well's patron saint (Figure 7.6), and attracted people from a distance. Protestant and Catholic, rural and urban, rich and poor alike visited holy wells, and holy well pilgrimages were generally supported by Catholic priests until the conservative "Devotional Revolution" in the second half of the 19th century (Read 1916:275). The "pattern," derived from the Irish *pátrún*, a term referencing the well's connection to a "patron" saint, was a circumambulatory religious ritual involving prayers and penitence, accompanied by drinking or washing with the well water. Pilgrims expressed religious devotion and sought cures for ailments. Carbonation in the water was said to confirm the well's supernatural power, possibly deriving from the legend of the Well of Segais's

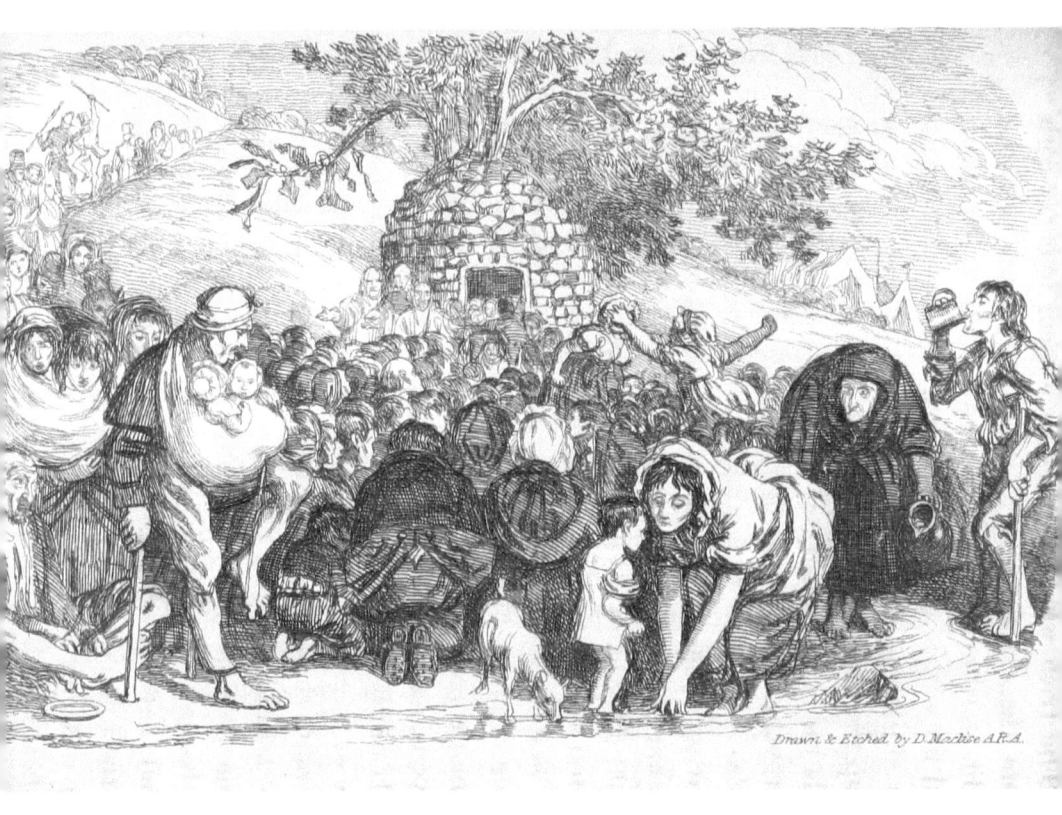

FIGURE 7.6. *"A Patron Day. Sketch taken at Ronogue's Well near Cork."* Drawn and etched by Daniel Maclise and published in *A Tour Round Ireland* (Barrow 1836:351). Note the man on the right drinking well water from a tankard and the older woman filling up a pitcher.

"bubbles of inspiration," while presence of a fish confirmed a request would be granted. Pilgrims often tied a piece of cloth to a nearby thorn bush as an offering and symbolic representation of the ailment or sin they were leaving behind to waste away (Read 1916:276; Ó Danachair 1955:195, 200; Brenneman and Brenneman 1995:14; Carroll 1999:19; Ray 2015:425–426).

Holy wells were said to be able to cure any ailment, but some wells were celebrated for their success at curing particular conditions. Ailments reported as curable by specific holy wells include: consumption, eye ailments, fairy possession, fevers, headache, infertility, insanity, pain, paralysis, scrofula, and skin problems.[42] The majority were conditions that did not respond well to popular remedies or physicians' prescriptions. For example, a schoolgirl in County Meath recorded that a certain well "cured a man named Walshe of consumption. After the doctors declared him dying, he drank a quart of the water every day and after a month it cured him" (NFCS 1938[713]:255).

Visitors sometimes brought holy well water home in their own containers for their own use or for "those who were too feeble to come in person" (NFC 1938[560]:543; Ó Danachair 1955:194) (Figure 7.6). Emigrants also brought bottles of holy well water with them on their journeys. A Donegal resident explained to a folklore collector in 1939 that "long ago when people used to go to America, they would take a bottle of the water [from a particular holy well] with them to cure the fever Ague. The fever Ague was a shivering the people would take when they would [words omitted] America" (NFCS 1939[1076]:431).[43]

A visit to a well on a pattern day was an important social experience that informed rural Irish immigrants' responses to American cities.[44] A festival-like atmosphere took place alongside the holy well patterns; participants traded, courted, arranged marriages and local or nationalist alliances, danced, drank, and fought, all in the outdoors near the well (Coyne and Willis 1841; Evans 1957; Carroll 1999; Ó Cadhla 2002). Pattern days also offered important opportunities for market exchange that were otherwise rare because reciprocity governed exchange in villages (Arensberg 1937). Fairs were also occasions to cultivate valued negotiating skills: "It was at the fair that a man proved his adult status by his ability to hold his own at buying and selling," but Evans (1957:261) notes they rarely bargained alone, believing a fair price was beneficial to all. Most Irish workers brought a similar philosophy to labor in the

U.S., refusing to adopt what they saw as American workers' every-man-for-himself approach (Roney 1931:180; Stott 1990:137). Faction fights sometimes occurred at holy-well patterns and such groups were precursors to urban and workers' gangs in the U.S. It is thus not surprising that in New York Irish immigrants engaged in fair-like behavior that middle-class New Yorkers were quick to criticize: dancing, parading, drinking, fighting, and spending time out in the streets. These uses of exterior space are crucial for understanding social dynamics in the city (Rothschild and Robin 2002).

Holy wells were also venues for the fight for independence from British rule. The large number of people gathered at holy wells presented Irish nationalists with opportunities to organize resistance. Daniel O'Connell organized his largest "monster meeting" to gain support for repeal of the 1801 Act of Union in 1843 at Tara, the seat of ancient Irish kings and location of St. Patrick's Well (Owens 1998). According to legend, it sprang up where St. Patrick first converted an Irish king. Many nationalists, including O'Connell, also supported the temperance movement, important for assessing soda water as a temperance drink in New York City. During the 1840s and 1850s, Father Theobald Mathew, an Irish Capuchin priest, who had once been the director of the workhouse in Cork city, gained hundreds of thousands of members in Ireland, England, and the U.S. for his temperance movement. Membership required a pledge of total abstinence from alcohol. Before Father Mathew, most temperance leaders were Protestants, and Catholics rejected them (Malcolm 1986:59; Kelly 2000). Nationalists subsumed Father Mathew's movement in Ireland by the mid-1840s, such that pledging temperance and nationalism were intertwined (Malcolm 1986:126–128). A teacup with a transfer-printed design showing Father Mathew administering the pledge was recovered from Feature J at 472 Pearl Street. Its owner might have considered it as much a nationalist symbol as a symbol of temperance.

These activities around holy wells presented people with opportunities for personal transformation outside of daily life and revitalizing social bonds. Diarmuid Ó Giolláin (1998:212–213) suggests that the pattern was a liminal occasion in which pilgrims existed in a sacred state outside the ordinary and engaged in communal rituals to leave sickness and sin behind, to create new selves. The journey to a holy well, through villages and countryside less familiar to the pilgrim, increased the ritual's transformative potential. The qualities of water also made it a critical element in the holy well pattern. "Water is the ultimate metaphor of fluidity" (Strang 2005:98, 105, 108, citing Lakoff and Johnson 1980). Michael Carroll (1999:42) argues the Irish linked holy well pilgrimages to the legendary pilgrimage of St. Columba, who exiled himself as penance. This legend may have been comforting for Irish immigrants, the vast majority of whom never returned to Ireland, possibly encouraging them to frame their emigration as a pilgrimage, in contrast to Kerby Miller's (1985) thesis that they coped by framing it as exile.

Some springs in Ireland were regarded as places to obtain fresh water for ordinary tasks: drinking, cooking, washing, etc. These "ordinary" springs were vital nodes of daily community activities, landscape features important to their identities, and sources for the preparation of home remedies. NFC manuscripts contain thousands of popular cures employing ordinary spring water. Some examples include: drinking large quantities of plain spring water for headaches, hangovers, and colds; infusions of herbs in spring water for consumption, constipation, jaundice; and soaking in, or making poultices with water as an ingredient, for bruises, cuts, and sprains.[45] A widespread home remedy for heartburn and headaches was to drink a few teaspoons of baking soda in water (NFC 1935[265]:597; NFCS 1937[624]:250; NFCS 1938[35]:133; Logan 1994:33).[46]

Given all these Irish uses of spring water and the layered cultural and social importance of this substance, Irish immigrants' reactions to bottled water in the U.S. must also have been complicated. The bottles of soda water found at the Five Points thus cannot be simple indicators of middle-class desires or even a strategy of relatively low-cost healing. Instead, the next section proposes that soda water was a commodity that was attractive to Irish immigrants because the resonances it triggered enabled them to use it to address a variety of their concerns: physical, social, economic, and emotional. Soda water facilitated Irish immigrants' ability to cope with the traumas of emigration and the ills of immigration.

Soda Water as Medicine in 19th-Century New York City

In 19th-century New York, Irish immigrants lacked access to the holy wells and springs of Ireland, yet as detailed throughout this book, they experienced great need for healing. Soda water was clearly not an equivalent replacement for these sources, but it was arguably the purest form of water available in New York City. Most natural springs and ordinary wells in the developed portions of the city were polluted by the early 19th century. Clean water piped in from upstate via the Croton Aqueduct became accessible in Lower Manhattan by 1851, but property owners were responsible for connecting individual buildings to the water mains and some older buildings were still supplied by public wells (Milne 2000:349–350).[47] Soda/mineral water manufacturers emphasized the purity of their water. These advertisements, combined with the facts that soda water was initially sold by druggists and utilized by American neighbors, likely inspired Irish immigrants to have confidence in soda water's healthfulness as a reasonable urban substitute for Irish spring water. The material qualities of soda water, particularly bubbles and mineral flavors, triggered connections to holy wells, and likely further enticed Irish immigrants to try this substance as a cure.

Given the wide variety of illnesses the Irish treated with holy well and spring water, it is likely they also considered soda water broadly applicable. Hospital records show some Irish immigrants chose soda water as a treatment for poisoning. In 1852, for example, New York Hospital admitted two Irishmen one month apart suffering from colic after lead exposure. George was a 31-year-old physician, and John was a 52-year-old waiter (NYHMCB 1852–1853:cases 23 and 60). Both stated they had imbibed soda water to prevent lead poisoning prior to admission. The soda water could have improved or exacerbated their symptoms, depending on the source of the water (see note).[48] Water with beneficial minerals could additionally help to prevent other ailments as well. Vitamin and mineral deficiencies caused by malnutrition have been found to increase the severity and the risk of developing respiratory infections, including pulmonary tuberculosis, as well as intestinal parasites, measles, and diarrhea (Cohen 1989:167). Sources of iron would have been particularly important for individuals with late-stage pulmonary consumption, who regularly lost blood through hemoptysis. Physicians at New York City hospitals prescribed iron for patients with advanced phthisis by the 1860s (NYHMCB 1865:C88, C349).

It is also possible that the Irish patients at New York Hospital suffering from lead colic hoped soda water could purge the lead from their bodies. Water from the Congress Spring at Saratoga Springs, New York,

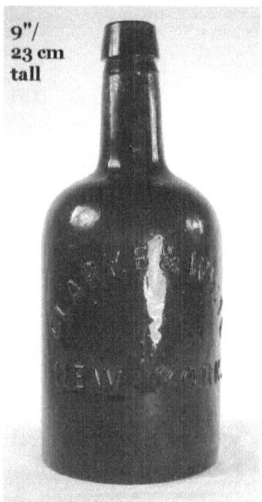

FIGURE 7.7. Photograph of a Clarke & White mineral water bottle, ca. 1856 to 1866 (Lindsey 2021b).

was advertised to have this ability. It was described as "a weak dilution of magnesia, with a dash of Epsom salts" (*HW* 1857:483), both substances that physicians and druggists prescribed for purging. Two of the 31 soda bottles embossed with brand names that were found in Irish deposits at 472 and 474 Pearl Street were marked with John Clarke and William White, proprietors of Congress Spring (Bonasera 2000a:381).[49] Figure 7.7 shows a typical Clarke & White soda water bottle circa 1856–1866. At prices of as much as $2 per pint, this water from a genuine spa was not likely bought on a whim.

It is possible that Clarke's water was recommended by a druggist or a neighbor, because of the good reputation of Congress Spring. A correspondent for *Harper's Weekly* wrote that among those who sought a cure at the Congress Spring were "men and women, crippled and crooked from hard work, hard fare, disease, and the infirmities of age; young maidens wasted and pale from those constitutional debilities to which, on this continent, they are so liable" (*HW* 1857:483). The correspondent continued, "We see among them too, the same expressions of faith, doubt, hope deferred, and incredulity, that we may believe marked the wretched groups which of old gathered about the Pool of Siloam," a spring-fed pool in Jerusalem that healed a blind man after Jesus told him to wash in the pool's water (John 9:1–11). For an Irish immigrant who could not afford a "pilgrimage" to Saratoga, or to the springs of Jerusalem or Ireland, a few days' wages might have seemed a reasonable price for a bottle of healing water.

For Irish immigrants who suffered from so many ailments in a new unfamiliar urban environment, soda/mineral water must have been a welcomed healing substance and a reasonable urban substitute for spring water. Like cod liver oil, it was a product that they could readily understand because of its familiar material properties and some similar recommended uses. Some bottled waters contained minerals that could have helped to restore health. For the seriously ill, who were physically removed from sources of healing in the Irish landscape, the therapeutic connection to the homeland and the hope that soda water offered was priceless. The experience of drinking cold, bubbly, and mineralized bottled water likely sent them dreaming, as it sent Mary MacLean in Quebec (see Introduction), of healing experiences at home in Ireland.

SODA WATER AND COMMUNITY HEALING: TEMPERANCE, NATIONALISM, AND HOSPITALITY

The experience of drinking whiskey likely had effects similar to these on Irish men and women in New York who longed for their homeland, relief from illness and injury, and/or camaraderie. But despite all the positive uses and meanings of whiskey discussed in previous chapters, it also had negative impacts upon many Irish immigrants—upon their reputations, relationships, finances, and health. As middle-class Americans embraced temperance, beginning in the 1830s, the perception that the Irish were heavy drinkers exacerbated preexisting ideas of Irish difference. Much of this stereotype of the Irish as prone to alcoholism was based on misunderstanding and prejudice. The delirium caused by typhus fever in the 1840s and 1850s fed into these stereotypes, as did the long-lasting importance of the pub as the center of social and political life and the persistence of whiskey-based cures. Yet, historical records show there were many Irish immigrants who struggled with alcoholism that exacerbated (if not caused) domestic disputes, loss of jobs and savings, injury (including accidents), sickness (including *delirium tremens* and alcohol-exacerbated tubercular illness), and even death (NYHMCB 1849:C65; NYHMCB 1852:C787; Stansell 1986:77–81).[50] Irish and Irish

American reformers themselves noted alcohol abuse to be a problem among the Irish poor. All of this considered, another important reason why soda/mineral water was so attractive to Irish immigrants was because it could act as a positive and culturally appropriate substitute for whiskey without the drawbacks of alcohol.

According to John Francis Maguire, Father Mathew's biographer and friend, one of the reasons why his temperance society grew so quickly was because the hard drinkers who abstained from alcohol after joining his society looked and felt so much better. People began to regard him as a healer (Kelly 2000:265–267; Maguire 1864:113). The transfer-printed teacup picturing Father Mathew administering the temperance pledge that was uncovered at 472 Pearl Street suggests that a resident was part of his society (Kelly 2000:265). This same deposit also contained soda water bottles that might have helped that resident to fully experience Father Mathew's healing. Using soda water as a replacement for whiskey could have enhanced a resident's reputation among middle-class native-born Americans, who saw soda water as a healthy and responsible beverage, and among Irish peers who connected it to the springs and political struggles of the Emerald Isle. Irish consumers seem to have deliberately accentuated this connection between soda water and Ireland through their choices of brands. Almost half of the embossed soda bottles found at 472 and 474 Pearl Street are marked with Irish surnames and an additional third with Scottish surnames.[51] The only embossed bottle of any kind from Ireland in the deposits was a soda water bottle embossed with "CANTRELL & COCHRANE// DUBLIN /&/ BELFAST" (Bonasera 2000a:381–383).

By the last quarter of the 19th century, there were scores of soda water companies from which to choose in the New York City area. Many of the more popular brands, including J. Boardman, W. E. Brockway, J. & A. Dearborn, W. Eagles, and George Spreitzer & Co. had English or German names. A comparison of brands of soda water found at the Five Points, Greenwich Mews, 25 Barrow Street, and Sullivan Street in New York City, and Paterson, New Jersey, shows that while Irish immigrants in the Five Points and Paterson preferred Irish-sounding brands, native-born Americans and German immigrants did not (Linn 2010:93–97). William Eagles Superior Soda Water, for example, was present in all non-Irish contexts and absent in all Irish contexts surveyed, likely because of a perceived connection with American nationalism, often symbolized by an eagle, during this period of high anti-Irish Catholic sentiment (Berger 1946).

Residents might have selectively purchased bottles with Irish names to express their support of and trust in their fellow countrymen, when newspapers questioned the purity of particular brands (*Harper's Weekly* 1886:446). A soda water bottle embossed with an Irish name might have been a desirable object to keep for entertaining guests. Remains of fancy tea wares found in the same deposits as the soda bottles show that providing good hospitality was important to Irish people in the Five Points, as it was in Ireland (Brighton 2000). Soda water might have replaced the whiskey bottle in a household with temperance leanings or a cup of tea during hot New York summers. The conversations provoked and social ties established over sharing a (soda) bottle would have been critical for the survival of most immigrants, constituting a kind of social medicine.[52]

Outside the home, soda fountains were important venues for social interaction, particularly the lively atmosphere of soda fountain shops that might have evoked memories of holy well fairs. Strutting up to the counter and paying for a soda displayed the attractive qualities of maturity and means men also asserted at fairs. For women, soda fountains were an alternative social venue to the pub, from which respectable women were traditionally excluded, excepting female bartenders (Malcolm 1998). Publicly purchasing a particular brand of bottled water, such as Clarke & White, at a drugstore could not only show support for Irish business owners but also convey awareness of the fashionable spa at Saratoga Springs. Because of soda/mineral water's positive associations with healing, nationalism, and hospitality, purchasing a reputable mineral water bottle like this would have been a subtle and acceptable way to assert sophistication, without inciting dangerous jealousy or animosity in friends and neighbors.

THE SODA WATER BUSINESS: A "CURE" FOR ECONOMIC AND SOCIAL ILLS

The soda water bottles embossed with Irish names attest to Irish ownership of businesses, and historical records show Irish involvement in soda water manufacture and the soda fountain business. Two Irish-born men admitted to New York Hospital in 1852, for example, declared their occupations to be "soda water vendors" (NYHMCB 1852–1853:C113, C198), while three Irish-born brothers at 472 Pearl Street reported their occupations as "soda water makers" to the 1850 U.S. census taker (USBC 1850). Given that according to the census, Dennis, Michael, and James O'Kelly were only 25, 23, and 16 years of age respectively, it is likely that they were lower-level employees. They might have worked at William Gee's Soda Water Apparatus Manufactory, advertised at 66 Gold Street in the *New-York Daily Times* (1852c), at one of many popular soda fountain shops on Broadway, or from a street cart. A Bellevue Hospital record notes that an old woman named Mrs. Shaw kept a soda water stand "on the corner of the block"; a boy's mother took him to see the woman after he had been bitten by a rabid dog, and he drank soda water (Bellevue Hospital 1874:347–349). It is possible that Mrs. Shaw was recognized in the community as a healer, and that soda water was part of her cure for the boy's sickness.[53]

One of the pioneers of the soda fountain shop in New York City was an Irishman named George Usher. George and his wife Sofia, who took over his business after his death, opened one of the first soda fountains in New York City by 1809. They might have incorporated their memories of holy well fairs into how they fashioned their shop. They chose a location next to a park to encourage outdoor socialization and advertised the health benefits of their water kept in copper casks.[54] Unlike their competitors, they were open on Sunday and invited both men and women to their establishment. Their water, like Irish spring water, was said to be exceptionally cold and bubbly (Funderburg 2003:13). Subsequent immigrants also invested successfully in the soda fountain business. For example, John Gelston, who emigrated from Belfast in the 1840s and made a fortune in finance, purchased the thriving soda water business of A. J. Delatour at 25½ Wall Street in 1865. Delatour had previously bought the business in 1808 from none other than Clark & Lynch, proprietors of Saratoga's Congress Spring, and had turned it into "a favorite resort for the business men of Wall-street," including "members of the Stock Exchange." By the time of Gelston's death in 1883, he had "long [been] one of the best-known men in Wall-street" (*NYT* 1883:3).

Involvement in the soda water business thus provided important economic and social opportunities for Irish immigrants, helping some to make ends meet and others to become wealthy and renowned.

Participating in the American marketplace as producers as well as consumers of a respectable product enhanced Irish immigrants' status in the eyes of middle-class native-born Americans. Individuals like George and Sofia Usher and John Gelston would have been able to establish helpful social connections with influential customers. Their positive reputations as successful business owners might have improved their patrons' opinions of other Irish immigrants as well. The understandings that these Irish business owners and workers brought to soda water were different and more complex than those of Americans, however. The connections between soda water and Irish spring and holy well water provided them with some relief from the more difficult aspects of acclimating to a new country, a new life, and a new identity.

NOSTALGIA THERAPY AND ADJUSTMENT AID

Experiences of emigration can trigger profound psychological stress, particularly in the context of a diaspora. Even Irish immigrants who left under more voluntary circumstances were often troubled that they almost certainly would never see their native land or certain family members and friends again. Unlike individuals from subsequent immigrant groups, only a very small percentage (less than 10%) of Irish immigrants during this era ever returned to Ireland (Miller 1993:265). Irish communities dealt with this reality with the "American wake," a funerary celebration commemorating the social death of the emigrant the night before his/her departure. Many immigrants additionally witnessed horrors of eviction, death, and abuse, which would have profoundly affected them psychologically, and then they encountered prejudice and poverty in New York City on top of all of this. These experiences contributed not only to cases of alcoholism, as mentioned previously, but also to other illnesses. From ancient times to the present, physicians have noted that a positive outlook increases chances of recovery. In the 19th century, physician Sir William Osler remarked, "If you want the prognosis of a case of tuberculosis it is as important to know what is in the patient's head as what is in his chest" (Dormandy 1999:247). Others believed that the chief causes of consumption were "affections of the mind, particularly ungratified desires, the principal of which is nostalgia" (Dormandy 1999:247). Immigrants who were able to find hope in New York City stood a better chance of surviving consumption, and the other health problems that beset them, than those who remained consumed by memories of their homeland. Soda water helped to soothe and even transform some difficult memories.

One of the characteristics of diasporic communities is a nostalgic "homing desire" (Brah 1996:180). Nostalgia is different from homesickness in that the nostalgic person yearns for a home that is displaced both in space and time; it is a place to which the person can never fully return (Matt 2007). According to sociologist Stuart Hall (1990:236), this longing transforms itself into a powerful creative force, "a renewable source of desire, memory, myth, search, [and] discovery." These feelings prompt the nostalgic to fashion a new home "from the materials at hand," most of which "are not mementos of their actual homes so much as items associated with the romantic image of home" (Matt 2007:497). Soda water might have reconnected Irish immigrants with positive memories of their old homes, possibly acting as a portal to romanticized past landscapes and a substance to help create new hybridized Irish American identities and communities.

While a variety of commodities could have functioned similarly for Irish immigrants, the physical and sensory qualities of soda water and the soda fountain were uniquely resonant with both events in everyday life in Ireland (such as collecting ordinary spring water) and occasions that were particularly memorable and out of the ordinary (especially holy-well patterns). Objects (such as soda water) can establish continuities with the past, because "as material symbols rather than verbalized meanings they provide a special form of access to both the individual and group unconscious process" (Rowlands 1993:144). While symbolism is important, objects are more than just symbols. As argued previously for patent medicines, objects have material presences that elicit important sensory responses. In the case of soda water, the coldness and distinctive tastes of particular brands could have unconsciously prompted powerful sensory effects causing Irish immigrants to remember cold and mineral-y Irish spring waters. Soda water's physical properties of being bubbly and shape-shifting could evoke memories of holy wells, where bubbling well water was a sign of supernatural presence, and personal transformation was the goal. The fact that soda water defies categorization by being neither fully water nor fully air, neither wholly artificial nor wholly natural, enhances its conjuring power. People often regard substances that cannot be easily categorized as magical (Dupre 1993). Anthropologist Veronica Strang (2005:111) notes that because water is integral to life on many levels, "water is the ultimate symbol of energy, potency, and the ability to extend human agency outwards into the world." Because of its material and symbolic qualities for Irish immigrants, soda water was a particularly powerful commodity from which to create magical material connections between new and old homes.[55]

FROM CONSUMPTION CURE TO ELIXIR OF EMIGRATION

This case study suggests that the surprisingly large numbers of soda water bottles found in Irish archaeological layers at the Five Points, in Paterson, New Jersey, and in San Francisco, California, are remains of more than an ordinary drink or even a consumption cure. Irish immigrants' previous experiences with spring water, combined with soda water's physical characteristics, transformed it from a simple commodity into a powerful hybrid substance, an elixir of sorts, which provided relief for physical and emotional illnesses caused by emigration and offered opportunities for personal and social transformation. Soda water's characteristics, including coldness, bitterness in taste, and effervescence, acted upon the senses of Irish immigrants. These qualities triggered memories of specific moments when Irish immigrants had drunk mineralized well water in their homeland, from ordinary water found in the community well to extraordinary water from holy wells promising healing and absolution. In a new land severed from these important nodes in the Irish landscape, soda water was a substance that resonated with their traditions, bringing comfort and perhaps even enabling Irish immigrants to frame their emigration as a sort of pilgrimage.

Soda water did more than elicit memories, however. It provoked Irish immigrants to use it in creative ways to remedy interconnected social, economic, and physical ills. For the Irish in New York City, soda water acted as a medicine to alleviate conditions, including consumption, iron-deficiency anemia, lead poisoning, alcohol addiction, and emotional trauma. It could act as a symbol of Irish pride and nationalism in a hostile American nativist environment; a form of social glue to create vital bonds of reciprocity among new community members through hospitality; a means of economic support for men and women trying to make ends meet; and a substance facilitating the transformation of an Irish immigrant into a "respectable" Irish American. New York City was brimming with many conditions beyond tuberculosis that consumed Irish immigrants; other epidemic and endemic diseases, dangerous labor, terrible housing, vicious prejudice, and more swallowed them up by the thousands. Soda water was likely so popular among the Irish in the U.S. because it could soothe, at least temporarily, so many kinds of wounds. It was a medicine for all these forms of "consumption," an elixir of emigration.[56]

Conclusion

When Archbishop Hughes described consumption as "the natural death of the Irish immigrant," he appears to have been commenting that the almost unfathomable number of Irish immigrant deaths from this disease was a "natural" outcome of the poor living and working conditions available to them in New York City. Irish immigrants were aware of the threat that consumption posed and utilized multiple strategies to counter it, detailed in this chapter. Documentary and archaeological records together reveal they tried popular Irish remedies, including strengthening foods, such as meat and fish, purifying herbs, whiskey, and consulting healers. They also employed new American resources, including soda water and certain patent medicines that conformed to their own cultural ideas about how to relieve symptoms and address the cause of illness. As in Ireland, they looked to the natural, supernatural, and social worlds for aid. In this process, the Irish strengthened ties with not only their compatriots but also with native-born Americans, expanding their social networks and safety nets.

For the Irish, consumption reinforced the importance of community and playing a cooperative role within it, both in their explanations of its causation and in their search for cures. Irish immigrants' adherence to Irish social codes at times irritated Americans—foremen were frustrated by Irish workers' disinclination to compete with one another, middle-class mistresses of households worried that their Irish domestic workers would give away their larder to relatives and friends, reformers thought the Irish wasteful for treating friends to drinks and meals instead of saving earnings, and Nativists and elites were irate at the favors politicians traded with their Irish supporters. It was through these sharing actions, however, that the Irish built vital connections that enabled them to collectively endure consumption as well as myriad other issues that threatened to consume their communities.

Personal interactions with non-Irish neighbors, druggists, and physicians—particularly when suffering from this illness that had already made such a mark on so many American lives—were also important and encouraged Americans to view the Irish as people not so different from themselves. These interactions enabled Americans to get to know more Irish immigrants as real individuals and not stereotypes or caricatures. Purchasing popular patent medicines and soda water as well as producing and selling the latter enabled the Irish to better integrate themselves into American commerce, an aspect of life vital to American identity, and arguably nowhere more important than in New York City, whose urban history began as a trading colony initiated by the Dutch West India Company.

Consumption and other forms of tubercular disease tragically took the lives of many Irish immigrants in New York, including the individuals recorded in the hospital case records presented in this chapter, and it decimated many families, such as the McPeakes. Nevertheless, the Irish community survived and even thrived. Emigration from Ireland continued throughout the century, reinfusing the community with new members and Irish worldviews and practices. These new immigrants required help to adjust to life in a new country too, but they were able to benefit from the gains made by those who came before them. Immigrants who arrived in the 1870s and later also faced fewer threats to their health because of increased public health measures that lowered death rates in New York City and other U.S. cities (Haines 2001). Additionally, as newcomers from Eastern and Southern Europe began to arrive in larger numbers and prejudice against African Americans continued to fester in the wake of the Civil War and Reconstruction, White native-born Americans focused more of their fear and ire toward those groups. The Irish found greater acceptance in comparison and sometimes themselves fomented anti-Black and anti-immigrant violence.[57]

Slowly, the Irish became integrated into American society, and they changed it in the process. None of this happened overnight, however. It was a long and complicated history, and one in which illness, injury, and healing—physical, social, and emotional—were deeply interwoven. The last traceable chapter of the McPeake family story illustrates this complexity and how one woman chose to manage it. In 1875, Ella Louise, the surviving daughter of James McPeake, who had been only an infant when her "affectionate and dutiful" father died from a "lingering consumption," graduated from the Normal College of the City of New York (Board of Education 1876:280). After her father's death, William L. Cole—her maternal uncle, editor of the *Irish American Weekly,* and author of her father's obituary—took Ella and her mother Emmeline into his household, where Ella lived on and off again until the 1880s (USBC 1860, 1870, 1880). It was likely with her uncle's support that she earned her license to teach "grammar and primary school," from the Normal College's rigorous five-year program, the only teacher-training program approved by the city, founded by Irish immigrant Thomas Hunter. Almost 20% of her 149 graduating classmates appear to have been of Irish descent, having surnames such as Brennan, Cassidy, Corrigan, Coghlan, Doherty, Gallagher, Geary, Grady, Harrigan, Kelly, Mahony, McGovern, Murphy, Neely, O'Brien, and Raferty (Board of Education 1876:280). They went on to teach the city's children, while many of their sisters went into nursing and cared for the city's sick; and their brothers increasingly policed the city's streets and controlled the city's government. By the 1870s, there was no doubt that Irish immigrants and their daughters and sons were both taking care of their own and shaping the city.

It appears that Ella Louise was successful in her career. In 1889 she loaned her uncle the considerable sum of $4,000 dollars for a mortgage on a property on Broome Street (*Real Estate Record and Builders Guide* 1889:996). Ella might have viewed this as reciprocating the aid he had provided to her in her youth, a gesture that likely would have pleased her father and paternal grandparents. But, the story of this last surviving member of the McPeake family took an interesting turn sometime around 1870 when she was about 16 and before she began Normal College: Ella Louise changed her surname from McPeake to Van Peake. And, it was not a passing teenage whim. She kept the Van Peake surname through at least 1899, when her uncle repaid his debt (USBC 1880; *Real Estate Record and Builders Guide* 1899:859).[58]

Did Ella Louise make this change to divorce herself from her family's tragic history, to make a definitive break from a lingering shadow of consumption? Taking on a new name is a strategy many people have used to leave behind a difficult past and to reinvent themselves. In shedding the most recognizably Irish part of her family name, Mc, it appears that Ella Louise might have considered her Irish heritage to be a difficult part of her past. Despite the success of her Irish immigrant uncle, other gains made by Irish immigrants, and Americans' more positive assessment of Irish consumptives that helped to counter ideas about essential Irish difference, anti-Irish prejudice was still not uncommon in 1870. As the daughter of one of consumption's victims, she had experienced some of the bitter costs of the disease, but as a young and healthy Irish American woman, she could not personally take advantage of social benefits associated with suffering from it.

In the absence of surviving family members from her father's side to offend, Ella Louise decided to style herself as Ella Louise *Van* Peake. She did not choose a different Irish surname, nor did she choose an English one nor one that evoked American heroes. Instead, Ella Louise chose a Dutch and Irish hybrid. She chose a name that simultaneously acknowledged she was *van* (from) the (Mc)Peake family and evoked the Dutch colony of New Amsterdam. With this new name perhaps Ella Louise Van Peak aimed to assert that she was formed both by Irish blood and American soil, a daughter of Ireland and the U.S., with no less right to the city than any other native-born New Yorker.

CONCLUSION

Looking Backward to Move Forward

THIS BOOK HAS FOCUSED on illness and injury among Irish immigrants in New York City from the 1840s through the early 1870s. It has pieced together different kinds of evidence—documentary, material, and oral—to better understand how Irish immigrants experienced and responded to life-threatening ailments—typhus fever, injuries, and tuberculosis—with remedies from Ireland and new healing resources in New York. It has also investigated how native-born Americans read the visible aspects of these conditions as evidence supporting—or in the case of consumption, challenging—preexisting anti-Irish prejudice. On a broader level, this book is about the interpretation of people and things from different, historically situated cultural perspectives and the roles of appearance and materiality in those interpretations. It is also about how medical ideas are intertwined with culture, history, and power.

Objects, Bodies, and Immigrant Encounters

This project began as a small study aiming to understand why Irish residents of 472 and 474 Pearl Street might have acquired the soda water and patent medicine bottles archaeologists discovered there. It is a project ultimately rooted in material things and sensory experiences and an historical archaeological approach that appreciates historical contexts and power structures but prioritizes the cultural perspectives, needs, and agency of the people who engaged with those things. In order to understand the perspectives of mid-19th-century Irish immigrants with regard to healing commodities, this project took a deep dive, inspired by cultural and medical anthropologists' ethnographic approaches and social and economic historians' "history from below," into historical documents and folklore collected from "ordinary" Irish people. Folklore records, despite the time lapse between the famine-era migration and their collection, provide insight into mid-19th-century popular views that are otherwise inaccessible. These records, collected from all over the country by and from Irish women and children as well as men, are also an important counter to the male, elite, and urban bias of many of the usual documentary sources available to historians. My resulting analysis of Irish popular ethnomedicine, as well as an overview of 19th-century American professional ethnomedicine gleaned from histories of medicine, I presented in Chapter 1: an examination of the 1847 encounter between Mrs. Huxley and Dr. Townsend and their differing perspectives about how to care for Mrs. Huxley's sick grandson, suffering from a fever and respiratory infection.

This encounter in Mrs. Huxley's boardinghouse was just one of innumerable meetings between Irish immigrants and native-born Americans in New York City, each of which shaped the larger engagement between this group of newcomers and their American hosts. My interpretation of both these micro and macro encounters was inspired by cultural and medical anthropological and historical studies of colonial entanglements between Europeans and Indigenous people outside of Europe, as well as sociological studies of the importance of bodily appearances and objects in the meetings between strangers in European or American contexts.[1] Although the contexts and dynamics of the meeting of the famine-era Irish and native-born Americans were different, such inspiration was important for keeping in view the importance of materiality (which I elaborate upon below) and how the British and many Americans had constructed the Irish as colonial subjects fundamentally different from themselves. Because the Irish were successful in becoming part of the American mainstream by at least the mid-20th century, it is often difficult from today's vantage point to fully appreciate how many Americans considered the famine-era Irish to be strange and undesirable not only because of their impoverished circumstances or differing religious faith. This study proposes that Americans suspected these traits to be symptoms of deeper, natural, essential, and perhaps unchangeable difference between the Irish and the English and Anglo-Americans. As described in Chapter 2, Americans responded viscerally to the dreadful appearances of many just-landed Irish newcomers and fell back upon an old, familiar theory to understand an unfamiliar epidemic. They read the symptoms of typhus fever—high temperature, rash, and delirium—as a surfacing of overheated sanguine Irish interiors and imagined typhus as a predictable "Irish fever." Similarly, they interpreted bodies of Irish immigrant laborers and domestic servants made muscular by labor and red-faced by exertion and the elements as evidence of the same humoral temperament which supposedly imbued them with energetic, passionate, and irrational characters that made them unsuitable for intellectual work but naturally suitable to manual labor, as detailed in Chapter 4. These prejudicial views carried more authority because they were underpinned by humoral theory, a long-dominant holistic medical theory, as well as new "scientific" ideas about human variation also informed by humoral theory.

In the 19th century, supposed differential temperaments, susceptibility to specific illnesses, and proclivities for particular kinds of work were observed by race scientists and early physical anthropologists in their quest to understand variability among human groups and, often, to justify slavery, white supremacy, and later, eugenics (Jacobson 1998; Harris and Ernst 1999; Watkins 2012; Blakey 2020). Race scientists were erroneous in their ideas about essential human difference and hierarchy of so-called races. Subsequent research has proven that while race is a powerful social construction, it has no biological basis. There is only one human species; there is greater variation within any of the so-called races than between them; physical variations in supposed racial traits, such as skin color, tend to occur gradually, not abruptly; and the range of one trait does not predict the presence of others. Work in physical anthropology, dating to Franz Boas's (1910, 1912) project to show changes in bodily form of descendants of immigrants, and more recently in bioarchaeology, has revealed how life experiences, including diet, illness, injury, and activity, shape human bodies in ways that are visible on the interior and the exterior (Larsen 2000; Blakey and Rankin-Hill 2004; Warner-Smith 2022).

This study has taken seriously the idea that the bodies of Irish immigrants were indeed sometimes different than those of middle-class native-born New Yorkers, not because of essential differences between these groups but instead because of their different life experiences in Ireland and New York. Chapter 4 explored how Irish men and women's hard work sculpted leaner bodies, and how injuries at work and medical and surgical interventions to remedy them resulted in additional visible differences that Americans read as proof of Irish stereotypes of brutish, belligerent, bogtrotting, and whiskey-besotted Bridget and Pat. Such interpretations were not limited to lay strangers who judged Irish newcomers from a relative distance but were shared by some employers who supervised and even approved of Irish male laborers' work, others who oversaw female domestic servants in their own homes, and physicians who closely examined Irish immigrants in hospitals and dispensaries.

Such assumptions, initially sustained even during close encounters, were aided by the way that extreme events often have disproportionately large and lasting impacts on public opinion. In the case of Irish immigration, scholars have pointed out how the relatively small percentage of very poor Irish immigrants whose migration was assisted by landowners or poorhouses greatly contributed to the impression that all famine-era migrants were poor, and how the high death rates on a few emigrant ships during a few months of the famine led to the characterization of all emigrant ships carrying Irish famine refugees as "coffin ships," or how the participation of some Irish immigrants in the atrocities of the 1863 Draft Riots convinced many that all Irish immigrants were not only brutish but also racist (Kenny 2006; McMahon 2015a, 2021; Hirota 2017).

In this book, I have argued that as an unfamiliar epidemic interpreted through such entrenched ideas about the nature of bodies, illness, and human variation, typhus fever had an outsized effect on native-born Americans' interpretations of famine-era Irish. It further fogged the already biased lens through which Americans viewed Irish labor, bodies, religious and cultural practices, and potential. In a sense, it was Americans who were infected with "Irish fever." Americans' fevered responses created a "second epidemic" of prejudice with ramifications for Irish immigrants that ranged from being passed over for better jobs to violent clashes on the streets to what might be characterized today as malpractice in hospitals. As Chapters 2 and 4 detail, physicians' views of the Irish were clouded such that they appear to have misdiagnosed some Irish patients with typhus fever, subjecting them to dangerous and ineffective therapies, and to have withheld anesthesia for painful surgeries, assuming alcoholism or brutishness or both made Irish (especially male) patients poor candidates for this new technology. Nativist attitudes that branded the Irish as insensitive and ignorant usurpers of public charity also facilitated experimentation on Irish bodies, alive and dead, justifying it as a means of repaying their "debt" to society (Warner-Smith 2022). Once anchored to humoral theory and the extreme event of an outbreak of an unfamiliar epidemic disease, stereotypes of Irish immigrants that had originated decades earlier in England became cemented in the U.S. These stereotypes proved to be a shared vocabulary and set of images that Americans could (and still can) dredge up whenever there was interest in censuring or degrading individuals of Irish descent, from Mary Mallon, a.k.a. Typhoid Mary, to John F. Kennedy and beyond.

Ideas about disease and/or physical abnormalities have been used since ancient times to characterize outsider groups as different and lesser, and they continued to be utilized in this way in the U.S. against subsequent immigrant groups, most recently stigmatizing Chinese Americans as carriers of COVID-19 (Farmer 1993; Kraut 1994). Nevertheless, the relationship between disease and anti-immigrant and/or ethnic or racial prejudice is not always so straightforward. As shown in Chapter 6, tuberculosis, an endemic disease in New York in the mid-19th century, did not elicit the same surge of anti-Irish bigotry as typhus fever when tuberculosis became an epidemic among Irish immigrants. This was not because Americans did not notice an outbreak among the Irish but because of how Americans (mis)understood the disease as affecting only individuals with a sensitive predisposition, enabling them to give meaning to and cope with terrible suffering the disease inflicted upon their own loved ones. This perspective, combined with the physical impacts of the disease on Irish immigrant bodies, enabled some Americans to recognize Irish consumptives beyond the stereotypes and as individuals not so different from themselves. Thus, when investigating the impacts of ailments on prejudicial views, it is critical to employ a nuanced approach that considers the intersection between ideas about the particular condition, stereotypes of the group in question, and the broader historical context.

This book has also focused on the perspectives and reactions of Irish immigrants themselves in their encounters with conditions in the U.S. and the country's native-born inhabitants. It has sought to highlight the experiences of particular individuals in each chapter and to excavate their strategies to manage and heal illness and injury through interpretation of documents, including hospital records and manuscripts of orally collected folklore, and reinterpretation of the archaeological deposits of 472 and 474 Pearl Street, with an approach informed by 19th-century Irish popular medical ideas and practices. Such an approach makes visible the remains of possible home remedies in floral and faunal assemblages and in wine bottles previously interpreted as evidence of diet, environment, or respectable entertainment, as detailed in Chapters 3, 5, and 7. Insights from medical anthropology—including the importance of materiality in healing and the powerful anxiety-reducing impacts of culturally competent care—and ethnobotany suggest that some of these remedies could indeed have brought physical relief and draw attention to the importance of the material qualities of medicines (Van der Geest et al. 1996; Moerman 2002; Allen and Hatfield 2004). Also informed by these insights, I proposed different interpretations of new healing commodities discovered in these Irish immigrant archaeological deposits, namely patent medicines and soda water, that appreciate how the material qualities of particular products (greasy, aromatic, fizzy, green, etc.) and symbolism in advertisements resonated with Irish consumers' cultural medical perspectives and needs in New York (see Chapters 5 and 7).

My approach throughout this book has presupposed some degree of Irish immigrant agency, even in the most difficult of circumstances, and considered the cultural perspectives and practices they brought with them from Ireland as wellsprings of inspiration. It has also recognized the characteristic resourcefulness of Irish popular medical approaches in incorporating compatible new local substances, knowledge, and people into healing efforts. Neighbors (Irish and non-Irish), priests, druggists, nurses, physicians, and surgeons were all potential healing resources the Irish could and did draw upon when home remedies or over-the-counter products failed. There were many conditions, including tuberculosis, that neither physicians nor Irish popular remedies nor healers could cure, however, and Irish individuals appear to have looked to soda water and/or patent medicines for miracles in the absence of holy wells or other sites of supernatural healing power in Ireland (see Chapters 5 and 7).

Irish immigrants saw hospitals and dispensaries as places to seek healing but usually as a last resort, especially hospitals, because of their known dangers to health and because of the cultural insensitivity that Irish and other non-native-born American patients often experienced there. Irish immigrants, as well as German, Jewish, and later Italian immigrants, worked to change both of these situations in New York. The predominantly Irish-born Sisters of Charity established St. Vincent's Hospital and a new standard of culturally competent, compassionate, and knowledgeable nursing care, while many Irish and Irish American individuals became physicians and nurses and changed existing New York City healthcare institutions from within. Among other factors, cultural and religious obligations to care for others, widespread experiences of suffering illness and injury within their communities, and desires for native-born Americans to recognize their positive contributions likely drew so many people of Irish descent into the field of medicine as it drew members of other immigrant groups who also established their own hospitals: the Jews' Hospital—later called Mt. Sinai (est. 1855), the German Dispensary—later Lenox Hill (est. 1857), and Columbus Hospital (est. 1892 by the largely Italian Missionary Sisters of the Sacred Heart of Jesus)—later Cabrini Medical Center.

Also like members of other immigrant groups, most Irish immigrants quickly became aware of American norms and used that knowledge to their advantage, as a number of historians have described in the context of machine politics and liquor-related businesses, for example. Chapter 7 draws attention to Irish success and ingenuity in the soda water business, while Chapter 5 highlights more mundane but potentially equally transformative efforts of Irish individuals to manipulate their appearances using commodities such as cosmetics, hair dyes, clothing, corsets, and braces to take control of how others viewed them. In some cases, this might have meant disguising Irish ethnicity and/or signs of stereotypical sanguinity, and in other cases, it might have meant projecting a higher-class status, and in still others, appealing to Irish ideals of beauty. For most Irish immigrants, their main audience was the Irish immigrant community. They brought with them a strong sense of mutual obligation and collectivism that had been formed in rural Ireland but was just as or even more important in urban New York, especially in the context of intense anti-Irish prejudice and Irish nationalists' efforts to construct a transnational Irish diasporic identity. Irish collectivism came in direct conflict with American individualism, and Irish immigrants' generosity in helping their friends triggered reproach from many native-born Americans as clannish, childish, or wasteful; but it was critical for the survival and success of so many who arrived with so few economic resources.

Similarly, the refusal of many Irish immigrants to renounce an Irish identity also provoked the ire of many Americans. In fact, the text that accompanies Figure 2.4, "The Irish Declaration of Independence That We Are All Familiar With" highlights this very issue, as does the cartoon, Figure 6.10, "The Mortar of Assimilation and the One Element That Won't Mix." Father Thomas N. Burke, a Catholic priest famous for his sermons, expressed the pride many had in their Irish heritage in a published sermon encouraging his flock to love thy neighbor: "Let me remind you that we are not a phlegmatic race, that we are not accustomed to conceal our feelings. The Irish heart is susceptible, the Irish temperament is sanguine, even demonstrative. We are people who have never been silent or contented under a great wrong or under great sorrow" (1872:49). Father Burke reappropriated the very humoral vocabulary that had been used to denigrate the Irish to assert the value of Irish difference. He was not unusual in that regard. Many Irish nationalists had by then long embraced a Celtic heritage distinct from, and in their view, superior to Anglo-Saxon heritage. They were not content with assimilating into culturally Anglo-dominant U.S., and instead avowed hybrid Irish American identities and the contributions Irish cultural practices and people could make to the U.S. and to the other countries to which the Irish dispersed (McMahon 2015a).

Looking Backward—and Forward

There are many opportunities for additional research on the topics covered in this book. First, more could be done to uncover additional and diverse experiences of Irish immigrants in New York City, examining records from Bellevue Hospital and Ward's Island Hospital from the famine period would be places to start. Greater attention to more individuals would help to increase the specificity of this study and highlight the divergent views that existed within the Irish community. The lives of the individuals mentioned in this book could also be traced further to better understand the long-term impacts of traumas they experienced.[2]

Additional research also could be done to examine the impacts of injured Irish Civil War soldiers upon native-born Americans' views of Irish laborers with visible injuries. The impacts of other ailments on Irish immigrant life could also be studied. Investigating diseases besides tuberculosis that caused great mortality among Irish children especially, including *cholera infantum*, could reveal more about food and childcare practices in New York. Examining the dangers affecting pregnant mothers might help to identify Irish midwives, a category of healer not focused on in this study, but one of great importance to communities in Ireland and the U.S. There is also much more to uncover in terms of Irish responses: how they shaped healthcare in the U.S. and their involvement in soda water businesses are just two examples.

This study could also be expanded in various comparative ways, such as enlarging the geographic scope beyond New York City, considering other locales in the U.S., and/or other major destinations of famine-era Irish immigrants: England, Canada, and Australia. The temporal frame could also be expanded to consider change over a longer period of time and how the advent of the germ theory affected attitudes toward Irish consumptives, for example, who later were stigmatized. Alternatively, the health-related experiences of the Irish in New York could be compared more extensively with those of other contemporary immigrant groups, such as German immigrants, and African Americans, who often lived in the same neighborhoods and worked in similar occupations, or subsequent immigrant groups, such as Italians, or with immigrant groups in the present.

There are many points of potential comparison between the famine-era Irish immigrants and present-day immigrants from a variety of regions in the world including Latin America, the Caribbean, Asia, and Africa, despite differences in culture and time. There are many positive things that have not changed, such as continued interest among individuals of many immigrant groups in health. Immigrants continue to utilize traditional medicines and preventive practices from their homelands, some of which have been shown to produce lower rates of illnesses endemic to the U.S. (such as heart diseases, cancers, and diabetes) among those groups (Chavez 2003). Many immigrants today also work in healthcare, from physicians, nurses, and hospital technicians to home healthcare providers. Networks of mutual assistance remain critical for many immigrant groups today, as do their assertions of the gifts their cultures bring to the U.S. and of hybrid identities that are simultaneously fully American and fully something else.

On the negative side, prejudice against newcomers remains prevalent, and many Americans react to immigrants in ways that are not well thought out and based on the most superficial appearances and rumors. Supposed natural connections between particular immigrant groups and diseases are still marshaled to support negative stereotypes. Immigrants are still overrepresented in low-paying and dangerous jobs and often limited in their access to safe housing or neighborhoods. Thus, they sustain more injuries and suffer from more environmental-borne illnesses than many native-born individuals. In hospitals and doctors' offices immigrants still suffer from unconscious (and sometimes conscious) bias in medical treatment and culturally incompetent care. Allegations that immigrants refuse to assimilate, spend their money unwisely, rely on insular networks and superstitious practices, and drain public resources still proliferate. And many Americans still believe that certain arbitrary visible characteristics are proof of natural, essential differences between people from different cultures and regions of the world. Those groups categorized as non-White suffer the intersecting prejudices of anti-immigrant and racial discrimination, along with gender and often class discrimination.

One of the many things that has changed over the last almost 200 years since the Irish Famine migration is how that group is widely regarded in the U.S. today. They, along with other "older" European immigrant groups, such as the Germans and Italians (Figure C.1), are commonly thought to have been culturally similar to native-born Americans, to have worked to assimilate quickly, to have pulled themselves up by their bootstraps, and to have joined the working or middle class with little assistance from the government or anyone else (Foner 2005:207–212). In taking a deep dive into how most native-born Americans considered the Irish to be essentially and naturally different, sometimes even unassimilable, how many Irish immigrants refused to assimilate, how many suffered and died, and how those who did succeed almost always did so with assistance from others within and outside Irish immigrant communities, assistance that Irish immigrants themselves deeply valued, I hope this book prompts readers to question present-day stereotypes of

338 Conclusion

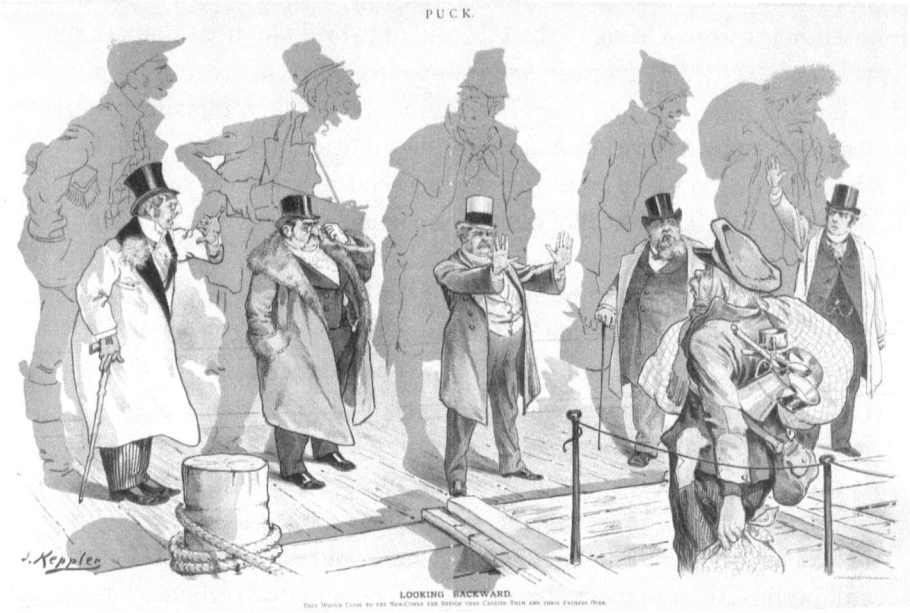

FIGURE C.1: Cartoon titled "Looking Backward: They Would Close to the New-Comer the Bridge that Carried Them and Their Fathers Over" by Joseph Keppler (*Puck* 1893). The image shows five wealthy men rejecting an Eastern European immigrant as he disembarks from a ship. Behind the men are shadows of their former selves or fathers who had been poor immigrants from Northern and Western Europe. In the center is an Irish American. Courtesy of the Art Institute of Chicago, Creative Commons Zero (CC0 1.0).

the "good old immigrants" as well as stereotypes of present-day immigrants. I hope that looking to this past promotes reflection upon what it means to be "a nation of immigrants" and how we might realize such a concept more fully and more compassionately going forward.

NOTES

Introduction

1. MacLean [1886–1900] notes how physicians were "baffled" by the illness, some believing it came over on ships, others that it was carried by the wind. To prove the latter, they "hoisted a long pole to the end of which was tied a leg of a lamb, into the upper air, certain . . . that the side of the leg on which the wind blew [would] turn putrid."

2. A note on the terminology I use to identify different groups: I use the term native-born Americans or simply Americans, throughout this book, although I recognize that is an imprecise, generalizing term, given that such a group was composed of people of different ethnicities, races, classes, and religions who had varying opinions about just about every issue. When referenced in this book, I usually mean the term to represent the majority view of the American public in which White middle-class men had the loudest and most influential voices. When I mean a more limited group, I will add specification, such as working-class (among which the voices of White men also predominated) or African American. I recognize that there was great diversity within these groups as well. I usually use the term African American following Black feminist historians who have argued that the majority of Americans of African descent in 19th-century New York felt a connection both to Africa and the U.S. (Alexander 2008). Many African Americans in 19th-century New York City (NYC) were native-born Americans, but some had been born in Africa or the Caribbean. To refer to Irish-born individuals, again a diverse group, I use the terms Irish emigrant, immigrant, newcomer, or refugee, depending on which aspect of their lives I intend to emphasize or how they are referred to in particular sources. Most hospital records, for example, use the term Irish-born. When I use the term Irish American, I usually mean people of Irish descent who were born in the U.S. or who immigrated as very young children and identified as equally or more American than Irish. I do recognize, however, that other Irish immigrants considered themselves to be equally or more American and Irish, that Irish-born naturalized citizens were legally U.S. citizens

(and thus legally Americans), and that American nativists' questioning of Irish immigrants' loyalty to the U.S. was a major point of contention.

3. Following Christine Kinealy (2006), most scholars consider the dates of the famine to range from 1845 until the blight-free harvest of 1852, and I have thus used these dates throughout. However, as Cian McMahon (2021:4) notes, numbers of migrants leaving Ireland did not return to pre-famine levels until 1855; from the perspective of immigration studies, the famine era ranges from 1845 to 1855.

4. In the U.S., this event is usually referred to as the "Irish Potato Famine" or the "Great Famine" (An Gorta Mór in Irish). Some historians have preferred to use the term "Great Hunger" to emphasize that the potato blight was not the sole cause of the famine, but that the ruling government failed to enact adequate relief measures (Cecil Woodham-Smith 1962). Some scholars, including Christine Kinealy (2006:8), have argued that "the famine became a tool [of the colonial government] in the long-desired aim to modernise and regenerate Ireland; . . . relief measures were driven by a moral, a financial, and an ideological imperative that gave priority to changing Ireland above the needs of a starving and desperate people." Historian James S. Donnelly Jr. (2001:21) also explains that British prejudices against the Irish were in part responsible for the government's inadequate response. "Irish problems were seen to arise mainly from defects in the Irish character"; many felt that "British policy during the famine must aim at educating the Irish people in sturdy self-reliance."

5. Many Irish families relied heavily on potatoes because of laws and customs that had impoverished them during the centuries of British rule. For example, among the many other economic, political, and religious restrictions of the Penal Laws (in effect between 1690 and 1829), was outlawing primogeniture among Catholics and nonconformist Protestants, forcing equal division of land among heirs. After a few generations, plots owned by any one family were tiny. Potatoes, especially a particular variety, were one crop that yielded enough to support a family. Additionally, many families had lost their land and rented plots from larger, often Protestant, landowners. The 1841 Irish Census categorized half of the rural population of Ireland (then composing 85% of the total population) as part of the lowest class, Class III, meaning that they lived in one-room mud huts and had no capital in either "money, land, or acquired knowledge" (Evans 1957:46; Keneally 1998:8). In some predominantly Catholic counties, such as Kerry and Cork, up to 80% of rural families were recorded as Class III (Evans 1957:46).

6. Diaspora, a term derived from the Greek word "to scatter," was initially applied to describe the multiple forced dispersals of Jewish people in history and then to forced dispersals of captive Africans. The classic criteria of a diaspora include: (1) a dispersal from a place of origin, (2) a history of traumatic and forced departure, (3) a collective, strong attachment to the homeland and desire to return, and (4) a relationship with a host society that is at some point troubled. Many scholars have described 19th-century Irish emigration as a diaspora (Kenny 2003; Brighton 2005:24–74; McMahon 2015a).

7. Factors put forth by historians include Irish immigrants' service and heroism in the Civil War; obtainment of greater political power, aided by machine politics; and favorable comparison, in the eyes of native-born White Americans, with African Americans and Asian Americans, as well as immigrants from Southern and Eastern Europe, who began to arrive in large numbers toward the end of the century. Over the past twenty years, scholars have debated how Americans racially classified the Irish and other European immigrants. This study follows the majority opinion that Americans always considered the Irish to be White in race, both legally and socially, as did the Irish themselves. Nevertheless, Americans used essentializing and naturalizing racist language to denigrate and assert prominence over Irish immigrants. Meanwhile, some Irish immigrants themselves embraced the idea that there were natural differences between the Irish and their English adversaries, styling the nationalist struggle for Ireland as an age-old battle between Celts and Anglo-Saxons (McMahon 2015a). Chapter 2 further addresses issues of race and how medical theories were part of racial thinking in the 19th century.

8. Sources about the history of medicine in Ireland that I draw upon include Fleetwood 1983, Malcolm and Jones 1999, Robins 1995, Jones 2001, Farmar 2004, and Preston and Ó hÓgartaigh 2012. For 19th-century American health-related ideas and practices, both professional and popular, I rely upon many sources, especially Risse, Numbers, and Leavitt 1977; Haller 1981a; Rosenberg 1974a, 1974b, 1977, 1987a, 1987b; Vogel and Rosenberg 1979; Hamlin 1992; Leavitt 1999; Humphreys 2006; and Brown 2009. For historical methods, I am inspired by the social history approaches of these authors, articulated by Roy Porter (1985) as "medical history from below," as well as by the work of social and labor historians, particularly Kerby Miller (1985), Christine Stansell (1986), Richard Stott (1990), Alan Kraut (1994), Kevin Kenny (1998), and more recently Cian McMahon (2015a, 2021) and Hidetaka Hirota (2017).

9. Invaluable published sources include those of contemporary ethnobotanists (Allen and Hatfield 2004), folklorists (Evans 1957; Buckley 1980; Glassie 1982; Mac Cárthaigh 1988; Logan 1994; Verling 2003; Ballard 2009), and anthropologists (Arensberg 1937; Scheper-Hughes 2001). The publications of early ethnographers and folklore collectors, many of whom were male medical doctors or well-educated women, are also informative and highlight what these middle- and upper-class collectors found to be unusual (Wilde, W. 1849, 1852; Egan 1887; Mooney 1887; Wilde, L. 1887a, 1887b, 1890; Purdon 1895a, 1895b, 1898, 1904; Barbour 1897; Doherty 1897; Pyne 1897; Gregory 1920). The National Folklore Collection (NFC) is largely composed of transcribed oral histories collected by trained staff of the government-sponsored Irish Folklore Institute (1930–1935), Irish Folklore Commission (1935–1971), and the Department of Irish Folklore UCD (1972–2005) (National Folklore Collection 2023).

10. The NFC Collections include two sets of manuscripts, the Main Manuscripts —2,400 bound volumes recording information collected by trained folklore collectors dating from the 1930s through the 1970s—and the Schools Manuscripts—1,128

bound volumes containing information schoolchildren collected from older community members as part of the national Schools Scheme Project between 1937 and 1939 (Dúchas Project 2022). Using the card catalog at the Delargy Center of University College Dublin, I surveyed and transcribed all the references to folk medicine in the Main Manuscripts collection written in English. These were collected in 24 Irish counties. Not represented in this sample were counties Down, Galway, Kilkenny, King's, Leitrim, Monaghan, Waterford, and Westmeath, although I did find cures from these counties in published sources. I also surveyed dozens of Schools Manuscripts from the western and southern counties of Galway, Kerry, Cork, and Clare, where there were many Irish speakers and from where many residents of the Five Points neighborhood originated. Unpublished theses from folklore students in the Department of Irish Folklore at University College Dublin (Farrelly 1979; McClafferty 1979; Fallon 1994) also aided my interpretations of material recorded in Irish. In addition, I consulted David Allen and Gabrielle Hatfield's 2004 ethnobotanical study of a broader sample of the Schools Manuscript Collection. I also consulted digitized versions of the many NFC and NFCS manuscripts now available online while revising the book (Dúchas Project 2022).

11. A challenge of using information collected from the abovementioned sources is that most postdate the famine by decades. They are thus more reflective of the points of view of subsequent generations. Nevertheless, I follow other folklorists in asserting that these records still capture famine-era beliefs and practices for several reasons (Ballard 2009:26). First, some informants specified that their grandparents had administered certain remedies, but they were no longer used. Second, some remedies were so widespread and well known that they likely had a long history. Third, some of the same information reported to Irish Folklore Commission collectors in the 1930s or even the 1970s had also been reported to independent collectors, such as Lady Wilde, in the late 1800s. Last, although ingredients in reported remedies varied, I was able to deduce general principles about healing and sickness that remained stable over time (see Chapter 1). This book thus presents a relatively comprehensive analysis of 19th-century popular Irish remedies and ideas about illness, injury, and healing.

12. By embodied, I mean a view widely accepted in anthropology and other fields that the mind and the body are inseparable and mutually influencing, counter to European Enlightenment ideas of separate entities (Scheper-Hughes and Lock 1987; Csordas 1994; Joyce 2005; Lock and Farquhar 2007). An embodied perspective helps to explain how ailments that are often categorized as mental can manifest physically, or vice versa, as well as how inert substances can elicit "placebo" or "meaning response" effects (Moerman 2000).

13. A total of 24 people who resided at 472 and 474 Pearl Street between 1850 and 1860 were identifiable in the records of the Emigrant Savings Bank and Transfiguration Church, using the databases of Anbinder et al. (2019b) and Yamin (2000[3]). This is only a small portion of the few hundred residents who lived in

the two buildings during those years, according to census records, but it nonetheless gives some sense of residents' origins. Thirteen of Ireland's 32 counties were represented in the sample, with the greatest number from Cork (17%), Sligo (17%), Galway (13%), Kerry (8%), Clare (8%), and Kildare (8%). One resident in the sample, or 4% each, hailed from Cavan, Kilkenny, King's, Meath, Mayo, Waterford, and Wexford.

14. My dissertation (Linn 2008) was a preliminary version of this study.

Chapter 1

1. Townsend was born in NYC and was a graduate of Columbia College. He studied with David Hosack (a founder of the Elgin Botanic Garden and the Lying-in Hospital of New York) at the College of Physicians and Surgeons. Townsend also was among the founders of the Lyceum of Natural History. He "was active in politics, serving on the NYC Common Council in 1829–1831. He died of tuberculosis (TB) on March 26, 1849. His publications include *A Dissertation on the Influence of the Passions in the Production and Modification of Disease* (1816); *An Account of the Yellow Fever, as it prevailed in the City of New-York, in the Summer and Autumn of 1822* (1823); and *Memoir on the Topography, Weather, and Diseases of the Bahama Islands* (1826)" (Augustus C. Long Health Sciences Library 2023).

2. Dr. Townsend's diagnosis, rationale, and treatment align closely with the ideas presented by his contemporary physician James Stewart (1846), a "Fellow of the College of Physicians and Surgeons, one of the consulting physicians of the Northern Dispensary of the city of New York, and late physician to the Orphan's Asylum, etc., etc.," in his book *A Practical Treatise on the Diseases of Children*.

3. Biomedicine became the dominant form of professional medicine throughout the world in the 20th century, but it too is shaped by local cultures and has regional differences (Lock and Nguyen 2018; Singer et al. 2020).

4. At the Bloomingdale Asylum in NYC during the 1840s, for example, doctors attempted to correlate mental illness with temperaments, hair color, and eye color (Earle 1845). The *Boston Medical and Surgical Journal* published a report about difficult obstetrical cases that tracked patients' temperaments (Ingalls 1860). Some life insurance companies requested customers indicate their temperament on applications through the third quarter of the 19th century. During the Civil War, insurance companies underwrote sanitary commission expenses in exchange for statistical information about how soldiers of different temperaments fared under certain diseases and environmental conditions. Companies used this information to revise their premium rates (Knobel 1986:21). Homeopathic medicine and phrenology also drew upon humoral theory (Little 2007).

5. Several investigations in the 1850s, most notably Dr. John Snow's in London, showed that cholera was transmitted by fecal and vomited matter from infected persons, and many theorized the involvement of a microorganism. It was not until

Robert Koch's discovery of *Vibrio cholerae* in 1883, however, that the specific source was identified (Rosenberg 1987a:193–200).

6. Moerman (2002:14–15) defines meaning response as "the psychological and physiological effects of *meaning* in the treatment of illness." He notes that it "includes most of the things that have traditionally been called the placebo effect" and "many things that are *not* part of the placebo effect as traditionally understood . . . meaning response is attached not only to the prescription of inert medications, but to active ones as well."

7. Physician James Stewart (1854:xxiii) warned about the dangers of children overheating in bed: "The child's bed ought to be composed of soft, elastic materials, but never of feathers in such quantities as to allow of its yielding to the pressure of the body, and rising up on each side; a most debilitating sweat is produced by being thus buried in the bedding."

8. Dr. Townsend's casebook does not explain why Mrs. Huxley and her husband took over care of Huxley, only that "this boy is the son of a Mr. and Mrs. McGuire, son of Mrs. Huxley by her first husband. The child was adopted as Huxley McGuire" (Townsend 1847:1).

9. Making the sign of the cross was a frequent element in a variety of Irish popular cures, including preventing harm to children by fairies or jealous humans (NFC 1941[782]:192, 255, 366; Logan 1994:71, 75; Verling 2003:86). See Chapter 7.

10. In Ireland, keeners, who praise and lament the dead with poetry and loud wailing, were often women (Ó Crualaoich 1998).

11. The *Paterson Evening News* reported in October of 1900 that Irish residents in Paterson, New Jersey, stated that fairies walked down the street there disguised as old women (Lees 1979:188). American folklorist Wayland Hand (1981) collected many other instances of immigrants' continued beliefs in fairies in the U.S. See Chapter 7.

12. Karl Reinhard (2000:403) found evidence of whipworm and roundworm infection in privies associated with Irish immigrant residents at the Five Points.

13. A number of Irish popular cures involved the sea. For example, a farmer in Cork stated, "If a person has fever it can be cured by carrying him to the seashore when the tide is in. Lay him down on the sand, and leave him there until the tide is going out, and the fever will leave and go away with the tide" (NFC 1941[782]:360).

14. Fairies are supernatural creatures in Irish mythology. Irish people described fairies to William Wilde and other 19th-century folklore collectors as fallen angels, guardians of the dead, or the *Tuatha Dé Danann*, the deities of pre-Christian Ireland (Wilde, W. 1852:124–125; Mac Cárthaigh 1988:90). Some fairies were said to be solitary (such as the female banshee, who mourns the deaths of people, and the pooka, who vandalizes property at night), others to dwell in troops, living together near thorn trees or in the ruins of old forts or tombs (thus they were sometimes called *aes sídhe*, "people of the mounds"). They were described as having human-like personalities and foibles, such as great senses of humor, appreciation of music and art, enjoyment of food and drink, and the ability to be generous and helpful or mischievous,

vindictive, greedy, easily offended, and ready to take advantage of the most vulnerable (Croker 1838; Dorian 2000:270; Glassie 1985; Wilde, L. 1887a, 1887b). Fairies were said to cause many of the same ailments as human-inflicted bewitching, including failure to thrive in infants and epilepsy and wasting diseases/consumption in children and young adults. See Chapter 7.

15. Historians of medicine have hypothesized that worms were one of the first distinct disease entities to be recognized in the ancient Mediterranean and Mesopotamia; and the Rod of Asclepius and later caduceus symbol that became the emblem of physicians is thought to originate from the treatment of wrapping an emerging guinea worm around a stick to reel it out, a technique still used today (Moran-Thomas 2013:211–212).

16. Irish popular methods of counteracting colds and respiratory ailments, for example, included applying ointments made of goose grease (Logan 1994:24; O'Regan 1997:21) or goose grease on its own (NFCS 1938[918]:179), camphorated oil (McClafferty 1979:63), or chopped garlic to the chest (Logan 1994:24); warming the body by placing compresses made of warm potatoes or oats on the chest or wrapping the head and feet or chest in a cloth (preferably red) (Morris 1937:178; Logan 1994:44); and feeding warm food, mustard (NFCS 1938[35]:247), blackcurrant jam (NFCS 1937[624]:249; NFCS 1938[35]:249; NFCS 1938 [45]:246), alcoholic beverages—such as whiskey, brandy, rum, or elderberry wine—(NFCS 1937[624]:249; McClafferty 1979:63), dandelion leaf juice (NFCS 1937[624]:556; Logan 1994:24), homemade cough medicines (NFCS 1938[345]:14; NFCS 1938[920]:70, and/or hot infusions of plants (such as garlic, onions) or carrageen, sometimes mixed with milk, thought to nourish the body or drive out sickness (NFC ca. 1929[36]:246; NFCS 1938[45]:197; NFCS 1938[345]:11; NFCS 1938[624]:79). These citations for Irish popular cures (as well as others included throughout this book) usually represent only a sampling of the sources that mention these cures. Many of the same cures for common ailments, such as colds and coughs, appear in dozens of NFC and NFCS manuscripts, as well as in some published sources.

17. A commonly reported method to purify the blood, and thus ward off fever and other illnesses, was to eat three meals of boiled nettles in May (NFC 1935[54]:368, NFCS 1938[35]:31; NFCS 1938[345]:8; Wilson 1943:182; Logan 1994:35; Allen and Hatfield 2004:85).

18. Henry Purdon (1895a:215), a medical doctor and folklore collector wrote in 1895, "for ascarides, a decoction of chamomile was used by forefathers as an enema, but now it is nearly obsolete." It is possible that Mrs. Huxley had, in fact, administered chamomile, which was not usually used by professional physicians of the time, who preferred senna or stronger-acting chemicals, such as turpentine (NYHMCB 1848:C670). In his case notes Dr. Townsend dismissed Mrs. Huxley's enema as not of the "proper kind "or "large [enough] in quantity" (Townsend 1847:5).

19. There are many similar versions of this charm recorded in NFCS manuscripts from Donegal, Cavan, Roscommon, Mayo, Westmeath, and Cork (and possibly other

counties). One version from County Donegal is: "When Jesus saw the cross he was to be crucified on, he trembled. The Jews asked Him if He had fever. 'No' said Our Lord Jesus Christ 'I have neither fever nor plague.' Anyone who keeps those words in memory or writing shall never take fever or plague" (NFCS 1938[1029]:16)

20. Metaphors link two things by perceived and often nonliteral similarities (a "wave" of nausea), whereas metonymy links two things by relationship. Metonymic connections can include part to whole, producer to product, object to user, controller to controlled, institution to people, place to event, and place to institution (Van der Geest and Whyte 1989:353–359). Many Irish popular cures appear to rely on connections of metaphor and metonym (Linn 2014:152–155).

21. The *Times* (1908:9) article describes how Father Adams had also rescued a drowning girl, gaining him local notoriety, and that he used the relics "too frequently," displeasing the Bishop. The Bishop likely feared he would attract negative reactions from American Protestants, and he removed Father Adams from his post around 1888 but reinstated him in 1893. An article in the *Brooklyn Daily Eagle* (1893:10) mentions that Father Adams had cured both "sick and disabled" people; "he said [his cures] were effected by the use of holy relics." Certain priests in Ireland were also said to have healed disabilities and incurable illnesses (NFC 1938[514]:30–37; NFC 1974[1838]:274–278).

22. Citations for this sentence about the healing powers attributed to certain kinds of individuals:

    priests (NFC 1938[514]:30–37; NFC 1974[1838]:274–278);

    seventh consecutively born son or daughter in a family (NFC 1930[80]:20; NFC 1941[782]:190; NFCS 1937[598]:433; NFCS 1938[345]:15; NFCS 1938[364]:146; Logan 1994:47);

    child born after his/her father's death ("posthumous child") (Blake 1918:222; NFC 1930[80]:12, 20; NFC 1938 [560]:534; NFCS 1937[598]:433; NFCS 1938[45]:61, 195, 197, 364; NFCS 1938[364]:146; Logan 1994:53);

    woman married to a man with the same surname as her maiden surname, or such a couple (NFC 1930[80]:11, 220; NFC 1935[54]:203; NFCS 1938[624]:80, 529; Logan 1994:42);

    blacksmith (NFCS 1938[35]:125, 140, 236; Wilson 1943:183; Logan 1994:68, 120; Westropp 2000:43);

    person who had licked a lizard or a frog (NFC 1930[80]:12; NFC 1941[782]:262; NFCS 1938[45]:201; NFCS 1938[345]:8; NFCS 1938[364]:219; NFCS 1938[624]:79, 249; Logan 1994:102–103);

    man riding a white horse (Pyne 1897:179; Blake 1918:223; NFC 1937[407]:142; NFC 1941[782]:353; NFCS 1937[598]:433; NFCS 1938[35]:33, 127, 236; NFCS 1938[45]:202; NFCS 1938[364]:219; NFCS 1938[624]:77, 251; Logan 1994:43; Westropp 2000:42).

23. These rumors likely reference contemporary Victorian-era concerns about grave robbing practiced by medical students and so-called "resurrection men" in 19th-century Europe and the U.S. in order to acquire anatomical specimens (Frank 1976), as well as physicians' centuries-old use of parts of deceased human bodies (especially Egyptian mummies) as medicine (Sugg 2015).

24. There is an oft-quoted Irish proverb that "[f]or every form of illness the Lord may choose to inflict on his people, He has also provided an herb to cure it" (MacNamara 1963:120). Legends suggest that in ancient times specialized healers knew the herbal cure for every disease, but that this knowledge was lost, and people have been slowly reassembling the knowledge since, bit by bit (Blake 1918:218).

25. Historians have critiqued Evans's and Scally's assertions that "throughother" characterized life in pre-famine Ireland as an exaggeration, noting that this land system (also known as the rundale system and involving periodic land redistribution to ensure fair shares to each family) was in decline and limited to small sections of the country by the early 19th century. They also argue that capitalist economic relations and social hierarchy (with Protestant estate holders at the top, middling and small farmers in the middle, and tenant farmers and landless laborers at the bottom) structured most rural areas as well as urban centers by the eve of the famine (Miller 1985:54–56). These are important critiques to avoid romanticizing or essentializing famine-era communities. Nevertheless, as historians point out and NFC and other folklore sources demonstrate, "most people living in Ireland at the time [of the famine] saw themselves as part of social networks bound by tradition, blood, and reciprocity," and they brought "strong notions of kinship and community" with them to the U.S. (McMahon 2021:4).

26. Irish surnames have been shown to be "remarkably consistent," enabling relatively accurate estimations of an immigrant's region of origin in Ireland (Sullivan 2013:6).

27. Anbinder et al.'s (2019a:1600–1604, 1607) study of Emigrant Savings Bank records highlights Cavan and Leitrim as sources of a significant number of famine-era immigrants to New York and the importance of previous arrivals' assistance. They were also able to identify previously invisible immigration from Dublin, as well as other southern Ulster counties of Tyrone and Monaghan. Dubliners dispersed throughout Manhattan, unlike former rural-dwellers who clustered in one or a few neighborhoods, mostly downtown. Their study also reconfirms that the southern and western provinces of Munster and Connaught were most represented among NYC's famine-era immigrants, especially counties Cork, Kerry, Limerick, Tipperary, Kilkenny, and Galway.

28. Anbinder et al.'s (2019a:1610) study details the concentration of Catholic Irish downtown. Irish Protestants more often lived in wards north of 14th Street. If they lived downtown, they tended toward the West side. Catholics tended toward the East side. Ulster Catholics were an exception; some lived uptown near Ulster Protestants.

29. The 1850 Federal Census as well as the 1855 New York State Census also record several African Americans who had been born in Africa, presumably all of whom were brought to the U.S. as captives. Captive and free people of African descent have been present in NYC since the very beginnings of the Dutch colony of New Amsterdam (Cantwell and Wall 2015).

30. Irish boardinghouse keepers who opened accounts at the Emigrant Saving Bank between 1850 and 1858 ranked 7th in terms of occupation in median and average account balances, $295 and $477, respectively (Anbinder et al. 2019a:1615).

31. The 1855 New York State Census shows John and Catherine Ward of 474 Pearl Street, who had two young children of their own, also adopted a daughter, Ellen Flyn, for example. Other arrangements, perhaps even that of Huxley McGuire, were less formal and/or more temporary. In times of desperation, parents also turned to Catholic orphanages and returned weeks or months later to reclaim their children (Fitzgerald 2006).

32. Historians have long had the impression that Irish and other immigrants in enclaves fared better in 19th-century cities than those who spread out. Anbinder et al.'s (2019a:1597) study of Emigrant Savings Bank records from 1850 to 1858 has provided quantitative support for this argument in the form of larger savings accounts among Irish who lived in enclaves.

33. The Marquis of Lansdowne, an English landowner of a 105-square mile property in County Kerry, assisted the emigration of 1,700 of his tenants to NYC in 1851. Almost all of them initially settled in the Five Points on Baxter, Worth, and Little Water Streets (Anbinder et al. 2019a:1610).

34. Crude death rates in the Third Ward were less than half of those in the Sixth Ward in 1855 (Baics 2016:Plate 7, 212).

Chapter 2

1. This fever is known as epidemic typhus fever today to distinguish it from endemic typhus fever, or murine typhus. Throughout this chapter and book, I use the terms typhus or typhus fever as shorthand for epidemic typhus fever.

2. The Irish usually were the most numerous steerage passengers on emigrant ships departing Liverpool during the famine period, although they often traveled with smaller numbers of emigrants from England (such as William Smith), Scotland, and Continental Europe. Overall, two-thirds of Irish immigrants to the U.S. in the 19th century departed from Liverpool (Miller 1985:198).

3. New York Hospital, which opened in 1791, did not list typhus fever as a diagnosis in annual reports between 1834 and 1841 (NYHAR 1835–1842). Dr. A. Sidney Doane, physician-in-chief to the Marine Hospital on Staten Island, was a rare dissenting voice against the view that typhus was new to New York. In his report to the NY State Commissioners of Emigration in 1851, he wrote that his study of the quarantine's own

records from as early as 1802 shows that immigrants had long been diagnosed with the "ship fever, . . . showing conclusively that this disease is by no means of recent origin" (Commissioners of Emigration 1861:83, emphasis in original). Doane's study does not seem to have changed views or lessened fears. Doane himself died from typhus fever he contracted treating patients (New-York Daily Times [*NYDT*] 1852a:2).

4. Rosenberg (1987a:129) further explains that from the 1840s onwards, physicians "categorized epidemic and infectious ills as 'zygomatic,' or fermentlike. The familiar process of fermentation and putrefaction provided plausible models for ways in which a small amount of infectious material could produce potentially pathogenic changes in a far larger quantity of material."

5. William Jenner distinguished typhus from typhoid by 1851. Some physicians accepted his findings quickly, but others, including London officials, did not until the 1860s (Hardy 1988:407–408). Pellagra, a deficiency of the B vitamin niacin, particularly afflicted the Irish during the famine who subsisted on cornmeal that was provided by poor relief. Pellagra causes a red rash, stomach pain, diarrhea or constipation, severe neurological disturbances, and can result in death (Hegyi et al. 2004). Severe symptoms of pellagra can result from eating cornmeal exclusively for several months (Crawford 1981).

6. McLeod advised a method of treatment consisting of cool baths, applications of cold and wet compresses and wraps, and as much water to drink as the patient desired, to bring down the fever (*Scientific American* 1847:43). Hospital case records from NYC suggest his advice made little impact upon treatment there.

7. The Commissioners of Emigration (1861:10) calculated the average number of sick per thousand passengers in 1847 was 30 on British ships, 9.6 on American ships, and 8.6 on German ships.

8. The Board of the Commissioners of Emigration was formed in the middle of 1847 and thus records for that year are incomplete and span from May to December. During those eight months, 52,946 Irish immigrants arrived at the Port of NY, along with 53,180 Germans, and 22,936 immigrants from other nations (Commissioners of Emigration 1861:288).

9. In 1847, the Commissioners (1861:10) sent another approximately 2,600 immigrants to other city institutions with unspecified illnesses, including 25 to New York Hospital.

10. Dr. Sidney A. Doane, Medical Chief of the Marine Hospital on Staten Island, explained in a report to the Commissioners left unfinished at his death from typhus fever, that "strong Westerly gales" had prevailed on the Atlantic during 1851, causing longer passages of many emigrant vessels from Europe. Some ships were forced to return to port because of storm damage and their passengers had to wait on the docks to start anew, using up precious supplies and energy. He attributed the greater number of sick immigrants than previous years to these delays and identified typhus fever as the "prevailing disease." Ice floes in the East River that winter also hindered regular communication, and presumably transfers to Ward's Island (Commissioners of

Emigration 1861:83–85, 115). Ward's Island Hospital was also routinely overcrowded, however. In 1853 inspectors found that two patients were often required to share one bed (Duffy 1968:496.)

11. *The Citizen* (1854a:225), for example, commented upon preferential treatment for new steamships and their higher-paying passengers: "Authorities at Quarantine at Staten Island, so well paid for their services, are according to their own confession, so lax in their duty as to allow the *steamship* to pass, on the mere statement of the doctors of these ships, that there is no sickness on board."

12. For example, in 1846 the Board of Aldermen found 100 sick immigrants lying on straw near the bodies of two deceased others in a 50-square-foot apartment on the city's outskirts (Maguire 1868:185–86).

13. In 1799, New York State passed a gradual emancipation law freeing the children of enslaved mothers born after July 4, 1799, but keeping them indentured until young adulthood. Then, in 1817, the state passed a law freeing enslaved people born before 1799, but not until 1827. July 4, 1827 has since been recognized as Emancipation Day in New York State and has been celebrated on the 5th of July to distinguish it from Independence Day.

14. Many were dressed in clothes that were seen by New Yorkers as poorly made, cheap, and ridiculously out of fashion (McMahon 2021:226). Immigrants themselves became aware of this immediately and some were warned ahead of time by guides or letters from friends (see Chapter 5).

15. As many historians have pointed out, the poorest of Ireland's poor very rarely emigrated to North America, because they could not make the journey physically nor could they afford it, unless assisted. Most thus stayed in Ireland and perished or, more rarely, survived. Some who were slightly better off migrated to Great Britain (Miller 1985:293–295; Hirota 2017:38; McMahon 2021:27–45). McMahon (2021:27-46) found that immigrants assisted by poorhouse guardians were generally better provisioned and protected than those who migrated independently, while cases of landlord-assisted emigration were variable. Hirota (2017:24) also explains that famine-era immigrants' relative economic standing in Ireland had little meaning in the U.S., because in the U.S. they generally occupied the poorest class.

16. Comparing people to apes as a form of disparagement has a long history in the West. As early as 4th-century-C.E. pagans were depicted as monkeys to convey their lack of reason. Since the Middle Ages, monkey metaphors have been used to condemn lascivious behavior and indicate lower position on the Great Chain of Being. Stories about apes mating with African women circulated in Europe and the Americas and functioned to support European supremacy and enslavement of Africans and African-descendant people (Hund 2015).

17. One of Nast's more famous cartoons of "Pat"—"The Usual Irish Way of Doing Things," published in the September 2, 1871, issue of Harper's Weekly—draws heavily from a cartoon John Tenniel drew of Guy Fawkes for *Punch* in 1867.

18. Morton and Nott's polygenist views challenged those of monogenists, who

believed in a single origin of humanity. Johann Friedrich Blumenbach was among the most influential of the latter and introduced the term Caucasian to describe people of European origin from whom he believed all other races descended.

19. Over the last several centuries, White Americans have interpreted real or imagined differential incidence of a number of diseases to support ideas of African American racial difference and inferiority. Such diseases include TB, syphilis, sickle cell anemia, and in the 1850s "Dysaesthesia Aethiopica," a supposed disorder fabricated by physician Samuel Cartwright said to cause "insensitivity 'to pain when subjected to punishment'" (Wailoo 2001:1).

20. Stereotypes are shared images that "distort . . . not just by generalizing to all what may be a characteristic of some. They are *selective* in their description, featuring and ignoring by applying some other mechanism than plain observation. They are evaluative. . . . They place the object of stereotyping in some kind of relationship to the stereotyper—usually in a flattering way, or at least useful, to the latter [emphasis in original]" (Knobel 2001:4–5).

21. Here Puckrein quotes William Harrison's *An Historicall Description of the Lland of Britaine* (1587) as cited in Furnival (1878:150–156) and Milton's *The History of Britain, the Third Book* (1670).

22. The British seem to have combined elements of the classical characterizations of the choleric and sanguine temperaments, the former previously understood to be bellicose and vengeful and the later to be good-natured (Puckrein 1981:1756; Feerick 2002:103). During the 16th century, some scholars, including Edmund Spenser, postulated that part of the Celtic lineage originated in Spain among the "Milesian" peoples, who had interbred with North Africans and/or Scythians (Garner 2015:204–205). This might have provided a rationale for incorporating choleric traits.

23. As Horsman (1976:406) notes, Knox's view of the Anglo-Saxon subset of the Scandinavian race was not wholly complimentary but complemented Irish nationalists' own counternarratives about the differences between Celts and Anglo-Saxons (McMahon 2015a). Knox "painted them as a vigorous, acquisitive, aggressive race, natural democrats, but lacking men of artistic genius or abstract thought. They were a race 'of all others the most outrageously boasting, arrogant, self-sufficient beyond endurance, holding in utter contempt all other races and all other men' . . . although no race perhaps exceeded them in a sense of justice and fair play, this was 'only to Saxons.'"

24. Paster (1998:423) also describes how, in the Early Modern Period, women were understood to be naturally phlegmatic in temperament, whereas men could possess any of the four temperaments. This difference, she argues, correlated with much greater constraints on women's behavior. The idea that women were naturally phlegmatic was still influential in the 19th century (see Chapter 6).

25. These tropes continue to have relevance into the 21st century. Edward Said (1978) has famously described the contours of Western Orientalism, within which feminization of Middle Eastern and Asian men is a significant feature. The idea that

African American women are too strong and are thus "pathological" has also had terrible longevity, most famously in the 1965 Moynihan Report (Spillers 1987). Such ideas are also a part of unconscious (and conscious) bias in hospitals today that result in greater deaths of Black mothers than mothers of other races and other poorer health outcomes for Black women.

26. Thomas (1830:15) explained that life experience cooled impetuous tempers and the aged were generally more phlegmatic. Stereotyping all Irish as sanguine in temperament thus additionally compared them to children, an idea visualized in several well-known British and American caricatures of the Irish, including Figure 2.4 (de Nie 2004:25).

27. Some race scientists explained the dark-haired phenotype as resulting from part of the Celtic lineage originating in Spain among "Milesian" peoples, who had supposedly interbred with dark-haired North Africans and/or Scythians (choleric types), an idea that supported ranking Celts below Anglo-Saxons (Wells 1866:286; Garner 2015:204–205).

28. Bellevue had a reputation for crowded and filthy conditions, inadequate nursing care, and high rates of patient deaths. During the 1851 typhus epidemic, eight of the twelve house staff at Bellevue became ill with the disease, leaving only two residents to care for 1,000 patients (Larrabee 1971:213). Dr. D. M. Reese increased the number of beds and qualified nurses in the late 1840s and early 1850s, but by 1860, deplorable conditions had returned (*New York Times* [*NYT*] 1860:8; 1877:8; Duffy 1968:485–488; Oshinsky 2016).

29. The hospital also had a marine ward for seamen, whose care was paid by assessments on the wages of sailors arriving from foreign countries. Nonpaying patients were supposed to be admitted only if they were judged to be "worthy poor" (Larrabee 1971:204). Such restrictions do not seem to have applied to cases of traumatic injury or severe illness, judging from case records.

30. Before 1844 and after 1860, U.S.-born patients were the largest group, with the increasing number of first-generation Irish Americans likely making a substantial contribution to the increased proportion of American-born patients after 1860 (NYHAR 1835–1866).

31. The second most frequent diagnosis that year, syphilis, amounted to about one-quarter of that number and U.S.-born individuals topped that list (NYHAR 1848).

32. Between 1845 and 1852, 10.7% of German-born patients, 6.4% of Irish-born patients, and 3.6% of U.S. born-patients were diagnosed with simple "fever" at New York Hospital. During the same years, 3.2% of German-born patients, 3.0% of Irish-born, and 4.2% of U.S.-born were diagnosed with "remittent fever" (NHYAR 1846–1853).

33. Several scholars have tried to account for inconsistent mortality rates among typhus sufferers in the 19th century by examining differences in gender, age, class,

previous exposure, ethnicity, and disease strain. According to a report on epidemic fever published in the *Dublin Quarterly Journal of Medical Science* (*DQJMS*) as early as 1849, wealthier people in Ireland experienced "worse" cases than those of poorer people (*DQJMS* 1849:340), likely because poorer people had been previously exposed. This observation is substantiated by modern studies showing that surviving typhus can generate immunity. In London and other English cities, rural immigrants—from Ireland as well as within England—had been especially susceptible to typhus fever, however, suggesting a relative lack of immunity among the rural poor. Anne Hardy (1988:423) suggests that poor urban areas in England harbored "submerged infection" that caused outbreaks during times of stress and among recent arrivals to the city. The "disappearance of typhus from Victorian cities [in England after the 1870s] constituted a significant improvement in the living conditions of adult urban populations, and marks something of a watershed in urban health history" (Hardy 1988:424).

34. The author of this comment was the British-born physician John Draper, who, according to historian David Oshinsky (2016:67), was well known for his anti-Irish views. Draper was largely responsible for the 1854 state law known as the "Bone Bill," which permitted the bodies of "all vagrants, dying unclaimed, and without friends" in public institutions to be used for dissection in medical schools. The bill reduced graverobbing from cemeteries to meet the demands for corpses but was premised on the idea that paupers owed a debt to society that they would repay with their bodies. Recent bioarchaeological research by Alanna Warner-Smith (2022) into Irish-born individuals in an anatomical collection made possible by this bill shows that institutions did not make much effort to contact relatives.

35. Cupping removed smaller quantities of blood than venesection. It involved placing a glass cup over a small incision in the skin and creating a vacuum to pull blood into the cup.

36. By the 1860s these treatments for typhus were recognized as ineffective and harmful. The English physician Charles Murchison (1862:265), who published an exhaustive study of typhus and relapsing fevers in 1862, noted that diaphoretics had little benefit for his patients and "increased prostration." Murchison and the eminent Irish physician Robert Graves also showed mercury to have no positive effects on typhus fever.

37. This cartoon also seems to reference and/or to have been inspired by an illustration contrasting Florence Nightingale with "Bridget McBruiser" in Samuel Wells's popular *New Physiognomy* (1866:537). The accompanying text, in part, notes, "Florence Nightingale . . . is developed in the 'upper story' while McBruiser lives in the basement mentally as well as bodily."

Chapter 3

1. The homesick Smith (1850:14) survived, the would-be priest died in his berth, the immigrant who dreamed of success jumped overboard, and the paranoid husband recovered.

2. Gerald Keegan, a schoolteacher from Sligo, for example, wrote about his ship that departed from Liverpool in 1847: "About half the passengers have no place to bed down for the night. There are no lights, no portholes and no ventilation except for what fresh air enters from the two hatchways" (Laxton 1996:57). Henry Johnson, from Antrim, described a storm at sea during his 1848 voyage to New York: "Anything I had read or imagined of a storm at sea was nothing to this. . . . The ship began to roll and pitch dreadfully . . . [and] the ship became unmanageable. . . . I was pitched right into a corpse, and there, corpse, boxes, barrel, women and children, all in one mess, were knocked from side to side" (Laxton 1996:117). Passenger acts required ship companies to provide a minimal amount of provisions for each passenger, but even when companies complied (not all did) and the food remained edible, immigrants stated that the food barely supported survival. Poor immigrants often could not afford additional provisions (McMahon 2021:61–62, 128, 183–184). Seasickness was common (McMahon 2021:103). Mary McLean (1886–1900), whose story is presented in the Introduction, wrote that she was seasick for the "entire voyage." Many ships did not have physicians. Either the captain performed such duties or a passenger was selected. Scottish cabin passenger James Sutherland, selected despite his lack of medical training, found "to be Ship Surgeon rather awkward berth, especially when you don't understand it" (MacShane 1958:309). On Robert Whyte's (1848:39) 1847 voyage from Dublin to Quebec, the captain's wife "dosed the sick with porridge containing drops of laudanum."

3. Mr. Vere Foster described to the British House of Commons in 1851 a sailor's abuse of John M'Corcoran, an older Irish man: He "gave him such a severe kick with his knee on his backside as he was stooping down that he threw him down upon the deck, since which he has been obliged to go to the water closet three or four times a day, passing blood every time." In 1860, a U.S. Act of Congress was passed to ensure better protection for female passengers; it imposed a one-year jail term or fine of $1,000 on anyone employed by a ship for "seducing" a female passenger (Maguire 1868:184). Henry Johnson described a leak in a porthole during his voyage. He complained that the 450 Catholics on board, "in the time of danger did nothing but sprinkle holy water, cry, pray, cross themselves and all sorts of tomfoolery instead of giving hand to pump the ship" (Laxton 1996:116). Another ship struck an iceberg and sunk in the North Atlantic. Passengers climbed onto the iceberg and were rescued by a passing ship (Laxton 1996:127–129).

4. Many sources have chronicled the history of the Great Famine in Ireland and its incalculable human suffering (McArthur 1956; Miller 1985; Neal 1998; Ó Gráda 2000; Kinealy 2006; Ó Murchadha 2013). Whole families perished from starvation in their homes. Others, evicted or in search of help, died along the sides of the roads. Workhouses and poorhouses overflowed. Ethics of hospitality broke down, so fearful

were people of the famine-related epidemics. The emotional toll on many of those who survived, whether they stayed or emigrated, was immense. Few famine-era migrants to America ever returned to Ireland, perhaps 10%, versus 40%–50% of Polish and Italian immigrants (Miller 1993:265).

5. Emigrants typically crossed the Irish Sea on small boats, sometimes with open decks also carrying animals such as fowl and pigs. It could take as few as seven hours and as many as a few days. Disasters could befall emigrants on this leg of their journeys. For example, in 1849 a ship sailing from Sligo to Liverpool in December carried 179 passengers, but only 102 survived the two-day crossing. Many died of suffocation and were trampled when panic set upon the seasick and frostbitten passengers (Neal 1998:69–84). On such ships, historian Frank Neal (1998:73) writes that "the fare for pigs was half that for a passenger but the pigs were better looked after because they were of value to someone."

6. "Victorian Liverpool . . . [was] one of the century's capitals of atrocity: organized daylight robbery on the quays, forced imprisonment in lodging houses, unburied corpses of whole families in unlit cellars, multiple suicides, mercy killings, and a plague of madness that filled the asylums and clinics to overflowing with emigrants crippled in mind and body" (Scally 1995:204).

7. Emigrants who were assisted by landlords and workhouses were sometimes given a set of suitable clothing for their journeys (McMahon 2021:64). There was a thriving secondhand clothing market in Ireland that would have been attractive to these suppliers to lower costs, as well as to individuals who purchased clothes for themselves. Guidebooks and immigrant letters advised purchasing sturdy and warm clothes but not to spend too much on them because they would be "altogether unsuited" to the U.S. Today, clothing is a known vector of typhus. It is possible that secondhand clothing contributed to typhus among Irish immigrants.

8. Upon the basis of his survey of nearly 5,000 immigrant letters, Miller has argued that while some letters created false impressions of prosperity in the U.S., many supplied cautious and even negative information in order to correct the image of America as promised land. "The Irish at home were not being deluded by the Irish overseas, rather, the Irish at home were deluding themselves" (Miller 1993:269).

9. Irish cities were small compared with New York. The population of Dublin and Cork in 1841, Ireland's two largest, were 232,000 and 80,000, respectively (Miller 1985:35). In 1840, the population of Manhattan was 312,710 (USBC 1840). By 1850, immigration had increased the population to just over a half a million (USBC 1850).

10. Dublin hospitals included: the Charitable Infirmary (est. 1718), Merchant's Key (est. 1728), Dr. Steeven's Hospital (est. 1733), Mercer Hospital (est. 1734), the Rotunda Hospital (est. 1745 as the first maternity hospital in the British Isles), St. Patrick's Hospital (est. 1757 for the mentally ill by a bequest from Jonathan Swift's Estate), the Sick Poor Institution (est. 1794), the Dispensary for Infant Poor (est. 1800), and St. Vincent's Hospital (est. 1834) (Fleetwood 1983:100; Malcolm and Jones 1999:1).

11. Prison reformer John Howard visited several county infirmaries in the early 19th century and found them to be seriously inadequate. In Tralee, for example, the roof of

the infirmary was falling in, and patients laid on straw they had collected themselves. The situation in Cavan was even worse, with a dirty upper room filled with fowl. None had any bathing facilities (Fleetwood 1983:104–8). The Medical Charities Act in 1851 created a national system of dispensaries, and in 1862 workhouse infirmaries were opened to the public, but neither had good reputations (Jones 2001:9).

12. Records from Dr. Joseph Edmundson show that he was the only dispensary doctor for 4,500 households in 1851. His district of Carrick-on-Sur encompassed three counties, Kilkenny, Waterford, and Tipperary (Farmar 2004:85).

13. Most physicians were Protestant because of policies limiting the number of Catholics admitted to Irish medical schools, a holdover from the Penal Laws. Some Catholics trained as physicians on the Continent, particularly in Paris, but many emigrated in search of better job opportunities (Froggatt 1999:64).

14. Kearns (1994:25) also found these values did not vanish when people migrated to cities, and they were embraced by tenement dwellers in early 20th-century Dublin.

15. Irish cures for a number of ailments involved transferring them to someone or something else (Logan 1994). These include passing warts to another person by touching them with a potato or pebble and putting the latter in a bag for another to pick up (NFC 1937[402]:141; Verling 2003:67). A cure for consumption was to sleep in the same bed as a healthy person, transferring the illness to them (NFC 1930[80]:19). A cure for mumps was to rub the child's face to the back of a pig or to lead the child around the pigsty reciting "A mhuic, A mhuic, chugat an leicneach seo" ["Pig, pig, here take the mumps"] (Blake 1918:223; NFC 1930[80]:15; NFC 1941[782]:352; NFCS 1939[705]:137; Logan 1994:54).

16. New York Hospital medical records from the 1840s and 1850s show that Irish immigrants also described colds and fevers beginning as a chilling sensation brought upon by exposure to a cold or wet climate. Examples include typhus patients, such as Ann, a 26-year-old woman who arrived in America two weeks previous to admission (NYHMCB 1848:C15), William, a 36-year-old Irish laborer who had been in the country for nine years (NYHMCB 1848:C107), and Joshua, a 28-year-old Irish physician (NYHMCB 1850:C758). This belief that a fever began with the sensation of a chill seems to have cut across gender, class, age, and length of time in NYC.

17. Allen and Hatfield (2004:272) write that this was said in the Forest of Dean in England, but records from Ireland indicate similar uses; throughout the British Isles, the elder tree was perceived to be connected to the supernatural.

18. Citations: whiskey, mint, chamomile, vinegar (Wilson 1943:182); poitín, tobacco (Dorian 2000:274); moss (Ó Súilleabháin 1970:312); cabbage and chamomile (Verling 2003:63); tea, cold water, cloth (NFCS 1938[35]:133; NFCS 1938[624]:250); goose grease (NFCS 1938[45]:247); crowfoot, pitch, mustard (Logan 1994:51); mint (Allen and Hatfield 2004:238); vinegar (NFCS 1937[598]:434; NFCS 1938[345]:9, 206).

19. Such backyard features are treasure troves for archaeologists. Privies can hold items residents lost or intentionally threw into the shaft while in use, as well as "night

soil" which can provide evidence about diet and intestinal parasites. Privies and cisterns no longer in use for their original functions, because of the introduction of sewers or running water, also served as convenient places for residents to deposit trash (Geismar 1993).

20. At 472 Pearl Street, Feature J, a stone-lined cesspool, and Z, an old cistern that was converted into a second cesspool, contained two deposits dating about 20 years apart. The initial cesspool (J) was created as the sump for the building's privy sometime after 1850 when the Irish-born building owner, Peter McLoughlin, upgraded the sanitation facilities in the rear yard. After his death in 1864, William Clinton bought the building and again updated the facilities. He began by covering the trash that had flowed into the cesspool via the privies with a layer of relatively sterile fill and bluestone slabs. He also placed the same slabs atop a layer of trash in the old cistern. Artifacts in the layer under these bluestone slabs indicate that the deposit was created sometime after 1850, while the presence of the bluestone slabs capped the layer in 1864, so nothing could have been added to it afterward. The completion of Clinton's project was delayed, however, and residents deposited trash on top of the bluestone, creating a second archaeological deposit in Features J and Z with a TPQ of 1870 (Yamin 2000[1]:98–102). At 474 Pearl Street, there was one archaeological deposit in Feature O, a stone-lined privy, relating to the period during which the building was occupied almost exclusively by Irish immigrants. In 1866, Irish immigrant carpenter and undertaker John Ward purchased the building, and sometime between 1873 and 1875, he built a brick tenement in the rear of the lot. During construction, workers filled the old privy hole in the yard with debris. Underneath the debris was a layer of refuse with artifacts dating between 1860 and 1875 that was deposited over time by building residents. Artifacts from this context generated a TPQ of 1860 (Yamin 2000[1]:104–115).

21. None of the names of typhus patients from New York Hospital medical casebooks in the years surveyed (1847–1853; 1865) match with residents who lived at 472 or 474 Pearl Street during 1850, 1855, 1860, or 1870, the dates of federal and state censuses. Additional research might uncover supporting evidence in records from other years or other institutions (e.g., Ward's Island and Bellevue). Some typhus sufferers never went to a hospital, however, and many immigrants moved frequently, such that they might not have been present in the buildings during a census year or might have been missed by a census taker.

22. In order to find botanical remains, archaeologists collected samples of soil from inside the privy shaft and cesspool features and separated plant remains (including seed, nutshell, husk, and stem fragments) from the soil using the technique of flotation. These remains had become part of the archaeological deposits either within human excrement, as garbage deposited in the privies, or by being blown in by the wind from the surrounding area. Thus, the plant remains represent the plants used by residents or available nearby (Raymer et al. 2000:199–200). They only reflect a portion of the total plants eaten, used, or nearby, however, because most fleshy or

leafy parts of plants decay rapidly and would no longer be present for archaeologists to find. Residents most certainly ate potatoes, for example, but neither remains of the peels nor digested potato flesh were present in the archaeological soils.

23. Conversely, absence of other ingredients used in Ireland to cure fever and that were available in NYC's markets, such as chamomile and cabbage, is not definitive evidence residents did not use them. Absence can also be explained by which kind of feature was excavated, how residents used the feature, and how depositional conditions affected the decomposition of remains.

24. I determined artifact vessel counts and percentages on the basis of the different totals presented in different sections of the site report, my own calculations from the report's general artifact inventory (Yamin 2000[1 and 4]) and from Bonasera (2000a), Ponz (2000), and Brighton (2005). For more detailed explanation, please see Linn 2008:673–675.

25. Dr. Townsend's Sarsaparilla claimed to cure the "ship fever" (Brighton 2008:143), and one bottle was found in association with Irish residences in Paterson, NJ (Yamin 1999). The brand name of the one sarsaparilla bottle found in Irish deposits in the Five Points could not be identified (Table 5.1).

26. Hardesty (1994) notes that similarly few liquor bottles are usually found in association with male-only residences in Western mining towns because it was acceptable for them to drink outside their homes.

27. There were five additional bottles from this deposit identified as "wine/liquor bottle, misc. unknown," presumably because they were too fragmentary to conclusively identify (Yamin 2000[4, part 2]:1056–1057).

28. New female immigrants from Ireland began to significantly outnumber males in the 1860s, and women were more likely than men to remain in NYC than to move on to other parts of the U.S. (Ó Gráda 2005).

29. Peter McLoughlin, originally from Sligo and the owner of 472 Pearl Street, ran a liquor store on the ground floor in the 1840s, and later rented it until his death in 1854. His brother, Michael, resided in the building by 1850. The 1850 Federal Census records James Keene was occupied in "liquors" and Michael Killoran as a distiller; both lived at 472 Pearl. James Doyle also worked in "liquors" and lived at 474 Pearl Street, where Daniel O'Connor owned a porterhouse and oyster bar in the 1850s, according to an 1851 city directory (Yamin 2000[3]).

30. Barrington (1832:34) also suggested wisewomen rarely had any teeth because they chewed the herbs used in their preparations, believing that contact with tools would destroy the purity of their charms. Another possible reason might have been to enhance the herbs' potency by breaking it down and by imbuing some of the saliva of the healer.

31. The ages of many individuals in these censuses must have been approximated, given the large number of people who are an even number of decades old, and the fact that the same individuals aged more or less from one census to the next than the number of years between censuses. Age approximations might have resulted from

the census-takers' own estimations or reporting by a family member or neighbor. It is also possible that those recorded, themselves, were not quite sure how old they were or did not wish to share specific information with the census taker. Ó Gráda (2005:11) notes, "it is well known that people with low literacy and numeracy rates are prone to age-heaping" (rounding to the nearest number ending in 0 or 5).

32. Occupations were only listed for five of these women. Two were laundresses, one was a porter, and two "kept house." The laundresses were in their early 50s, and the porter and women who kept house were in their early 60s. Only two of the 23 women over 50 were 70 years or older; neither had a recorded occupation. Both were also noted in the 1860 census; a boarder aged 70 lived at 474 Pearl, and an "in-law" aged 73 lived at 472. Older Irish men were fewer, represented by 12 individuals 50 years old or more, 5 of whom were 60 years old or more, and only 1 was 70 years old or more (USBC 1850, 1860).

33. Heather Griggs (2000:37) found that 36 of 74 Five Points Irish women who deposited money in Emigrant Industrial Savings Bank accounts in 1855 did not report an occupation. She suggests that these women were responsible for managing their family's money, but it is possible they had earned it themselves via a hidden home industry.

34. People in Ireland reported to folklore collectors that priests could cure fevers, epilepsy, and paralysis, especially if these conditions had been caused by fairies or bewitching. Lady Gregory (1920) was told that priests, like other traditional healers, had to pay a "price" for their power to heal, such that some misfortune or sickness would come upon them for each time they healed someone else. Another story about a healing priest (from Irish National Folklore Archive's card catalog referencing NFC 1940s?[979]:106, written in Irish) emphasizes the degree of personal risk taken on by the healer: "Boy cured at mass but priest dies." Another account from Armagh emphasizes the cosmic reciprocity of curing: a priest healed a dying girl, but afterward a sheep belonging to her family died. When the family complained, the priest restored health to the sheep, but the girl died (NFC 1974[1837]).

35. Priests and nuns were among the staff at Canada's Grosse Isle quarantine in the late 1840s (Maguire 1868:137). The Sisters of Charity, who were the city's first well-trained nurses and ran St. Vincent's Hospital, similarly volunteered for the dangerous task of staffing the Emigrant Hospital on Ward's Island during the 1866 cholera epidemic and the hospital on Blackwell's Island during the 1875 smallpox epidemic (McCauley 2005; Wall 2005:18). The Sisters also converted their own motherhouse into a hospital for wounded soldiers during the Civil War (Jolly 1927).

36. Examples include: To cure a headache, "take the sheet that the corpse was wrapped in and tie it around the head" or do the same around a leg to cure a swelling (NFC 1941[782]:247). The ends of candles used at a wake were said to cure burns (NFC 1974[1838]:73; Furey 1991:111), while snuff left over from a wake could cure a headache (Wilson 1943:181), and the water the deceased person was washed in could cure a sore: "They keep it and rub it to sores and say 'In the Name of the Father and of the Son and of the Holy Ghost" (NFC 1935[107]:487). The deceased person's body

was also said to be curative: Touch the hand of a dead person to warts or an area afflicted by rheumatism, and the dead person will take the warts or rheumatism with him/her (M'Clintock 1912:475). A toothache is cured by rubbing the tooth or the gum with the finger bone of a dead hand (Blake 1918:225; Westropp 2000:42). A "running evil" (tubercular ulcer) is cured by touching with a "dead hand" (Ní Bhrádaigh 1936:266).

Chapter 4

1. Other historians have found similar percentages of Irish males employed in manual labor in Jersey City, Philadelphia, and Buffalo in the 1850s and 1860s (Laurie et.al. 1977:140–144; Glasco 1977:154–55; Shaw 1977:87).

2. A few men over 40 were engaged in other occupations: brass turner, fish vendor, grocer, mason, and watchman. Most male residents were under the age of 40 and many worked as laborers; others worked in skilled or semi-skilled occupations (USBC 1850, 1860, 1870; NYSC 1855; Brighton 2009).

3. Frank Roney, for example, took his children on outings to parks and amusements in San Francisco whenever he could afford it. Roney, who wrote mostly about his work and debts in his diary, noted how his life's satisfaction centered on his children: "It[']s [a] charm for me in my anxiety to see my children in a fair way to become worthy citizens, honorable and honored. This is what I desire and accumulate for" (Shumsky 1976:249, 252).

4. The Hudson River between Albany and NYC froze an average of 89 days each winter; the Erie Canal was closed for six weeks longer (Stott 1990:111).

5. Thompson (1967:91) noted: "By the 1830s and 1840s it was commonly observed that the English industrial worker was marked off from his fellow Irish worker, not by a greater capacity for hard work, but by his regularity, his methodical paying-out of energy, and perhaps also by a repression, not of enjoyments, but of the capacity to relax in the old, uninhibited ways."

6. Adding to the obvious dangers of racing around without protective clothing carrying burning hot metal was the Irish popular belief that perspiring excessively in the heat was dangerous because it could induce a chill that could lead to fever or pulmonary TB (Logan 1994:27).

7. During the frigid winter of 1851–1852, for example, railroad contractors in upstate NY advertised high wages for twice the number of workers needed. When laborers assembled, contractors reduced the wage to 55 cents a day and called the state militia to force their terms on the men. Only half were permitted to stay while the remainder, according to one Irish American, "were pronounced troublesome, and driven off, with their families, to perish . . . in the midst of a fearful American winter'" (Miller 1985:322).

8. The case of *Farwell vs. Boston & Worcester Railroad* 1837, in which a railroad worker sued the railroad company for the loss of his arm in a train derailment, was

the leading case in common law of employer liability. The court found the railroad to be without fault (Tomlins 1988).

9. For example, people who run or walk long distances have femur bones that are oval in cross-section because more bone develops on the anterior and posterior sides of the femur in response to locomotor muscles exerting most of their force on those sides. Conversely, individuals who practice sedentary weight-bearing activities have more equal anterior-posterior and medial-lateral forces upon their femurs resulting in a rounder-shaped cross-section (Larsen 2000). Activity also places stress on sites where muscles, tendons, or ligaments insert into the periosteum and the underlying bony cortex, creating distinct skeletal markings that can be used as indicators of activity (Munson Chapman 1997). When a muscular insertion site is subject to stress, the number of capillaries increases, stimulating bone remodeling at the point of greatest stress, usually resulting in the hypertrophy of bone at that area. Size and placement of these musculoskeletal stress markers can thus be used to glean information about the type, frequency, and intensity of activities in life.

10. Hughes (1987:174) found that 80% of 465 men listed as escaped convicts at large in Hobart on Tasmania in 1850, many of whom were Irish, were under 5'8" tall and 15% were only 5'3".

11. Historical and archaeological records indicate that Irish immigrants eagerly partook of the more plentiful amount and variety of affordable food in NYC. Irish immigrant William Williamson wrote to his brother Hugh in County Armagh, for example: "I have not seen much of America yet, but I think if some of my countrymen were here that is living on potatoes and milk they would bless the day, before long that they left Ireland. In every house here there is no meal eaten without meat, and tea twice a day" (Harris 1989:v). Archaeological excavations at 472 and 474 Pearl Street show residents consumed a variety of animal foods but especially favored pork, which was typically more familiar and less expensive than beef or poultry (Milne and Crabtree 2000).

12. These figures were calculated directly from the ratio of Irish-born patients treated for fracture at New York Hospital to the number of Irish-born residents of the city, as ascertained by census records, and are thus overestimates. These calculations do not account for the unknown number of Irish immigrants missed by census takers. Nevertheless, the percent increase from 1845 to 1850 is probably roughly accurate because the numbers of Irish missed by census takers likely remained about the same.

13. These records were written by hospital physicians and thus present their view of each patient's case history. Information typically included was the patient's name, age, gender, occupation, place of birth, diagnosed ailment and explanation of its origin (sometimes including some acknowledgement of the patient's view), treatments prior to admission (occasionally), treatments administered in the hospital (including surgeries, medicines, and diet), and results. Results included the following categories: cured, relieved, not relieved, died, improper object (infected with an incurable disease, smallpox, the itch," or other "infectious distempers," and mothers with small

children, except in cases in which the child was also a patient) or discharged disorderly (Larrabee 1971:107).

14. NYC dispensaries recorded treating nearly 29,000 cases involving Irish-born patients in 1850 (Brighton 2005:251).

15. In order to protect the identities of individuals, only first names will be used when referencing medical and surgical case records.

16. *The Citizen*, an Irish American newspaper, reported two fires in their February 4, 1854, issue, one on Duane Street between Elm and Center and another at 14 and 10 Pearl Street. Both fires drove numerous families out to the streets. "These houses were occupied by about 50 families, some of whom lost their all. The Battery was strewn with furniture and household goods, among which women and children were moving and lying in the greatest state of distress, both of body and mind." A case record from two years previous details a heroic escape from a building fire. A 38-year-old Irish-born seaman named Cornelius jumped out of a second story window with his two children in his arms and his wife then jumped from the same window on top of him. He fractured a few ribs and sustained bruises and a cut to his arm but saved himself and his family (NYHSCB 1852:C579).

17. It is possible that this patient lived at 472 Pearl Street in the Five Points in 1860. A comparison of names, ages, and occupations between census and hospital records suggests that a few of the residents of 472 and 474 Pearl Street were treated at New York Hospital; but the evidence is not conclusive because New York Hospital case records do not include patients' addresses, and most patients had names that were relatively common among the Irish in NYC.

18. Miller (1985:54) writes that in pre-famine Ireland "Among the Catholic Irish especially, only family members were considered "friends" (*cairde*), while nonrelated neighbors, regardless of intimacy, were merely "acquaintances" (*lucht aitheantais*). Arensberg (1937:67) noted that in early 20th-century Ireland "friend" implied duty or obligation to reciprocal relations. "It is part of the 'friendliness' owed one's kinsmen to make up and serve food at wakes and weddings, to dig the grave, to carry the coffin, to keen over the dead. The conduct is reciprocal."

19. Although Joseph Lister's antiseptic surgical techniques, discovered in 1865, were adopted by Parisian surgeons by 1867, it was not until 1878 that Dr. Lewis Atterbury Stimson, who trained abroad, demonstrated Lister's methods in the U.S. at New York Hospital during an amputation at the knee. Physicians at New York Hospital and beyond remained skeptical, and it took several years for the techniques to be used routinely. As late as 1906, Dr. George Ludlam, superintendent of New York Hospital and President of the American Hospital Association, did not see the full value of antiseptic techniques. He commented on the difficulty of working with doctors trained in antiseptic methods: "Familiarity with these methods engenders a spirit of extravagance which permeates the whole establishment and which is exceedingly difficult to check or control." He criticized what he termed the "craze for rubber gloves" (Vogel 1979:113–114).

20. There were two main methods of amputation, both performed with hand saws, the circular method and the flap method. The circular method cut the limb straight across the bone, while the flap method left skin that was sewn to create a curved stump.

21. Mortality rates of 732 cases of amputation during the Crimean War are as follows: overall mortality 22.6%, fingers 0.5%, forearm and wrist 1.8%, arm 22.9%, shoulder 27.2%, tarsus 14.2%, ankle 22.2%, lower leg 30.3, knee 50%, lower third of thigh 50%, middle thigh 55.3%, upper thigh 86.8%, hip 100% (Gross 1861:84–85).

22. Inhaling the vapors of white phosphorus, used in making matches from 1840 through 1910, led to the deposition of phosphorus in jaw bones and could cause brain damage, painful and disfiguring jaw abscesses and deterioration of the jaw, and death. White phosphorus was finally replaced in the U.S. after a French chemist discovered a substitute. Diamond Match Company purchased the patent rights in the U.S. and then waived them, in an "extraordinary display of industrial generosity" (Kraut 1994:171–172).

23. From 1851 to 1857, the *New York Times* was called the *New-York Daily Times*. In 1858, the paper dropped "Daily."

24. A July 6, 1850 advertisement for a missing husband named Joseph Duglass in the Boston newspaper *The Pilot* provides a colorful description of the man that highlights visible work-related scars: "He is 5 ½ feet high, fair hair, cross eyed, and a bend in one of his fingers, and a scar on his hand and on the back of his neck; he got blown up in East Boston at the foundry; he has small ear-rings in his ears. He is from County Derry, Ireland, and says he's a Scotchman" (Harris and Jacobs 1989:496).

25. Mott (1862:5, 7–8) wrote, for example, "Most men fear pain even more than death. . . . Pain is positively injurious to the pained. If sufficiently acute and long continued, it will of itself produce death. . . . Whatever, then, may be the physiological necessity for pain, though its uses in the animal economy may be to prevent lesion and deter from danger, we are here to view the question merely in a therapeutic light, and to conclude that pain is only evil."

26. Chronic and acute alcoholism are still recognized today as increasing risks associated with anesthesia and complicating dosing (Chapman and Platt 2009).

27. When Mary McLean (1886–1900) passed out on the docks in Quebec, the captain of her ship came to her aid with cayenne-laced brandy (see Introduction).

28. Hirota (2017) also suggests that anti-Irish prejudice was generally greater in New England than in New York in the 19th-century.

29. MacNeven was born in County Galway in 1763 (MacNeven 1842b).

30. St. Vincent de Paul (1581–1660) was a French priest noted for his devotion to the poor. He founded charitable organizations and established the Daughters of Charity, an order of nuns devoted to helping the poor. The Sisters of Charity are an American order based on the Daughters of Charity, founded in 1809 by Elizabeth Ann Bayley Seyton, whose father had been the Chief Health Officer of the Port of New York and whose husband had died of TB (Walsh 1965; Fitzgerald 2006).

31. This assessment was not unbiased, however. McMahon (2015a:85) notes that the *New York Freeman's Journal* was the unofficial mouthpiece of Archbishop John Hughes.

32. Mott was President of the Medical College of the University of the State of New York, Professor of Surgery and Chief Surgeon at New York Hospital and Bellevue, and President of the New York Academy of Medicine. Van Buren taught surgery at the Bellevue Medical College and anatomy at the NYU Medical College (Walsh 1965:12–17).

Chapter 5

1. Toxic ivy berries were reportedly eaten in very small quantities to relieve pain (Allen and Hatfield 2004:180, Barbour 1897:388). Drinking whiskey was advised to relieve pains from consumption, cough, sciatica, and more (NFCS 1938[920]:70; Wilson 1943:182; McClafferty 1979).

2. Eel oil was also recommended for earaches (Wilson 1943:180) and deafness (NFC 1955[1389]:41). Olive oil was also recommended for burns (NFCS 1938[35]:129).

3. In County Donegal dog fat (Barbour 1897:387) and in County Laois groundhog fat (NFC:ca. 1929[36]:246) were thought to be especially useful for stiff joints. Irish household healers might have chosen to use goose grease as an ointment because it had a lower melting point than other animal fats, making it more conducive to massaging into skin.

4. Selected citations: NFCS1938[35]:139; NFCS 1938[345]:20; NFCS 1938[920]:325; NFCS 1937[598]:43; Wilson 1943:182; Logan 1994:51. Many of the same cures were repeatedly reported to folklore collectors, especially commonly known cures for everyday colds, cuts, aches, and pains. In such cases I have cited only a sample of these mentions.

5. "An old woman . . . from near Leighlinbridge, who had cures, used . . . old bread as a poultice on cuts which were slow to heal. She used to soften the bread with milk or water. Informant does not know if the bread kept until mold" (NFC subject card index, subject G, subsection Cerithe 7 Ungaithe).

6. Irish folklore sources indicate that boiled plantain juice was used to treat headaches, liver trouble, and sore eyes, while plantain poultices were used to staunch bleeding and treat cuts, burns, and varicose veins (Allen and Hatfield 2004:248). *Slánlus* was later the name of a patent medicine company in Ireland (Farmar 2004).

7. Physician and folklore collector Patrick Logan (1994:114) notes many people assured him that a poultice of salt and sugar would heal a wound infected by foreign matter, such as a thorn. Sugar alone or a sugar-salt mixture was also used to draw out boils and even the fluid in an infected joint (bursitis). Irish informants reported

that a bit of chewed tobacco was curative if applied to boils, cuts, sores, chilblains, hives, ringworm, or toothaches and could prevent blood poisoning from a cut (Egan 1887:13; NFCS 1937[598]:434; NFCS 1938[35]:139; NFCS 1938[45]:199–200; NFCS 1938[345]:11, 206; NFCS 1938[624]:249, 529; NFC 1941[782]:350; NFC 1974[1838]:66; Logan 1994:74).

8. Cow's urine was also recommended for cracked hands and chilblains in County Carlow (NFC 1935[265]:593, 601). Logan (1994:104) specifies mare's urine as a folk treatment for burns. Urine from both animals and humans has been used throughout the world for centuries to disinfect wounds. Its sterility, provided the urine supplier does not have an infection, makes urine a good choice for cleaning in the absence of sterilized water (Ortiz de Montellano 1990).

9. An informant from County Clare reported to a National Folklore Collector that ragweed "ha[d] been used in [the] family for at least one hundred years, carried on from generation to generation by the women of the family. The leaves of the *buachalán* [ragweed] are cut up and boiled for an hour, all the others (fresh butter, hog's lard, beeswax, Stockholm tar, resin, soap) are added to them and the whole boiled until thick and applied as a poultice" (NFC 1930s?[128]:231). Dock is one of the most well-known plants in the Irish folk medicine arsenal because it supplies the cure for nettle stings, which virtually every child experiences; it was also used for insect stings, burns, sunburns, and ulcers (Allen and Hatfield 2004:97–98; Logan 1994:67–68). The leaves of common ivy are high in acetic acid, and throughout the British Isles were the treatment par excellence for corns when used as a poultice after soaking them in vinegar or boiling them. In Ireland, household healers extend ivy's uses to burns, eczema, inflammation, cuts, chilblains, warts, boils, ringworm, and sprains (Allen and Hatfield 2004:179–180). Allen and Hatfield (2004) write that willow is curiously rarely mentioned in Irish folklore records as a pain remedy. In Great Britain it was common. According to Frank Brew (1990) "sally willow" (the word for willow in Irish is *saileach* and was Anglicized to "sally"; willow belongs to the Salix taxonomic genus) was used in County Clare to remedy pain. The NFCS manuscripts note willow bark was applied externally to relieve rheumatic fever and gangrene, and a poultice of the leaves was used to cure boils (NFCS 1938[289]:319; NFCS 1938[405]:465; NFCS 1938[849]:350). One informant recommended drinking an infusion of the bark for diarrhea (NFCS 1938[385]:55).

10. Citations: NFCS 1937[624]:137; Brew 1990:25; O'Regan 1997:12. Comfrey was also applied for the complexion, boils, toothache, rheumatism, and sprain, and taken internally for colds (Barbour 1897:389; NFC 1930[80]:21; NFCS 1938[624]:276–77; NFC 1941[782]:352; Logan 1994:77; Allen and Hatfield 2004:209).

11. Informants also reported that smoking a pipe was useful for toothaches and could relieve recurrent headaches when smoked in the morning (NFCS 1938[35]:139; Dorian 2000:114).

12. Elder has long been associated with the supernatural in Ireland, which likely

increased its reputation as a healing substance. A 48-year-old male publican in Tipperary gave a Christianized explanation for elder's powers: "The elder is the only tree that was never struck by lightning, because the Lord's cross was made out of elder" (NFC 1938[560]:16–17).

13. Selected citations: NFCS 1937[598]:105; NFCS 1937[624]:251; NFCS 1938[35]:139–140; NFCS 1938[45]:249; Wilson 1943:180; Logan 1994:51,55, 129; O'Regan 1997:6

14. Selected citations: NFC 1935[54]:78; NFCS 1937[598]:104; NFCS 1938[35]:130; NFC 1953[1364]:64; Logan 1994:124.

15. Nettles are a common weed in Ireland. Tiny hair-like spines on the stem contain histamine and formic acid and are irritating to the skin. Folklore informants specified that nettle was used as a counterirritant for sprains, chest colds, and rheumatism (Barbour 1897:389; NFCS 1937[598]:167; NFCS 1938[345]:8; Logan 1963:91). In Counties Cavan and Leitrim, people made an oil out of rotten bream fish from a nearby lake that they applied as a counterirritant for "rheumaticky pains" (Logan 1963:91). According to Logan (1994:73, 93), pitch acted as a counterirritant for pain when applied. Pitch was also used for rheumatism (NFC 1935[265]:597–599).

16. Other informants indicated to folklore collectors that the water in which a corpse had been washed could cure a sore (NFC 1935[107]:487) and touching the hand of a dead person to an afflicted area could cure rheumatism (M'Clintock 1912:475; Ó Crualaoich 1998). Red was said to have special healing power, and red-colored strings and flannel were used in many cures. Several sources mention a connection between the color red and Christ's blood; others connect red to fairies (Hutchings 1997:59; Linn 2014:153).

17. Soil from priests' graves was recommended to cure sore eyes. Logan (1994:59) wrote, for example, that before his death the Franciscan friar Father John MacKeon "is reputed to have said that people could take clay from his grave to cure sore eyes, and today it is evident that a considerable amount of clay has been taken. It is used in the same way as Jesus used it—mixing with spittle and applying on eyes."

18. Selected citations: NFCS 1938[45]:201; NFCS 1938[345]:8; NFCS 1938[364]:219; NFCS 1938[624]:79, 249; NFC 1941[782]:262; Logan 1994:102–103.

19. Selected citations: Wilde, W. 1852:128–129; NFC 1930[80]:10; NFCS 1938[229]:118; NFC 1974[1837]:121–122. Logan (1994:28–30) identified this condition as angina from heart disease and noted it was called *croí-chrá* or *feochair croí* in Irish, but folklore records suggest chest pain from other sources was also treated this way (see Chapter 7).

20. Logan (1994:91) notes that until the 17th century bonesetters were probably trained in Irish medical schools. When the schools were closed down by the Penal Laws, knowledge was transmitted by apprenticeship. Certain families, including the O'Hickeys or the O'Shiels are thought to be old medical families. Some bonesetters might have also acquired skills caring for sheep and other farm animals, becoming so skillful they were asked to assist humans (Logan 1994:97, 100). Particular Irish

families were renowned for bonesetting skills, some through the 1980s. They include the Castellos of Ballinahown, Westmeath (6 Feb 1943, *Westmeath Independent* cited in NFC subject card index G, subsection Dochtuiri, 7 Lucht Leighis); the Donaghys and the Teagues from County Leitrim; the Tuiles (anglicized Tully or Flood) in Counties Cavan, Leitrim, and Longford; the Lanes of County Cork; and the Actons in the Galway-Mayo area. Family lore associated with two of the families stresses how they came to the skill without asking for it (Logan 1994:95–100).

21. There is evidence that bonesetters were knowledgeable about the effects of TB on the bones and avoided treating those suffering from it. Any manipulation of a TB-infected bone or joint is likely to cause more damage. Tom Acton of Tuam, a bonesetter Logan (1994:94–95, 98) spoke with, said that he could distinguish a child with a broken knee from a child with TB of the knee by the overall appearance of the child.

22. Julia Lane, a 70-year-old widow, resided at 472 Pearl Street with the Sullivan family in 1855 (NYSC 1855).

23. Efforts to link particular residents of 472 and 474 Pearl Street with hospital records were relatively inconclusive, but for about ten possible cases. Two of these ten cases resulted from work-related conditions and were noted in Chapter 4—a fever from working on the Erie Railroad and a fall from a roof. Neither included details of any remedies used before admission.

24. According to census records, residents of 472 and 474 Pearl Street from 1850 to 1870 were engaged in a variety of occupations. They were artificial flower makers, blacksmiths, boatmen, bookbinders, brass turners, carpenters, cap makers, carriage drivers, caulkers, clerks, coachmen, cooks, coopers, distillers, dressmakers, drivers, glasscutters, grocers, housecleaners, laborers, laundresses, liquor dealers, machinists, masons, metal roofers, milliners, peddlers, printers, porters, sailmakers, seamen, seamstresses, servants, shoemakers, soap-boilers, soda water makers, speculators, storekeepers, tailors, tinsmiths, and undertakers (USBC 1850, 1860, 1870).

25. Selected citations: Egan 1887:12; Logan 1994:33; Allen and Hatfield 2004:141–142, 145.

26. Selected citations: Egan 1887:11; NFCS 1937[624]:251, 527; Allen and Hatfield 2004:323–324.

27. Remains of *Rumex* species, categorized by Raymer et al. (2000) as dock or sorrel, were found only in the 1850 layer of Feature J, and not in the 1870 layer or in Feature O. Selected citations: Egan 1887:12; NFC 1930[80]:20; NFCS 1937[598]:166; NFCS 1937[624]:137; NFCS 1938[35]:131; NFC 1941[782]:350; Harris 1960:65; Logan 1963:91, 1994:109–110; Allen and Hatfield 2004:95–100.

28. Selected citations: Barbour 1897:389; NFC 1935[54]:191; NFCS 1938[45]:246; NFC 1941[782]:352–353; Furey 1991:111; Logan 1994:74; Allen and Hatfield 2004:270–272. Brew (1990:25) points out that a patent medicine ointment containing elder tree leaves, called Zam-Buck Ointment, was popular in the early 20th century.

29. Citations: NFC 1938[560]:110; Logan 1994:34.

30. Allen and Hatfield 2004:90.

31. Remains of *Mentha* species, categorized by Raymer et al. (2000) as mint, were found only in the 1850 layer of Feature J, and not in the 1870 layer or in Feature O. Selected citations: NFCS 1938[345]:8; Wilson 1943:182; Furey 1991:111; Allen and Hatfield 2004:238.

32. Selected citations: Egan 1887:12; Purdon 1895a:216; Barbour 1897:388; NFC 1955[1389]:200; Allen and Hatfield 2004:306-307.

33. Remains of wheat (*Triticum aestivum*) were found only in the 1870 layer of Feature J, not in the 1850 layer of Feature J or in Feature O (Raymer et al. 2000). Selected citations: NFCS 1938[35]:134; NFCS 1938[364]:22; Logan 1994:107; 1 O'Regan 1997:21

34. Selected citations: NFCS 1938[624]:77; Logan 1994:87.

35. Selected citations: Wilson 1943:180; NFC 1953[1364]:52; NFC 1955 [1389]:41; Logan 1963:9; O'Regan 1997:21.

36. Selected citations: NFCS 1938[35]:130; NFCS 1938[45]:247; NFCS 1938[345]:8; NFCS 1938[918]:179; NFC 1941[782]:357; Logan 1994:24; O'Regan 1997:21.

37. Archaeologists found remains of rabbits, *Sylvilagus* species, only in the 1870 layer of Feature J and not in the 1850 layer or in Feature O (Milne and Crabtree 2000). Selected citations: NFCS 1938[35]:127; NFC 1955[1389]:177, 201; Logan 1994:86.

38. Selected citations: NFCS 1938[35]:33, 128-129; NFC 1940[80]:14; Logan 1994:114.

39. Selected citations: NFC 1937[407]:142; NFCS 1938[35]:132; NFCS 1938[624]:77; NFC 1955[1389]:209; Furey 1991:111; Logan 1994:6, 23; O'Regan 1997:20; Castleconnor Parish Development Group 2000:126.

40. Mint was used for healing and culinary purposes throughout Europe, so it is somewhat surprising that it was only found in one of the deposits associated with German families (AN TPQ 1860), but in the same deposit there was a bottle of Essence of Peppermint, a popular patent medicine (Ponz 2000:54). The Irish families at 472 and 474 appear to have preferred mint in the plant form. This is consistent with how the Irish traditionally used mint medicinally, either eaten raw or made into a medicinal tea or homemade cough syrup (NFCS 1938[345]:8; Allen and Hatfield 2004:238). One bottle of Essence of Peppermint was also uncovered in Feature AM, the feature at 110 Chatham Street associated with Conlon's Oyster Saloon (Bonasera 2000b).

41. The Irish physician Henry S. Purdon (1895a:216) reported that ragwort was kept on hand by Belfast druggists as a fluid extract at the request of older medical men in the area. Purdon attested to seeing jaundice healed by decoctions of the ragwort plant drunk three days in a row.

42. An informant from Cork described why "chickweed is a cure for burns. A drop of our Lord's blood is said to have fallen on one of the leaves. Now it is on every leaf. The

upper side of the leaf has the cure but the underside has not" (NFCS 1938[364]:220–221). Thomas Melody, aged 73 when interviewed by a schoolboy in 1938, noted a chickenweed poultice was good for a pain in the side (NFCS 1938[45]:366).

43. Selected citations: burns (NFCS 1938[35]:129; NFCS 1938[364]:221), heartburn (NFC 1930[80]:14), rheumatism (Barbour 1897:388; NFC 1930[80]:18; NFCS 1938[624]:81), sores (NFC 1941[782]:349), sore throat (NFCS 1938[35]:140; Logan 1994:55), sprain (Egan 1887:11), swelling (NFC 1938[560]:317; NFC 1941[782]:362), warts (M'Clintock 1912:475; NFC 1930[80]:8, 220; NFC 1935[265]:591; NFC 1953[1364]:54; Logan 1994:119; Verling 2003:67), and whitlow (NFC 1935[265]:595; NFCS 1937[598]:103; NFCS 1938[35]:31; Logan 1994:108).

44. Jimsonweed was present in several Irish-related, German-related, and brothel-related features at the Five Points (Features J, O, AM, AN, B, and AG—dating from the 1830s to the 1870s). Pokeweed stands out in one Irish-related deposit in the Five Points (Feature J AS IV, fill between the 1850s and 1860s strata) but was absent in soil samples from other Irish- or German-related features (Raymer et al. 2000).

45. Wilkie (2003:157) notes that jimsonweed is also a known abortifacient and has been uncovered archaeologically in deposits associated with former slave cabins in the South.

46. According to Covey (2007:106), herbalists today use pokeweed to treat high blood pressure, and the berries might stimulate the immune system.

47. Whiskey was also used externally to relieve headaches, toothaches, earaches, and breathing difficulty, likely because of its pungent smell and quick evaporation rate that brought a feeling of coolness (NFCS 1937[598]:43; NFCS 1938[35]:139; NFCS 1938[345]:20; NFCS 1938[920]:325; Wilson 1943:182; Logan 1994:51).

48. Green coffee pods are not poisonous, but recently, scientists have identified a few species of fungi (*Aspergillus ochraceus*, *A. carbonarius*, and strains of *A. niger*) that grow on coffee beans and produce poisonous toxins.

49. Selected citations: NFC 1935[265]:595; NFCS 1938[35]:33,128, 133; NFCS 1938[45]:255; NFCS 1938[345]:207; NFC 1941[782]:359; NFC 1955[1389]:210; Logan 1994:59.

50. Irish informants recommended carron oil by name as a cure for burns (NFCS 1938[35]:129; Logan 1994:104), as well as the ingredients alone (NFCS 1938[45]:249; NFCS 1938[916]:68). Linseed oil on its own was also recommended as a cure for burns and wounds (Logan 1994:104; O'Regan 1997:20).

51. Most "patent medicines" in the U.S. were not patented, because patenting required disclosing ingredients and demonstrating efficacy. Instead, the producers of these products registered the product's name, symbol, or bottle shape, making their product a proprietary medicine. In practice, few consumers made the distinction between patent and proprietary medicines, and instead, referred to all of them as patent medicines (Cramp 1912:9). This article employs the language of the period and refers to both types of medicine as patent medicines.

52. Europeans initially acquired Peruvian bark in the 17th century from a few species of trees in the *Cinchona* species native to the northern Andes. There is a long and complicated history of how the bark was used to treat malaria and other fevers (Harris 2012).

53. Friedrich Engels (1887:70) sounded the alarm in the 19th century about the damaging and deadly effects of Godfrey's Cordial upon children in England.

54. Patricia Laird (1998:3) describes how completion of the transcontinental railroad in 1869 enabled some businesses to become truly national and encouraged them to paint every boulder and barn along the train route from the East to the West Coast with an advertisement.

55. Patent medicine business owners had considerable power over editors, according to Adams (1912:5). Advertising contracts included "red clauses" that made it difficult for newspapers to support legislation against patent medicines. Such clauses rendered the advertising contract null if legislation affected a patent medicine company's ability to advertise or sell its product.

56. People with limited means used free posters and printed handbills as household decoration, and even the "better sort" of people used them to adorn kitchens, children's rooms, and laundry rooms (Laird 1998:63).

57. Medicine bottles composed about 33% of the total glass assemblage in the 1850 deposit associated with 472 Pearl Street, and 26% of the glass assemblage in the 1870 deposit in the same feature, and 41% of the glass assemblage in the 1860 deposit associated with 474 Pearl Street (see Figure 3.5). Soda water was also used medicinally in the 19th century, and these bottles are sometimes categorized as medicine bottles. Here they will be considered separately and discussed in Chapter 7.

58. The ratio of patent medicines to ethical medicines at 472 and 474 Pearl Street ranged from 0.7 to 3.1, whereas at 22 Baxter Street and Greenwich Mews, they were 0.3 and 0.22, respectively (Brighton 2008:144).

59. Evidence of turpentine was not found archaeologically at the Five Points, but it is possible that some of the liquor bottles found there were reused to store it. Turpentine and linseed oil were often sold in the U.S. in empty liquor bottles (Busch 1987:70). Hospital records indicate that some Irish immigrants used turpentine to manage their injuries. At New York Hospital, for example, a 19-year-old Irish-born farmer with a chronic inflammation of the knee joint reported applying turpentine to it prior to admission (NYHSCB 1852:C979).

60. Hostetter's Bitters was a very successful product selling between 500,000 and 1,000,000 bottles annually from 1859 through 1883 (Young 1961).

61. The metal syringes shown in Figure 5.4 were likely uncovered in the lower layer of Feature J (TPQ 1850), as the general artifact inventory lists two "pb/sn/ni alloy pewter" syringes in that context (Yamin 2000[4, Part 2]:675.) The syringes pictured closely resemble the type invented and popularized by Alexander Wood of the Royal College of Surgeons in Edinburgh, an early proponent of hypodermic medication in Scottish and English medical journals in 1855 and 1858 (Howard-Jones

1947). Historian Norman Howard-Jones (1947:217) notes that Dr. Benjamin Fordyce Barker was the first to use such a hypodermic syringe in the U.S. in 1856, having been given one while visiting Edinburgh. Dr. Barker was Chair of Obstetrics at New York Medical College from 1850 to 1857 and an obstetric physician at Bellevue Hospital in the 1850s (*National Cyclopedia of American Biography* 1893:157; *NYT* 1893:5). It is possible that a woman from 472 Pearl Street had been treated by Dr. Barker at Bellevue and sustained an injury during childbirth that required continued use of hypodermic morphine at home.

62. According to Logan (1994:111), a man from the Castlebar Hospital sought this woman to avoid a scheduled amputation of his hand. She took some blood out of her arm, mixed it with unsalted butter, applied it to the wound, and it quickly healed. James Mooney relates a similar story from County Kerry, where a swollen limb that physicians decided to amputate was saved by a traveling woman. The woman applied a painful poultice from a plant called *uarac-a-loc* or *greim a diabail*, "the devil's bit." The man was tied down so that he could not move from the excruciating pain of the poultice. In the morning the poultice fell off and he was cured (Mooney 1887:165).

63. There was a popular Dublin newspaper called the *Freeman's Journal* from which this NYC publication took its name. Similarly, there was a Dublin newspaper called *the Pilot* from which the *Boston Pilot* took its name.

64. Pharmacist James C. O'Neill, for example, arrived from County Sligo in 1852 and in 1855 was living at 84 Mulberry Street (Yamin 2000[3]:Appendix V)]. Groneman Pernicone (1973:156) notes that there was a female Irish druggist living in the Sixth Ward in 1855.

65. One bottle of Rowland's was found in association with the earlier deposit (TPQ 1850) in Feature J+Z at 472 Pearl Street, while one bottle of Batchelor's Hair Dye and two bottles of Lubin Perfume were found in the later (TPQ 1870) Feature J layer. One bottle of Lyon's Kathairon and one of Lubin Perfume was found the deposit (TPQ 1860) in Feature O at 474 Pearl Street (Ponz 2000).

66. Six bottles of Batchelor's Hair Dye were present in a privy at the Greenwich Mews Site associated with three American-born middle-class families (Geismar 1989:85). At least one bottle of Lubin Perfume was found at Van Cortland Manor, home to the old New York Van Cortland family (Amanda Sutphin 2015, personal communication). Advertisements for these brands ran in *Harper's Weekly*, the *New-York Daily Tribune*, and the *New York (Daily) Times*, and Irish immigrant papers, such as the *New York Freeman's Journal* and *the Citizen*. The same marketing strategies observed in patent medicine advertising are also common in advertisements for cosmetic products: repetition of key phrases, testimonials from satisfied customers, and claims of exotic ingredients, safety, and guaranteed efficacy (Laird 1998, Young 1961).

67. In the same deposit, archaeologists also found fragments of several lice combs and toothbrushes, showing residents' concerns about personal hygiene (Yamin 2000[1]:102, 153).

68. Lyon's Kathairon contained antibacterial and antifungal ingredients, such as alcohol, tannic acid, castor oil, and clove oil, that could have improved some ailments, including dandruff (Hiss 1900:190). Castor oil is used today as a popular cure for lice. The same company advertised an insect powder in the *NYT* (1868a:5) and the *NYFJ* (1854d:6).

69. Advertisements claimed Batchelor's Hair Dye turned hair "black or brown . . . instantly and permanently" (*NYT* 1868b:5). Lyon's Kathiron advertisements promised to restore the color to gray hair through repeated applications. It contained oils of clove and rosemary, natural hair darkeners (Hiss 1900:190).

70. An advertisement for Hoyt's Imperial Coloring Cream in *HW's* (1864:208) claimed it "changes light and red hair to a beautiful brown or black." An advertisement for Dr. Gouraud's Dye in the *NYFJ* (1855:8) similarly declared it "instantly converts red or grey hair to beautiful black or brown without staining the skin."

71. Fair complexions were also considered desirable in Ireland. Recipes for skin lightening include applying a mixture of oatmeal and buttermilk (Logan 1994:77) or washing the face with the liquid strained from boiled tansy on a May morning. An informant in County Longford shared this rhyme with collector Pádraig MacGréine: "Tansey fair and tansey bright will make a brown skin fair or white" (NFC 1930[80]:21).

72. In Ireland, red hair was also sometimes considered undesirable and linked to unluckiness, the evil eye, and witchcraft (Blake 1918; Wilde, L. 1887a:43, 1890:64; Doherty 1897:16; Dorian 2000).

73. Lyon Kathiron contained cantharides, a powerful blister-inducing irritant (Hiss 1900:190).

Chapter 6

1. Death rates from diagnoses of "consumption" and "phthisis," which do not capture all the possible forms of tubercular infection, in these cities hovered between 400 and 500 per 100,000 people for decades (Drolet and Lowell 1952:v; Barnes 1995:4). For comparison, the death rates of the four leading causes of death in the U.S. in 2020—heart disease, cancer, COVID-19, and unintentional injuries—were respectively 168.2, 144.1, 85, and 57.6 per 100,000 people (Murphy et al. 2021:4). The average death rate from TB in the U.S. from 1990 through 2006 was 1.16 per 100,000 (Jung et al. 2010).

2. Later in the century, typhoid fever was added to the list (Leavitt 1992).

3. Scrofula can be caused by either *Mycobacterium tuberculosis* or *Mycobacterium bovis*, another related bacterium that affects cows. Humans most often contract the latter from drinking unpasteurized milk or eating meat from infected cows. *Mycobacterium bovis* can also cause disease in joints (Hayes 2009:155). Pott's disease is a tubercular infection of the spine that erodes the vertebrae (usually the thoracic)

and creates a characteristic "gibbus" (hump) in the back. TB of the skin can produce open sores, most often appearing on the face (Dormandy 1999:23–25).

4. "Walling off" causes the bacteria to enter a dormant phase for years or even decades. Factors that decrease the strength of an individual's immune system include other illnesses, traumatic injuries, malnutrition, aging, exposure to the elements, and certain drugs, such as today's steroids and chemotherapies.

5. Available NYC mortality reports do not provide much information about the extent of tubercular disease among the Irish in the city; they do not list causes of death by place of birth. The statistical report analyzing mortality schedules from the 1850 Federal Census does. It shows a higher rate of death attributed to consumption among Irish-born than native-born New Yorkers, 326 versus 254 per 100,000 (De Bow 1855:180–181). However, these figures seem to be too low, when compared with Drolet and Lowell's (1952:iii) average estimate of 431 per 100,000 for the years 1849 to 1853, perhaps because the mortality schedules are incomplete.

6. New York Hospital's policy of rejecting or quickly discharging "incurable" patients (Larrabee 1971:107) might have contributed to lower numbers of patients hospitalized there with tubercular diseases. The 1848 case of a 12-year-old Irish girl diagnosed with *morbus coxarius* and discharged as incurable is an example (NYHMCB 1848:C517). Individuals with advanced phthisis were also frequently considered incurable, but a number of patients with advanced phthisis were treated at the hospital and died there, so the admission criteria for tubercular patients is unclear.

7. Pathologist and medical historian Thomas Dormandy (1999:14–16) notes that physicians occasionally bled pulmonary TB patients well into the 1860s. It apparently quickly reduced coughing fits.

8. Physicians' liberal prescription of opiates for a variety of ailments was a major cause of drug addiction in the 19th century, as it continues to be today (Dormandy 1999:49). At least one case at New York Hospital supports this link: an Irish woman suffering from debility and a fractured arm explained to the admitting physician that "three years ago while a patient in this hospital she contracted the habit of taking opium and since then has been unable to break herself of it" (NYHSCB 1862:C287).

9. The hospital treated fewer patients overall during the latter period, so the number with phthisis represents a greater percentage of total hospital patients.

10. Future research into the reports of other dispensaries could help to assess the extent of tubercular illness among the Irish in other parts of the city.

11. There were no official training programs for nurses until the Bellevue School of Nursing opened in 1873, in consultation with Florence Nightingale and her school of nursing at St. Thomas Hospital in London. Before then, at Bellevue and New York Hospital most nurses were men, and they did more janitorial work than nursing. The work was difficult and nurses were constantly exposed to disease. Nursing thus frequently attracted less educated people and was thought to be unsuitable for respectable women, unless they cared for other women or children. Nurses thus had

poor reputations. In contrast, care of the sick was part of the Sisters of Charity's religious devotion. They were required by their order to be compassionate, disciplined, selfless, and obedient to doctor's orders. They quickly achieved notoriety in the city, especially during the Civil War, when they nursed many wounded soldiers in the city and throughout the warring states (Jolly 1927). The dedication of the Sisters of Charity at St. Vincent and in other hospitals in Europe influenced later nursing programs, including those at Bellevue and St. Thomas. Florence Nightingale, in fact, was initially trained by the Sisters of Charity in Paris (Walsh 1965:225–228).

12. Other illnesses in the top three at St. Vincent's Hospital in 1859, 1860, 1863, and 1874 fluctuated somewhat in order but included rheumatism, typhus and/or typhoid fever, and malaria. In 1881, the top diagnoses were contusion, fracture, and *ebrietas* (drunkenness) (SVHAR 1861, 1864, 1875, 1882).

13. Fewer patients with nonpulmonary TB were treated at New York Hospital than St. Vincent's, perhaps because physicians at New York Hospital considered them to be incurable and refused to admit them. The number of patients treated for *morbus coxarius* at New York Hospital never reached more than 11 per year between 1835 and 1865. Between 1845 and 1854, only a couple of patients with this ailment were admitted to the hospital. Then, between 1855 and 1861, cases ranged between 0 to 11 per year (NYHAR 1836–1866).

14. TB mortality began to decrease in England in the 1830s. Leonard Wilson (2005) has argued that this was not a result of better standards of living, as suggested by other historians, but an unintended consequence of the 1834 Poor Laws that isolated the poor in workhouses. This law effectively quarantined the population most affected by the disease long before doctors understood that it was contagious. In the 1860s, death rates in NYC, Boston, and Philadelphia were over 400 per 100,000, compared with 275 per 100,000 in England in 1850 and 219 per 100,000 in Ireland in 1861 (Drolet and Lowell 1952:ii–vi, Feldberg 1995:29).

15. Upon arrival in 1827, the McPeake family consisted of seven, headed by John and Rachael and including their four children and John's mother, Allay. About three years later, the 1830 U.S. Census lists an additional male child under the age of five in their household. This child does not appear in subsequent censuses and thus might have passed away during infancy.

16. By 1840, the family took in two boarders, one male and one female, both between the ages of 20 and 29 (USBC 1840).

17. It is possible that his mother and his wife also died from the disease. The death notices of Allay and Rachael McPeake do not specify cause of death (*New-York Evening Post* 1830; NYC Municipal Deaths Records 1861).

18. A Patrick McPeake, a builder residing at 32 Wooster, next door to John McPeake and family, from at least 1828 to 1830 might have been a relative of John's who had arrived earlier and advised him to settle in this neighborhood (*LAA* 1828, 1829, 1830).

19. According to the 1841 Irish Census, many relatively well-off Irish farmers lived in one- or two-room homes, and it was common for Irish families to live in one-room

semi-subterranean mud huts. These were the dwellings of more than 50% of the overall rural population, and as much as 67% and 81% in Counties Kerry and Cork, respectively (Evans 1957:46), where many of the Irish in New York had originated (Anbinder et al. 2019a).

20. According to Bishop John Hughes, himself an immigrant, "their [Irish immigrants'] abode in the cellars and garrets of New York is not more deplorable nor more squalid than the Irish hovels from which many of them had been exterminated" (Dolan 1975:37). Despite Hughes's comments, designed to emphasize how bad conditions had been for the Catholic Irish in Ireland, Irish immigrants were not accustomed to the kind of darkness and filth they encountered in tenements and gladly exchanged it for better accommodations when possible. They resorted to living in tenement apartments in order to pay bills with meager wages and remain near friends and family.

21. Beginning in 1848, directories list James and Thomas's painting business at 28 Wooster and their residence at the same address; by 1849, the family had moved their residence back to 30 Wooster (Doggett 1848, 1849).

22. Additionally, 1851 was a peak year of Irish immigration with accompanying outbreaks of typhus and typhoid fevers and smallpox, likely also contributors to increased tubercular disease among the Irish in New York.

23. An Irish widow explained to physicians at the New York Orthopaedic Hospital and Dispensary that her funds were so limited that she could only afford to use fuel for cooking and not for heating, for example (NYODAR 1872:14).

24. In the month of August of 1864 alone, for example, 576 infants died in the city from *cholera infantum* (Keeney 1865:41), understood today as acute gastroenteritis with many possible causes. Those who survived were more susceptible to tubercular infection.

25. This pattern was recognized to a degree in the 19th century. Physicians then noted that few dyspeptics became consumptives (Stillé 1994:108). Today, medical researchers note a correlation between obesity and dyspepsia (Ho and Spiegel 2008).

26. Because of New York Hospitals' agreement with the Port of NY to take care of sick and injured seamen, a large number of seamen were treated for phthisis. They are excluded from this discussion because most were not residents of NYC.

27. This birthrate data comes from Philadelphia. Leavitt (1999:330) writes that there Irish immigrant women bore an average of 7 children from the 1880s through 1900, while there had been a reduction from between 5 and 7 live births in the 18th century to 3.5 births by 1900 among White native-born American women.

28. This appears to have been what happened to Irish-born Hannah, another 12 year old, treated at the same hospital a few years prior. Hospital physicians diagnosed her with severe *morbus coxarius* and tried to treat her with cathartics and liniments, but to no avail, and then offered her opiates to assuage her "paroxysms of pain giving great suffering," before discharging her as "incurable" (NYHMCB 1848:C517).

29. NYC Inspector's Reports, from at least 1853 through 1863 show higher TB

mortality among men over 50 than among women of the same age group (City Inspector's Department 1855, 1858; Board of Aldermen 1864:226).

30. Citations: tobacco for headache (Dorian 2000:114), wounds (Egan 1887:13; NFC 1941[782]:350), and toothache (NFCS 1937[598]:434; NFCS 1938[35]:139; NFCS 1938[45]:200; NFCS 1938[345]:11, 206; NFCS 1938[624]:249, 529; NFC 1974[1838]:66).

31. In summary, the Irish used whiskey for many purposes, including as a medicine, painkiller, work aid, nationalist symbol, social lubricant, stress and sorrow reliever, marker of hospitality, alliance builder, celebratory beverage, and source of income.

32. After her own children died, Rachael McPeake lived at 30 Wooster with James and David Agnew, identified in the census as nephews. In 1855, James Agnew was a 31-year-old painter and naturalized citizen, who had arrived in the U.S. around 1847. Daniel Agnew was a gilder who had arrived around 1852 and was not yet naturalized. It is likely the McPeake family helped these relatives to come to NYC, and the Agnews seem to have supported Rachael after her children's deaths (NYSC 1855; Trow 1859:26).

33. Other Irish folk cures also could have facilitated the transmission of TB throughout the Irish community. During the early 20th-century crusade against TB in Ireland, public health officials decried the technique used by midwives of breathing "heavily down the throats of newborn babies" to clear their breathing passages (Farmar 2004:105). Similarly, a cure for thrush involved a healer, usually a son born after his father's death, blowing into the mouth of a sick child (Blake 1918:222; NFCS 1937[598]:97, 433; NFC 1938[560]:534; NFCS 1938[35]:237; NFCS 1938[45]:197; NFC 1941[782]:190, 356; Logan 1994:53).

34. Mortality rates from TB peaked in NYC during the beginning of the 19th century. In 1804, the rate was 688 per 100,000 and in 1812 it was 697 per 100,000. By 1838, the rate dropped slightly to 500 per 100,000. It plateaued to an average of a little over 400 per 100,000 from 1839 to the late 1870s. In the 1880s, rates finally began to decline more rapidly, such that by 1900 it was 237 per 100,000 (Drolet and Lowell 1952:ii–vi). In contrast, the rate in England was only 275 per 100,000 in 1850 and 140 per 100,000 in 1895. In Ireland, it was 219 per 100,000 in 1861. Rates in Ireland *increased* until 1904 (Smith 2008:27).

35. In contrast, in southern Europe, the populace believed consumption to be contagious and often shunned foreign consumptives seeking a cure from the Mediterranean climate (Hayes 2009:158).

36. Physicians at New York Hospital in the 1840s and 1850s, in contrast, did not record this kind of probing (NYHMCB 1847–1853 and 1865 and NYHSCB 1848, 1852–1853, 1861–1862, 1865). Support for the idea of contagion grew after experiments in the 1860s and 1870s. The French physician Jean-Antoine Villemin demonstrated TB's contagion in animal experiments in 1865, for example, but his work was not accepted as accurate until the 1890s (Barnes 1995:13). Annual reports from the New York Orthopaedic Dispensary describe many of their young patients as tenement

dwellers suffering from tubercular conditions, including scrofula, Pott's disease, and "insidious" hip disease (NYODAR 1867:6; 1869:19,22; 1872:14; 1876:21).

37. Arthur Boylston (2013) unpacks the history of this discovery, which he shows was based initially on several country doctors' observations of dairy farmers' and milkmaids' unusual responses to smallpox inoculation and not on the myth that Jenner was inspired by the beautiful unmarked skin of milkmaids.

38. Lack of natural immunity also contributed to a rise in TB mortality rates in Ireland in the late 19th and early 20th centuries, when rates had subsided in England, leading the British to then link the Irish and TB (Jones 2001).

39. As the century progressed, a stigma of weakness began to be attached to families who had consumptive members. People often declined to marry children from these families, fearful they would not live long. Physicians then used other less stigmatizing diagnostic terms—such as nervous decline, respiratory weakness, convulsions, and bronchitis—especially if they were uncertain the patient had pulmonary consumption. When tubercular patients had to be registered in Britain after 1870, there was a 100% increase in diagnoses of bronchitis (Dormandy 1999:77).

40. Physicians identified physically or mentally draining conditions, activities, or states as exciting causes. Nineteenth-century physicians "Cartwright, Donaldson, Flint, and others of their generation explained" that "overindulgence and other city habits deprived the tissues of proper nourishment and of an adequate source of oxygen or pure air, which rendered them tuberculous" (Feldberg 1995:33). Physicians identified "overindulgence" in material goods, such as fashionable dresses with low-cut bodices, alcohol, tobacco, food, and sex as problematic. "Other city habits" likely included unhygienic living conditions, damp environments, "dusty" trades, overwork, anxiety, ungratified desires, corsets, nostalgia, and inadequate clothing, food, and rest (Kunzle 1982:92; Bowditch 1994a, 1994b; Stillé 1994; Dormandy 1999:247). Fresh air was thought to be important not because of infection but because of the supposed negative effects of rebreathed air upon respiration (Jones 2001:17).

41. For similar reasons some physicians in the middle of the 19th century believed African Americans to be immune to pulmonary TB; stereotypes of African Americans also did not conform to the consumptive diathesis (Ott 1996:18–19).

42. This story draws upon Psalm 23 "The Lord is My Shepherd" in the Old Testament and the parable of the Good Shepherd (John 10:1–21) in the New Testament. The image caption "He Giveth His Beloved Sleep" references Psalm 127.

43. Beginning in 1854, Charles Loring Brace and his Children's Aid Society sent supposedly orphaned children west on "orphan trains" to be adopted by farming families. Some of the children were neither orphans nor given up voluntarily by their parents, however (Fitzgerald 2006).

44. The Draft Riots made a lasting negative impression in NYC. The *New York Times* claimed the mob—who protested conscription to fight in the Union Army by beating and murdering African Americans and their allies and attacking property, including burning down the Colored Orphan Asylum—was composed of "almost

exclusively Irishmen and boys." The newspaper described the rioters as a "tribe of savages" and a "race of miscreants," while the *New York Tribune* called them a "savage mob," a "pack of savages," and "incarnate devils." *Harper's Weekly* initially guarded against blanket assumptions, stating "there was nothing peculiar . . . to the Irish race in this riot." As the violence continued, *Harper's Weekly* editors declared "the impulsiveness of the Celt . . . prompts him to be the foremost in every outburst, whether for a good or an evil purpose" and their limited education in Ireland made them susceptible to being "misled by knaves." Later in the summer the same paper noted the "riotous propensities" of the Irish (Jacobson 1998:54–55; McMahon 2015a:131). New Yorker George Templeton Strong commented that the Irish "came from a land 'populated by creatures that crawl and eat dirt and poison every community they infest'" (Kenny 2006:373). The Draft Riot continued to be a touchstone for anti-Irish sentiment. Some scholars have pointed out that while the heinous acts of the Irish rioters were inexcusable and worthy of the strongest condemnation, there also were many Irish New Yorkers, including policemen, who attempted to stop the mob and who helped rescue the African American orphans (McMahon 2015a:131). Irishman James T. Brady commented in *Harpers Weekly* in August of 1863 that instead of rekindling "Know-Nothing prejudices," Americans should bear in mind that "riots are natural and inevitable diseases of great cities, epidemics, like small-pox and cholera, which must be treated scientifically, upon logical principles" (McMahon 2015a:131).

45. The text that accompanies this cartoon, Figure 6.10, as well as Figure 2.4 complains about the refusal of Irish immigrants to renounce their Irish identity (*Puck* 1883, 1889).

46. Typhus fever research during the Civil War also chipped away at Irish stereotypes, in questioning the presumed link between Irish immigrants and the disease. For example, Joseph Jones, a Confederate physician, wrote "I supposed that if typhus fever existed anywhere in the Confederate States if would be found at Andersonville [Prison] and especially amongst the foreign element of the Federal armies, which had been but recently imported from the bogs of Ireland," but typhus was not to be found. He opined that its absence "strongly sustains the view that typhus and typhoid fevers are dependent upon the actions of special poisons, the conditions for the origin and the action of which are definite and . . . limited" (Humphreys 2006:280). According to Humphreys (2006:280), "the absence of major typhus outbreaks drove the evolving theories of infectious disease toward belief in the specificity of causation, paving the way for the specificity of bacteriology."

Chapter 7

1. Also like the English term "consumption," these Irish terms were sometimes applied to other wasting conditions in the 19th century that today would not be identified as tuberculosis.

2. According to folklorist Crístóir Mac Cárthaigh (1988:39), "Despite there being evidence to suggest that the fairies comprised a community which mirrored our own in all respects . . . a basic flaw was thought to exist in the fairy make-up with respect to procreation. Thus, their undoubted interest in mortal women and children."

3. William Wilde (1856:455) identified "scrofulous tubercular diseases, chiefly of the abdominal cavity, many of *tabes mesenterica*, and very many of *chronic peritonitis*" as the main inspirations. Another possibility could have been Tay Sachs Disease, a rare genetic disorder more common in people of Irish descent today that typically affects children around the age of 6 months, before which they appear to develop normally. The disease deteriorates the nerve cells causing progressive degeneration and death, usually before the age of four.

4. John Grenham points out in an *Irish Times* (2015) article that today the word begrudgery is exclusively Irish. He describes it as a "very specific kind of scepticism, more irreverence than envy. . . . It is peasant anger at inequality, egalitarianism in its raw, uncooked state. . . . In Ireland, you can be as different as you want, once you recognise you're no better than the rest of us."

5. Selected citations: making the sign of the cross (NFC 1941[782]:191), invoking the Holy Trinity (NFC 1935[54]:204), imbibing or applying holy water (NFC 1937[463]:44–45), and visiting holy wells (NFC 1941[782]:255). According to folklore collector Michael J. Murphy, in county Tyrone, baptismal "sponsors had curative powers applicable to the child for which they had acted. . . . I am told by Annie McCrea . . . 'The child would have to get flour from them and have it baked at a running stream, between townlands . . . and eat that, and that was supposed to be a cure'" (NFC 1951[1220]:45).

6. Allen and Hatfield (2004:256–257) note foxglove was recognized as dangerous and more typically used in Ireland in a tea for coughs and as an all-purpose topical salve for wounds, swellings, burns, ulcers, festering bruises, and other skin-related ailments. One of Lady Gregory's (1920:151) informants, Mrs. Ward, claimed "lusmor" could bring long life: "If you put a bit of this with every other herb you drink, you'll live forever. My grandmother used to . . . and she lived to be over a hundred."

7. A more extreme cure was to place the changeling upon a shovel before a fire. It was said that "a fairy imp" would fly up the chimney and disappear, but "while waiting for the solution of the question, the baby is often so dreadfully burned that it dies in great torture, though its cries are heard with callous indifference by the family around" (Wilde, L. 1890:49). A husband burned his wife to death in 1895 in Ballyvadlea, County Tipperary, claiming she was a changeling. His wife, Bridget Cleary, had been ill with a respiratory illness. Her husband was convicted of manslaughter, although he swore that he did not kill his wife, because she was away with the fairies (*NYT* 1895:4).

8. Evidence of other protective measures and cures for fairy capture and bewitching is often impossible to detect archaeologically. Many do not leave material traces

at all, or they do not survive in the archaeological record (e.g., spitting three times or sprinkling holy water). Additionally, other remedies use materials that archaeologists typically interpret as traces of more mundane activities, such as iron nails as remains of buildings or furniture, rather than possible apotropaic practices. If archaeologists become more familiar with popular medicinal and protective practices, they will be more aware of what to look for (Fennell 2000; Linn 2014; Manning 2014).

9. Selected references: dandelion (Gregory 1920:149; NFC 1935[96]:309; NFCS 1937[598]:101; NFCS 1938[364]:276; Logan 1994:22), chamomile (NFC 1935[117]:65; Verling 2003:62), carrageen (Allen and Hatfield 2004:34), garlic (NFC ca. 1929[36]:246; NFC 1930[80]:33; Logan 1994:22), mint (NFCS 1938[345]:8), myrtle (NFC 1953[1364]:49, 51), watercress and chickweed (O'Regan 1997:8), and nettles (NFCS 1938[710]:47; Logan 1994:35; Allen and Hatfield 2004:85).

10. Dandelion sap, leaves, and/or infusions of leaves were also used to cure anemia (Brew 1990:25), bronchitis (NFCS 1938[624]:556; Logan 1994:24), whooping cough (NFCS 1937[598]:436), cold (NFCS 1938[624]:79), indigestion (NFC 1930[80]:21; NFCS 1937[598]:100; NFCS 1938[345]:205), heart problems (NFCS 1938[624]:137, 276; Wilson 1943:182), kidney (NFCS 1938[45]:366; NFCS 1938[624]:79; NFC 1953[1364]:59; Logan 1994:37) and liver problems (Egan 1887:12; NFCS 1938[45]:67, 164; NFCS 1938[345]:13; NFCS 1938[364]:221), nerves (Castleconnor Parish Development 2000:126), rheumatism (NFCS 1937[598]:100), styes (Logan 1994:59), and warts (NFCS 1938[35]:33; NFCS 1938[45]:197).

11. Healer Bridget Ruane claimed that dandelion and plantain were herbs that Mary, Mary Magdalen, and Joseph administered to Jesus to bring him back from the dead (Gregory 1920:150), an unorthodox interpretation of the resurrection.

12. Selected citations: milk (NFC ca. 1929[36]:250; NFCS 1937[598]:101; NFC 1953[1364]:49; Logan 1994:23), eggs (Logan 1994:22–23), snails (NFC 1955[1389]:205), and salted snails in milk (Purdon 1904:41). Eating fish brains was said to ensure an easy labor for pregnant women (Logan 1994:15).

13. Citations: goat's milk (Castleconnor Parish Development Group 2000:126, Logan 1994:23), donkey's milk (NFC ca. 1929[36]:250; NFC 1953[1364]:49), and milk of a Kerry cow (Logan 1994:22–23).

14. Selected citations: bogbane and dandelions (NFC ca. 1929[36]:249; NFC 1935[96]:309; NFCS 1937[598]:101; NFCS 1938[364]:276; Logan 1994:22; Allen and Hatfield 2004:287), burdock (Purdon 1895:214; Allen and Hatfield 2004:282); dock (Wilde, L. 1890:28; Harris 1960:65; Allen and Hatfield 2004:97), flaxseed (Logan 1994:22), furze and knapweed (Allen and Hatfield 2004:284, 163), garlic (NFC ca. 1929[36]:246; NFC 1930[80]:33; Logan 1994:22), nasturtiums (Logan 1994:22), and sorrel (NFCS 1938[345]:11; Allen and Hatfield 2004:173–4). Informants told Lady Wilde (1890:47) that "duckweed [dock] boiled down, and the liquid drank three times daily, is an excellent potion for the sick."

15. Selected citations: NFC 1935[54]:368; NFCS 1938[35]:31; NFCS 1938[345]:8; Wilson 1943:182; Logan 1994:35; Allen and Hatfield 2004:85.

16. Selected citations: NFC 1930[80]:11–12; NFC 1935[117]:106–107; NFCS 1937[598]:433; NFC 1941[782]:190; Logan, 1994:61–63. An informant told an NFC collector in Antrim in 1953 that "the seventh son they reckoned always had the cure for that [scrofula]. You never hear of that now at all" (NFC 1953[1364]:65. The belief that the seventh son in the family had special powers is not unique to Ireland; it is common in many places in Europe and North America (Leach 1949:999; McClafferty 1979:4), possibly related to powers attributed to the number seven in the Bible.

17. Another Irish cure for scrofula included touching the wound with the rope that had been used to hang a criminal. The "king's evil" was a popular term for scrofula, which caused "running sores," or "evils." From the Middle Ages through the 18th century, it was believed that being touched by a monarch could cure this disease. Kings and queens of England and France held ceremonies to touch to their afflicted subjects and sometimes distributed commemorative medals (Grzybowski and Allen 1995:1473). For more about scrofula and Irish cures involving magic, see Linn 2014.

18. Selected citations: buttercup (Barbour 1897:388), burdock (Allen and Hatfield 2004:282), walnut leaves (Purdon 1895:296), watercress (Egan 1887:13; Allen and Hatfield 2004:118), wren's blood (Mooney 1887:157), holy well water (Mooney 1887:157), meadowsweet (Egan 1887:13; Allen and Hatfield 2004:140). In response to a questionnaire distributed in County Cavan in 1960, an informant reported a special cure for scrofula made by his great-great grandmother and great grandmother for which people came from all around. The cure was a pill made of hemlock and oatmeal plus the application of turpentine to the sores. Patients started with a small amount of hemlock and gradually increased the dose. Great care was taken so that the patients were not poisoned (Harris 1960:65).

19. Selected citations: NFCS 1938[35]:127; NFCS[345]:14; NFCS 1938[920]:70; NFC 1953[1364]:59; Allen and Hatfield 2004:153.

20. Selected citations: mugwort (Allen and Hatfield 2004:298), mullein (see next endnote), ox-eye daisy (Allen and Hatfield 2004:221), self-heal (Allen and Hatfield 2004:221), elderberry (NFCS 1938[45]:246; McClafferty 1979), thyme (Allen and Hatfield 2004:225), and foxglove (Allen and Hatfield 2004:254–257).

21. Mullein as a remedy for consumption is noted in a number of sources, including: Egan 1887:12; NFC ca. 1929[36]:250; NFC 1937[598]:102; NFCS 1938[45]:201; NFCS 1938[773]:125; O'Regan 1997:9; Allen and Hatfield 2004:250.

22. Additional Irish popular cough remedies included visiting a sweathouse (NFC 1974[1837]:228) and breathing in air near freshly ploughed earth (NFCS 1938[35]:236) or a freshly tarred road (Logan 1994:24, 44). The last remedy was likely from a later date and related to Isoniazid, an important mid-20th-century TB drug prepared from coal tar (Dormandy 1999:368).

23. Unfortunately, Michael's case did not end well. Surgeons at New York Hospital diagnosed him with necrosis of the femora. They surgically removed the necrotic bone, but Michael suffered from bouts of diarrhea, likely caused by a postoperative

infection, and then several hemorrhages. He died within a few weeks (NYHSCB 1852:C183).

24. Mary passed away after about a month in the hospital (NYHMCB 1848:C622).

25. Morphine and opium were available at drugstores and not yet regulated; the possibility of overdose and addiction were known but not well understood (Haller 1981b:1677; Schablitsky 2006:17).

26. Two bottles of bitters/tonics were found at 472 and 474 Pearl Street, one Hostetter's and one Brown's (Tables 5.1 and 5.2). Containing alcohol and botanicals, bitters resembled popular medicinal preparations of herbs and alcohol, as discussed in Chapter 5. Producers claimed bitters were strengthening tonics and renovators of the blood, but they walked a fine line between alcoholic beverages and medicine. Lindsey (2021c) writes that bitters were invented in England in the 18th century to avoid tax on liquor by adding herbs to gin and calling the concoction medicinal, the latter a strategy used by the Irish American proprietors of Duffy's Malt Whiskey in the 19th century.

27. One bottle of sarsaparilla was found in Feature J at 472 Pearl Street (Tables 5.1 and 5.2). Sarsaparillas contained extracts from plants of the genus *Smilax* and alcohol, as well as additional plant extracts. They were so popular during the middle of the 19th century that "druggists called the era of the 1840s the 'sarsaparilla era'"(Lindsey 2021c). Patent medicine makers marketed sarsaparillas as blood purifiers, useful for respiratory congestion and scrofula, but they were also commonly understood and used as an alternative to mercury for syphilis (Young 1961:61–63, 187; Estes 1995:7–8; Howson 1993:149).

28. Balsams were very popular in the U.S. in the 1840s and 1850s when they were recommended for respiratory ailments. True balsams could have been somewhat effective in treating congestion because they act as expectorants, and in treating wounds because they have antibacterial properties (Blasi 1974:vi–vii; Marsalic et al. 2007; Jones and Vegotsky 2016:40). See Chapter 5.

29. Red flannel, for example, was said to possess curative power to resolve earache (NFCS 1938[45]:200), rheumatism (NFC 1935[265]:599), cough, whooping cough (pertussis), and sprain (Morris 1937:178; Logan 1994:44, 124). The University of California, Los Angeles's Online Archive of American Folk Medicine (2001) reported continued use of red flannel among Irish Americans to cure coughs in Tennessee and California (Hilliard 1966:123). De Craen et al. (1996) suggest the power of red substances is probably universal because of the color's association with blood. While this might be broadly accurate, specific meanings vary by culture and context. The Irish associated red with fairies and Jesus's blood (Hutchings 1997:59).

30. Bottles made of so-called "black glass" were mass produced and ubiquitous in the U.S. and Britain in the 19th century. This darkest of glass colors was actually a very dark olive green (Lindsey 2020).

31. Samuel Hopkins Adams (1912:5), the journalist who drew attention to the dangers of many patent medicines in support of the Pure Food and Drug(s) Act

of 1906, noted these testimonials were very successful in getting customers to try products.

32. There are precedents in Ireland for taking the healing advice of strangers. Female strangers from the north of Ireland were said to possess strong cures (Ó Súilleabháin 1977:84). A frequently reported cure for whooping cough was to ask a man riding a horse and encountered accidentally what to do, and then to do whatever he said. Some specify the color of the horse (usually white); some specify that the man's hair cannot be red (Pyne 1897:179; Blake 1918:223; NFC 1937[407]:142; NFCS 1937[598]:433; NFCS 1938[35]:33, 127, 236; NFCS 1938[45]:202; NFCS 1938[364]:219; NFCS 1938[624]:77; NFC 1941[782]:353; Logan 1994:43).

33. The 1851 Irish census lists only 648 licensed apothecaries and 260 unlicensed druggists for a population of 6.5 million people. The number of physicians and surgeons was 2,439 (Farmar 2004:82–83).

34. These references to cod liver oil from the late 1930s might reflect influence from 19th- and early 20th-century professional medicine, but fishing (including cod) and fish oil production has a centuries-old history in Ireland.

35. Physicians published ideas about how to best disguise the strong fishy flavor of cod liver oil. Oil of peppermint, lemon juice, anise, cinnamon, and coffee were recommended. Some also suggested patients shut their eyes and hold their nostrils closed, and still others skipped oral administration and administered it by enema (Grad 2004:109). The taste might have increased patients' credibility in the medicine, and thus improved its results, because of the popular idea that bad-tasting medicines are more powerful than pleasant-tasting ones.

36. The 1850 layer of Feature J (472 Pearl Street) contained 6 soda water bottles (about 3% of the glass bottle assemblage) in that stratum, while the 1870 layer contained 27 bottles (14% of the glass assemblage) in that stratum. The 1860 deposit in Feature O (474 Pearl Street) yielded 7 bottles, composing about 7% of the glass assemblage (Bonasera 2000a:373). Thirty-one of the bottles were embossed with brand names.

37. For a comparison of the numbers and percentages of soda water bottles as well as brief descriptions of each site, see Linn 2010:77–78.

38. Sulphate and magnesium act as laxatives, bicarbonate eases indigestion, iodide can remedy goiter, and iron can remedy iron-deficiency anemia, counter lead poisoning, and strengthen consumptives, for example.

39. Soda water was an inappropriate name because it did not contain soda. "Aerated water, marble water, and carbonic acid water were also promoted as more precise terms, but the public was accustomed to soda water and didn't care that it was a misnomer" (Funderburg 2003:19).

40. Lemon and sarsaparilla, both of which were also used medicinally, were among the first flavors available (*NYT* 1866b:2). In August of 1870, the *New York Times* estimated that "not less than 100,000 glasses per day" were sold from NYC's 280 fountains in drugstores and Brooklyn's 150, plus confectionery shops and stands

(*NYT* 1870b:6). An 1871 article further specified that Hegeman & Co.'s three stores on Broadway sold an average of 250 glasses per day, while Bigelow Manufacturing Co. at nearby 309 Broadway, which specialized in cold drinks, sold about 1,000 cups a day (*NYT* 1871:2)

41. Documentary, oral, and archaeological sources suggest costly bottled water was not often used in the Irish countryside (Scally 1995:29; Dorian 2000:113; Hull 2004; Brighton 2005). Excavations of houses of families evicted during the 1840s in the villages of Mulliviltrin, Gortoose, and Ballykilcline in County Roscommon revealed a paucity of glass remains and no soda water bottles, for example (Hull 2004; Brighton 2005).

42. Citations: consumption (NFCS 1938[844]:156; NFCS[1938]713:200A), eye ailments (NFCS 1937[598]:433; NFCS 1937[624]:271), fairy possession (NFC 1941[782]:255), fevers (Logan 1994:8), headache (NFCS 1938[35]:239–240), infertility (Logan 1994:16), insanity (NFC 1941[782]:363; Robins 1986:12–13), pain (NFCS 1937[598]:434), paralysis (NFC 1937[463]:44–45; NFCS 1937[624]:271), scrofula (Mooney 1887:157), skin problems (NFCS 1938[345]:6–7), and "illness" or "disease," in general (NFC 1935[54]:71, 100; NFCS 1937[624]:273; NFCS 1938[35]:238; NFCS 1938[345]:8; NFCS 1939[1076]:431). A recent Trinity College Dublin study found that a holy well in County Kerry, *Tober na nGealt*, renowned for its ability to cure insanity, contains forty times the normal concentrations of lithium, a chemical used to treat bipolar disorder today (Foley 2015:15).

43. Ó Danachair (1955:215) writes that some emigrants took pebbles used to mark pattern rounds: "A girl going to America took pebbles from the well [in County Limerick]; during a storm she threw the pebbles into the sea; the storm ceased and the pebbles returned to the well."

44. Estyn Evans (1957) wrote that "a countryman found any excuse to go to the fair," while Conrad Arensberg (1937) noted that rural Irish people marked the passage of time by fairs.

45. Selected citations: for headaches, hangovers, and colds (NFCS 1938[35]:126; NFC 1955[1389]:205); for consumption, constipation, jaundice (NFC 1941[782]:343, 347; Logan 1994:46–47; Allen and Hatfield 2004: 163, 181, 218, 221, 275, 284, 287); for bruises, cuts, and sprains (NFC 1935[265]:595; NFCS 1937[598]:104; NFCS 1938[35]:130).

46. People also visited forges for the iron-laden water blacksmiths used to cool their work, a kind of mineral water (Linda-May Ballard 2010, pers. comm.) thought to cure skin ailments, including abscesses, sores, chilblains, and warts (NFCS 1938[35]:125, 236; Wilson 1943:183; Logan 1994:68, 120), as well as sore throats (NFCS 1938[35]:140), rickets (Ballard 2009:32), and other complaints.

47. *Harper's Weekly* (1877:387) published a short satirical piece describing the poor condition of natural springs in nearby, less populated Brooklyn. The paper reported that a man discovered a spring near Newtown Creek and took a sample to a "German chemist for analysis, telling him he should advertise the result, and convert the place into a regular Baden-Baden." The German chemist wrote his report in "common

language" so all could understand. He said the water consisted of "salt-water, coal oil, extract of dead dog, precipitate of cat, oxide of hoop-skirt, sesquioxide of barrel hoops, quintessence of glue, decomposed bone, infusion of soot, triturated paint screenings, boarding-house butter, fish residuum, conglomerated sediments, other nasty things 1000."

48. According to Dr. H. Ogden Doremus (1854a; 1854b), some soda fountains were poorly tinned or used lead solder that could leach lead into the water. Water from such fountains would have worsened patients' conditions. Water from a better-quality fountain or bottled from natural springs could have improved their conditions. The waters of Bath, England, for example, were a well-known cure for paralysis from lead poisoning (Heywood 1999:101). Bath's waters were high in iron and calcium. People with inadequate amounts of these minerals are more susceptible to lead poisoning, because their bodies absorb and retain more lead. During the famine in Ireland and during periods of hardship in NYC, many Irish suffered from iron-deficiency anemia, a common result of malnutrition (Maletnlema 1992). If John and George drank soda water high in iron and/or calcium, it could have helped them to recover from lead poisoning, particularly if they were iron-deficient.

49. Both Clark & White bottles were found in Feature J at 472 Pearl Street (Ponz 2000:52,55).

50. Another example of troublesome drinking is suggested by a note in the margin of an Emigrant Savings Bank account: "Michael is drinking, his wife desires that he get no money, October 12, 1862" (Griggs 2000:45).

51. Of a total of 31 embossed soda water bottles found in Irish contexts at the Five Points, 42% have (Anglicized) Irish or Anglo-Irish surnames embossed upon them, including Walsh & O'Neill, Seely & Bro., Lynch & Clarke, Clarke & White, P. Kellet, and G. Cassidy. An additional 35% were embossed with Scottish surnames, such as Tweedles Celebrated Soda & Mineral Waters. The brand most represented at the Five Points, Seely & Bro. (Figure 7.4), was also uncovered in Irish contexts in Paterson, NJ. Several other brands found in Paterson had potentially Irish surnames, such as McKenna & Connolly, McGovern Bros., Boyle Bros., William S. Kinch, and William T. Allen (Bartlett 1999; Yamin 1999; Linn 2010).

52. It is possible that residents retained these bottles for reuse. Jane Busch (1987) noted that durable soda bottles were so often reused for homemade "exhilarating drinks" and sauces that there were shortages in bottle supplies for soda manufacturers. Irish immigrants might have used them for such purposes and, along with wine bottles (see Chapter 3), as convenient receptacles for popular Irish cures.

53. This possible remedy evokes a cure for fairy capture noted earlier in the chapter: give a changeling a cup of holy well water or "spring water to drink . . . [with] the sign of the cross . . . made over it" (NFC 1941[782]:255).

54. At the time, a prominent physician had stated that ingesting small amounts of copper acted as an excellent tonic (Funderburg 2003:16).

55. Mark Weiner (2002) found that another carbonated commodity, Coca-Cola,

similarly connected World War II servicemen with their previous civilian lives. In his study of soldiers' letters in the company's archives, he concluded that "Coke was a potent, even Proustian conjurer of the social life of the drug store soda fountain." "The ole 'Coke' sign," a serviceman penned from Sicily, "brings every soldier back to moments in his favorite drug store, where he sat and conversed with his friends." Another soldier wrote that "the shape of the bottle, the memory of the refreshing taste, brought to mind many happy memories" (Weiner 2002:133).

56. The importance of Irish immigrant involvement with soda water does not end there. In 1891, reporter Mary Gay Humphreys wrote in *Harper's Weekly* that "soda-water is the American drink. It is as essentially American as porter, Rhine wine, and claret are distinctively English, German, and French. . . . The millionaire may drink champagne while the poor man drinks beer, but they both drink soda-water" (Humphreys 1891:923). Irish immigrant preference for this beverage and participation in this business aided in soda becoming an important part of American culture.

57. As scholars have shown, the Irish in the U.S. felt they were in competition with these other groups for jobs, neighborhood territory, and status. Some (though certainly not the majority of) Irish actively denigrated other groups—particularly Chinese Americans in the West and African Americans throughout the country—and participated in shameful racist rhetoric and violence. Among the worst examples was the 1863 New York City Draft Riots, but groups of Irish immigrants and Irish Americans committed intermittent violence upon African Americans well into the 20th century in Northern cities, especially when African Americans attempted to gain employment, housing, and education during the Great Migration (Grossman 1989; Sugrue 2014). Irish immigrants and their American-born children and grandchildren recognized the benefits of being considered White in a society built on white supremacy.

58. William Cole died in 1910 and left his estate to his two daughters. He did not name Ella Louise in his will (New York County Surrogate's Court 1910: 224–225).

Conclusion

1. Some of the works that inspired my thinking about such entanglements included: Wirth 1938; Goffman 1959; Crandon-Malamud 1991; Duden 1991; Thomas 1991; White, R. 1991; Taussig 1993; Burke 1996; Sahlins 2000; White, L. 2000; and Rothschild 2003.

2. Mary MacLean (Introduction) lived to an advanced age in Ontario, Canada. Ella McPeake, the surviving granddaughter of John and Rachael McPeake (see Chapter 7), was assisted by her uncle, the author of her father's obituary, and trained as a teacher at Hunter Normal School (established by an Irish immigrant). By 1897, she had purchased a house in Ridgewood, NJ, still standing as of 2022 (Bergen County Division

of Cultural & Historic Affairs 1984–1985:41, 90). So far, I have been unable to discover more about Huxley McGuire (see Chapter 1) or Mary the match seller (see Chapters 4 and 5), and I have not tried to track William Smith (see Chapters 2 and 3) or the many other individuals mentioned in the surveyed hospital records, other than cross-referencing them with Five Points census records.

REFERENCES CITED

Adams, Samuel Hopkins
1912   *Great American Fraud: Articles on the Nostrum Evil and Quackery*, 5th edition. American Medical Association, Chicago, IL.

Alexander, Leslie M.
2008   *African or American? Black Identity and Political Activism in New York City, 1784–1861*. University of Illinois Press, Urbana.

Allen, David E., and Gabrielle Hatfield
2004   *Medicinal Plants in Folk Tradition: An Ethnobotany of Britain and Ireland*. Timber Press, Portland, OR.

Anbinder, Tyler
2001   *Five Points: The Nineteenth-Century New York City Neighborhood That Invented Tap Dance, Stole Elections and Became the World's Most Notorious Slum*. Free Press, New York, NY.
2002   From Famine to Five Points: Lord Lansdowne's Irish Tenants Encounter North America's Most Notorious Slum. *The American Historical Review* 107(2):351–387.

Anbinder, Tyler, Cormac Ó Gráda, and Simone A. Wegge
2019a   Networks and Opportunities: A Digital History of Ireland's Great Famine Refugees in New York. *The American Historical Review* 124(5):1591–1629.
2019b   "Emigrant Savings Bank Depositor Database, 1850–1858," version 3.0, 13 September. <https://scholarspace.library.gwu.edu/work/ok225b85w>. Accessed 27 March 2023.

Arensberg, Conrad M.
1937   *The Irish Countryman: An Anthropological Study*. MacMillan, New York, NY. Reprinted 1968 by Natural History Press, Garden City, NY.

Arnesen, Eric
2001 Whiteness and the Historians' Imagination. *International Labor and Working-Class History* 60:3–32.
Atlanta Constitution
1872 Rheumatism Cure. *Atlanta Constitution* 25 February:1. Atlanta, GA.
Augustus C. Long Health Sciences Library
2023 Peter S. Townsend Daily Register of Medical and Surgical Practice finding aid. Archives and Special Collections. Augustus C. Long Health Sciences Library. Columbia University, New York, NY. <https://www.library-archives.cumc.columbia.edu>. Accessed 27 March 2023.
Baics, Gergely
2016 *Feeding Gotham: The Political Economy and Geography of Food in New York, 1790–1860.* Princeton University Press, Princeton, NJ.
Baldwin, Peter C.
2012 *In the Watches of the Night: Life in the Nocturnal City, 1820–1930.* University of Chicago Press, Chicago, IL.
Ballard, Linda-May
2009 An Approach to Traditional Cures in Ulster. *Ulster Medical Journal* 78(1):26–33.
Banks, Ann
1980 *First-Person America.* Alfred A. Knopf, New York, NY.
Barbour, John H.
1897 Some Country Remedies and Their Uses. *Folklore* 8:386–390.
Barnes, David S.
1995 *The Making of a Social Disease: Tuberculosis in Nineteenth-Century France.* University of California Press, Berkeley.
Baron, Ava
2006 Masculinity, the Embodied Male Worker, and the Historian's Gaze. *International Labor and Working-Class History* 69(1):143–160.
Barrett, James R.
2012 *The Irish Way: Becoming American in the Multiethnic City.* Penguin Books, New York, NY.
Barrington, Jonah
1832 *Personal Sketches of His Own Times.* Vol. 3. Henry Colburn and Richard Bentley, London, UK <https://www.gutenberg.org/files/49794/49794-h/49794-h.htm>. Accessed 22 December 2018.
Barrow, John
1836 *A Tour Round Ireland through the Sea-Coast Counties, in the Autumn of 1835.* John Murray, London, UK. Internet Archive <https://archive.org/details/tourroundireland00barr>.

Bartlett, Alexander B.
1999   A Functional Analysis of the Glass Assemblage from Selected Features on Blocks 863 and 866 in Paterson's Dublin Neighborhood. In *With Hope and Labor: Everyday Life in Paterson's Dublin Neighborhood, Vol. 1, Data Recovery on Blocks 863 and 866 within the Route 19 Connector Corridor in Paterson, New Jersey*, Rebecca Yamin, editor, pp. 116–124. John Milner Associates, West Chester, PA.

Bayor, Ronald H., and Timothy J. Meagher (editors)
1996   *The New York Irish.* Johns Hopkins University Press, Baltimore, MD.

Beaudry, Mary C.
1993   Public Aesthetics versus Personal Experience: Worker Health and Well-Being in Nineteenth-Century Lowell, Massachusetts. *Historical Archaeology* 27(2):90–105.
1998   Farm Journal: First Person, Four Voices. *Historical Archaeology* 32(1):20–33.
2013   Foreword—City Lives: Archaeological Tales from Gotham. In *Tales of Gotham, Historical Archaeology, Ethnohistory, and Microhistory of New York City*, Meta F. Janowitz and Diane Dallal, editors, pp. vii–xiii. Springer, New York, NY.

Beaufoy, Mark
1828   *Tour Through Parts of the United States and Canada.* Longman, Rees, Orme, Brown, and Green, London, UK. Internet Archive, Original from the Library of Congress <http://hdl.loc.gov/loc.gdc/scd0001.00141073898>. Accessed 20 December 2019.

Bedford, Gunning S.
1863   *The Principles and Practice of Obstetrics*, revised and enlarged 3rd edition. William Wood and Co., New York, NY.

Beggs, C. B., C. J. Noakes, P. A. Sleigh, L. A. Fletcher, and K. Siddiqi
2003   The Transmission of Tuberculosis in Confined Spaces: An Analytical Review of Alternative Epidemiological Models. *International Journal of Tuberculosis and Lung Disease* 7(11):1015–1026.

Bellevue Hospital Casebooks (BHMCB)
1866–1868   Bellevue Hospital Medical Casebooks. Archives & Special Collections, Augustus C. Long Health Sciences Library, Columbia University Medical Center, New York, NY.
1873–1875   Bellevue Hospital Medical Casebooks. Archives & Special Collections, Augustus C. Long Health Sciences Library, Columbia University Medical Center, New York, NY.

Bergen County Division of Cultural & Historic Affairs
1984–1985   *Bergen County Historic Sites Survey: Village of Ridgewood*.
             Courtesy of Department of Parks, Division of Cultural and Historic
             Affairs, Bergen County, NJ. Bergen County History Archives
             <https://ppolinks.com/bergencountyhistory> Accessed March 27,
             2023.

Bergen, Fanny
1899   *Animal and Plant Lore: Collected from the Oral Tradition of
             English Speaking Folk*. Houghton, Mifflin, and Company for the
             American Folk-Lore Society, New York, NY.

Berger, Max
1946   Irish Emigrant and American Nativism as Seen by British Visitors,
             1836–1860. *Dublin Review* 219(438):174–186.

Blackmar, Elizabeth
1995   Accountability for Public Health: Regulating the Housing Market
             in Nineteenth-Century New York City. In *Hives of Sickness: Public
             Health and Epidemics in New York City*, David Rosner, editor, pp.
             42–64. Rutgers University Press, New Brunswick, NJ.

Blake, R. Marlay
1918   Folklore with Some Account of the Ancient Gaelic Leeches and the
             State of the Art of Medicine in Ancient Erin. *Journal of the County
             Louth Archaeological Society* 4(3):217–225.

Blakey, Michael L.
2020   Archaeology under the Blinding Light of Race. *Current
             Anthropology* 61(supplement 22):S183–S197.

Blakey, Michael L., and Lesley M. Rankin-Hill
2004   *The New York African Burial Ground: Unearthing the African
             Presence in Colonial New York*. Vol. 1, Skeletal Biology of the New
             York African Burial Ground, Parts 1 and 2. US General Services
             Administration, Washington, D.C. <https://www.gsa.gov/about-us
             /regions/welcome-to-the-northeast-caribbean-region-2/about
             -region-2/african-burial-ground/introduction-to-african-burial
             -ground-final-reports>. Accessed 27 March 2023.

Blasi, Betty
1974   *A Bit About Balsams: A Chapter in the History of Nineteenth
             Century Medicine*. Mrs. Eugene J. Blasi, Sr., Louisville, KY.

Board of Aldermen
1864   *Annual Report of the City Inspector of the City of New York,
             for the Year Ending December 31, 1863*. Edmund Jones and Co.,
             New York, NY. HathiTrust Digital Archive, Original from
             University of Michigan <https://babel.hathitrust.org/cgi/pt?id=
             mdp.39015065233838>. Accessed 20 December 2018.

1866   *Annual Report of the City Inspector of the City of New York, for the Year Ending December 31, 1865.* Edmund Jones & Co., New York, NY. HathiTrust Digital Library, Original from University of Michigan <https://babel.hathitrust.org/cgi/pt?id=mdp.39015065233820>. Accessed 20 December 2018.

Board of Education

1876   *Thirty-Fourth Annual Report of the Board of Education of the City and County of New York, for the Official Year Ending December 31, 1875.* Board of Education, New York, NY. Internet Archive, Original from the New York Public Library <https://archive.org/details/annualreport11educgoog>. Accessed 8 July 2018.

Boas, Franz

1910   *Changes in Bodily Form of Descendants of Immigrants.* United States Immigration Commission. Senate Document 208.

1912   *Changes in Bodily Form of Descendants of Immigrants.* Columbia University Press, New York, NY.

Bodie, Debra C.

1992   The Construction of Community in Nineteenth Century New York: A Case Study Based on the Archaeological Investigation of the 25 Barrow Street Site. Master's thesis, Department of Anthropology, City University of New York. New York, NY.

Bonasera, Michael

2000a   Good for What Ails You: Medicinal Practices at Five Points. In *Tales of Five Points: Working-Class Life in Nineteenth-Century New York, Vol. 2, An Interpretive Approach to Understanding Working-Class Life,* Rebecca Yamin, editor, pp. 371–390. John Milner Associates, West Chester, PA.

2000b   Condiments and Related Serving Pieces. In *Tales of Five Points: Working-Class Life in Nineteenth-Century New York, Vol. 2, An Interpretive Approach to Understanding Working-Class Life,* Rebecca Yamin, editor, pp. 250–264. John Milner Associates, West Chester, PA.

Bonasera, Michael, and Leslie Raymer

2001   Good for What Ails You: Medicinal Use at Five Points. *Historical Archaeology* 35(3):49–64.

Bond, Kathleen H.

1989   The Medicine, Alcohol, and Soda Vessels from the Boott Mills Boardinghouses. In *Interdisciplinary Investigations of the Boott Mills, Lowell, Massachusetts, Vol. 3, The Boarding House System as a Way of Life,* Mary C. Beaudry and Stephen A. Mrozowski, editors, pp. 121–139. *Cultural resources Management Study,* No. 21. U.S. Department of Interior, National Park Service, North Atlantic

Regional Office, Boston, MA. Report prepared by Center for Archaeological Studies, Boston University, Boston, MA.

Bord, Janet, and Colin Bord
1985   *Sacred Waters: Holy Wells and Water Lore in Britain and Ireland.* Granada, New York, NY.

Borst, Charlotte G.
1999   The Training and Practice of Midwives: A Wisconsin Study. In *Women and Health in America*, Judith W. Leavitt, editor, pp. 425–443. 2nd edition. University of Wisconsin Press, Madison.

Boston Pilot
1863   Events of the Week. *Boston Pilot.* 28 March 1863:5. Boston, MA.

Bourdieu, Pierre
1984   *Distinction: A Social Critique of the Judgement of Taste*, Richard Nice, translator. Harvard University Press, Cambridge, MA.

Bowditch, Henry I.
1994a   Consumption in America. In *From Consumption to Tuberculosis: A Documentary History*, Barbara Rosenkrantz, editor, pp. 57–96. Garland Publishing, New York, NY.

1994b   Is Consumption Ever Contagious, or Communicated by One Person to Another in Any Manner? In *From Consumption to Tuberculosis: A Documentary History*, Barbara Rosenkrantz, editor, pp. 43–56. Garland Publishing, New York, NY.

Boyarin, Daniel, and Jonathan Boyarin
1993   Diaspora: Generation and the Ground of Jewish Identity. *Critical Inquiry* 19(4):693–725.

Boylston, Arthur
2013   The Origins of Vaccination: Myths and Reality. *Journal of the Royal Society of Medicine* 106(9):351–354.

Brace, Charles Loring
1873   The Little Laborers of New York City. *Harper's New Monthly Magazine* 47 (August):321–332. New York, NY.

Brah, Avtar
1996   *Cartographies of Diaspora: Contesting Identities.* Routledge, London, UK.

Breathnach, C. S., and J. B. Moynihan
2003   An Irish Statistician's Analysis of the National Tuberculosis Problem: Robert Charles Geary. *Irish Journal of Medical Science* 172(3):149–153.

Brenneman, Walter, and Mary Brenneman
1995   *Crossing the Circle at the Holy Wells of Ireland.* University of Virginia Press, Charlottesville.

Brew, Frank
1990	Rural Medicine in Former Times—Medicine in Rural Ireland in the 1800s. *The Other Clare* 14:25-26.

Brickman, Jane Pacht
1983	Public Health, Midwives, and Nurses, 1880-1930. In *Nursing History: New Perspectives, New Possibilities*, Ellen Condliffe Lagemann, editor, pp. 65-88. Teachers College Press, New York, NY.

Brighton, Stephen A.
2000	Prices That Suit the Times: Shopping for Ceramics at Five Points. In *Tales of Five Points: Working-Class Life in Nineteenth-Century New York, Vol. 2, An Interpretive Approach to Understanding Working-Class Life*, Rebecca Yamin, editor, pp. 11-30. John Milner Associates, West Chester, PA.
2004	Symbolism, Myth-Making and Identity: The Red Hand of Ulster in Nineteenth-Century Paterson, New Jersey. *International Journal of Historical Archaeology* 8(2):149-164.
2005	*An Historical Archaeology of the Irish Proletarian Diaspora: The Material Manifestations of Irish Identity in America, 1850-1910*. Doctoral Dissertation, Department of Anthropology, Boston University, Boston, MA.
2008	Degrees of Alienation: The Material Evidence of the Irish and the Irish-American Experience, 1850-1910. *Historical Archaeology* 42(4):132-153.
2009	*Historical Archaeology of the Irish Diaspora: A Transnational Approach*. University of Tennessee Press, Knoxville, TN.
2011	Middle-Class Ideologies and American Respectability: Archaeology and the Irish Immigrant Experience. *International Journal of Historical Archaeology* 15(1):30-50.

Brooklyn Daily Eagle
1893	Father Adams Restored. *Brooklyn Daily Eagle* 15 February:10. New York, NY.

Brown, Kathleen M.
2009	*Foul Bodies: Cleanliness in Early America*. Yale University Press, New Haven, CT.

Buchli, Victor
2002	Introduction. In *The Material Culture Reader*, Victor Buchli, editor, pp. 1-22. Berg, Oxford, UK.

Buckley, Anthony D.
1980	Unofficial Healing in Ulster. *Ulster Folklife* 26:15-34.

Burke, Thomas N.
1872　　　*Lectures and Sermons by the Very Reverend Thomas N. Burke*. P. M. Haverty, New York, NY. <https://www.google.com/books/edition/Lectures_and_Sermons/MtM3AQAAMAAJ>.

Burke, Timothy
1996　　　*Lifebuoy Men, Lux Women: Commodification, Consumption, and Cleanliness in Modern Zimbabwe*. Duke University Press, Durham, NC.

Burn, James
1865　　　*Three Years Among the Working-Classes in the United States during the War*. Smith, Elder and Co., London, UK.

Busch, Jane
1987　　　Second Time Around: A Look at Bottle Reuse. *Historical Archaeology* 21(1):67–80.

Cantwell, Anne-Marie, and Diana diZerega Wall
2015　　　Looking for Africans in Seventeenth-Century New Amsterdam. In *The Archaeology of Race in the Northeast*, Christopher N. Matthews and Allison Manfra McGovern, editors, pp. 29–55. University Press of Florida, Tallahassee.

Carroll, Michael P.
1999　　　*Irish Pilgrimage: Holy Wells and Popular Catholic Devotion*. Johns Hopkins University Press, Baltimore, MD.

Casella, Eleanor Conlin
2000　　　Bulldaggers and Gentle Ladies: Archaeological Approaches to Female Homosexuality in Convict-Era Australia. In *Archaeologies of Sexuality*, Robert A. Schmidt and Barbara L. Voss, editors, pp. 143–159. Routledge, New York, NY.

Castleconnor Parish Development Group (editor)
2000　　　*Castleconnor Parish: An Historical Perspective*. Castleconnor Parish Development Group, Sligo, Ireland.

Chaloner, E. J., H. S. Flora, and R. J. Ham
2001　　　Amputations at the London Hospital 1852–1857. *Journal of the Royal Society of Medicine* 94(8):409–412.

Chapelle, Francis H.
2005　　　*Wellsprings: A Natural History of Bottled Spring Waters*. Rutgers University Press, New Brunswick, NJ.

Chapman, Richard, and Felicity Platt
2009　　　Alcohol and Anaesthesia. *Continuing Education in Anaesthesia Critical Care & Pain* 9(1):10–13.

Chavez, Leo R.
2003　　　Immigration and Medical Anthropology. In *American Arrivals: Anthropology Engages the New Immigration*, Nancy Foner, editor, pp. 197–228. School of American Research, Santa Fe, NM.

Chicago Press and Tribune
1858a   Cure for Consumption. *Chicago Press and Tribune*. 12 August 1858a:3 Chicago, IL.
1858b   Throw Physic to the Dogs—Soda the Grand Catholicon. *Chicago Press and Tribune*. 28 August 1858a:2 Chicago, IL.

The Citizen
1854a   Untitled (Comments about lax authorities at the Staten Island Quarantine). *The Citizen* 15 April:225. New York, NY.
1854b   The Family Drug Store: Advertisement. *The Citizen* 2 January:18 New York, NY.

City Inspector's Department
1855   *Annual Report of the City Inspector of the City of New York for the Year Ending 1854*. City Inspector's Department, New York, NY. HathiTrust Digital Library, Original from The Ohio State University <https://catalog.hathitrust.org/Record/100633557>.
1858   *Annual Report of the City Inspector, of the City of New York for the Year Ending December 31, 1857*. New York, NY. HathiTrust Digital Library, Original from University of Chicago <https://babel.hathitrust.org/cgi/pt?id=chi.102195959>.

Coates, John Boyd (editor)
1963   *Internal Medicine in World War II, Vol. 2, Infectious Diseases*. Office of the Surgeon General Department of the Army, Washington DC. HathiTrust Digital Archive, Original from University of Michigan <https://babel.hathitrust.org/cgi/pt?id=mdp.39015072234571>.

Cohen, Lisbeth
1990   *Making a New Deal: Industrial Workers in Chicago 1919–1939*. Cambridge University Press, New York, NY.

Cohen, Mark Nathan
1989   *Health and the Rise of Civilization*. Yale University Press, New Haven, CT.

Cohn, Raymond L.
1984   Mortality on Immigrant Voyages to New York, 1836–1853. *Journal of Economic History* 44(2):289–300.
1987   The Determinants of Individual Immigrant Mortality on Sailing Ships, 1836–1853. *Explorations in Economic History* 24:371–391.

Coley, Noel G.
1990   Physicians, Chemists and the Analysis of Mineral Waters: "The Most Difficult Part of Chemistry." In *The Medical History of Waters and Spas*, Roy Porter, editor, Medical History, Supplement No. 10, pp. 56–66. The Wellcome Institute for the History of Medicine, London, UK.

Commissioners of Emigration (State of New York)
1861   *Annual Reports of the Commissioners of Emigration of the State of New York, From the Organization of the Commission, May 5, 1847 to 1860 Inclusive.* Commissioners of Emigration of the State of New York, New York, NY.

Condran, Gretchen A.
1995   Changing Patterns of Epidemic Disease in New York City. In *Hives of Sickness: Public Health and Epidemics in New York City*, David Rosner, editor, pp. 27–41. Rutgers University Press, New Brunswick, NJ.

Connell, Kenneth Hugh
1968   *Irish Peasant Society: Four Historical Essays.* Oxford Clarendon Press, Oxford, UK.
1975   *The Population of Ireland, 1750–1845.* Greenwood Press, Westport, CT.

Covey, Herbert C.
2007   *African American Slave Medicine.* Lexington Books, Lanham, MD.

Coyne, J. Stirling, and N. P. Willis
1841   *The Scenery and Antiquities of Ireland: Illustrated in One Hundred and Twenty Engravings, from Drawings by W. H. Bartlett.* Virtue & Co., London, UK.

Cramp, Arthur Joseph (editor)
1912   *Nostrums and Quackery: Articles on the Nostrum Evil and Quackery*, 2nd edition. Press of American Medical Association, Chicago, IL.

Crandon-Malamud, Libbet
1991   *From the Fat of Our Souls.* University of California Press, Berkeley.

Crawford, [E.] Margaret
1981   Indian Meal and Pellagra in Nineteenth-Century Ireland. In *Irish Population, Economy, and Society.*, J. M. Goldstrom and L. A. Clarkson, editors, pp. 113–134. Clarendon Press, Oxford, UK.
1999   Typhus in Nineteenth-Century Ireland. In *Medicine, Disease, and the State in Ireland 1650–1940*, Elizabeth Malcolm and Greta Jones, editors, pp. 121–138. Cork University Press, Cork, Ireland.

Crellin, John K., and Jane Philpott
1989   *Herbal Medicine Past and Present, Vol. 2, A Reference Guide to Medicinal Plants.* Duke University Press, Durham, NC.

Croker, Thomas Crofton
1838   *Fairy Legends and Traditions of the South of Ireland.* J. Murray, London, UK.

Croutier, Alev Lytle
1992   *Taking the Waters: Spirit, Art, Sensuality*. Abeville Press, New York, NY.

Csordas, Thomas
1994   *Embodiment and Experience: The Existential Ground of Culture and Self*. Cambridge University Press, Cambridge, UK.

Curley, James Michael
1957   *I'd Do It Again: A Record of All My Uproarious Years*. Prentice-Hall, Englewood Cliffs, NJ.

Curtis, L. Perry, Jr.
1997   *Apes and Angels: The Irishman in Victorian Caricature*, revised edition from 1971 original publication. Smithsonian Institution Press, Washington DC.

Dales, R., H. Zwanenburg, R. Burnett, and C. A. Franklin
1991   Respiratory Health Effects of Home Dampness and Molds among Canadian Children. *American Journal of Epidemiology* 134(2):196–203.

Daniel, Thomas M.
1997   *Captain of Death: The Story of Tuberculosis*. University of Rochester Press, Rochester, NY.

Darwen, Lewis, Donald M. MacRaild, and Liam Kennedy
2020   'Irish Fever' in Britain during the Great Famine: Immigration, Disease and the Legacy of 'Black '47'. *Irish Historical Studies* 44(166):270–294.

Davies, P. D. O., W. W. Yewb, D. Ganguly, A. L. Davidow, L. B. Reichman, K. Dheda, and G. A. Rook
2006   Smoking and Tuberculosis: The Epidemiological Association and Immunopathogenesis. *Transactions of the Royal Society of Tropical Medicine & Hygiene* 100(4):291–298.

Dawdy, Shannon Lee
2005   Thinker-Tinkers, Race, and the Archaeological Critique of Modernity. *Archaeological Dialogues* 12(2):143–164.

De Bow, J. D .B.
1855   *Mortality Statistics of the Seventh Census of the United States, 1850*. 33rd Congress, House of Representatives, Ex. Doc. No. 98. United States Census Bureau, Washington, DC <https://www.census.gov/library/publications/1855/dec/1850b.html>. Accessed 27 March 2023.

de Craen, Anton J. M., Pieter J. Roos, A. Leonard de Vries, and Jos Kleijnen.
1996   Effect of Colour of Drugs: Systematic Review of Perceived Effect of Drugs and Their Effectiveness. *British Medical Journal* 313:1624–1626.

de Nie, Michael Willem
2004   *The Eternal Paddy: Irish Identity and the British Press, 1798–1882.* University of Wisconsin Press, Madison.

Desborough, Michael J. R., and David M. Keeling
2017   The Aspirin Story–from Willow to Wonder Drug. *British Journal of Haematology: Historical Review* 177:674–683.

Dietert, R. R., and M. S. Piepenbrink
2006   Lead and Immune Function. *Critical Reviews in Toxicology* 36(4):359–385.

Diner, Hasia, R.
1983   *Erin's Daughters in America: Irish Immigrant Women in the Nineteenth Century.* Johns Hopkins University Press, Baltimore, MD.

1996   "The Most Irish City in the Union": The Era of the Great Migration, 1844–1877. In *The New York Irish*, Ronald H. Bayor and Timothy J. Meagher, editors, pp. 87–106. Johns Hopkins University Press, Baltimore, MD.

2001   *Hungering for America: Italian, Irish, and Jewish Foodways in the Age of Migration.* Harvard University Press, Cambridge, MA.

Doggett, John, Jr.
1844   *The New-York City Directory for 1844 & 1845.* John Doggett, Jr., New York, NY. HathiTrust Digital Archive, Original from The Ohio State University <https://babel.hathitrust.org/cgi/pt?id=osu.32435056191521>.

1846   *Doggett's New-York City Directory for 1846 and 1847.* John Doggett, Jr., New York, NY. New York Public Library Digital Collections, New York, NY <https://digitalcollections.nypl.org/items/e1081b90-8225-0136-88d6-376951526e42>.

1848   *Doggett's New-York City Directory for 1848–1849.* John Doggett, Jr., New York, NY. New York Public Library Digital Collections, New York, NY <https://digitalcollections.nypl.org/items/e7e02690-820c-0136-405f-5b8aa44a1b41>.

1849   *Doggett's New York City Directory for 1849–1850.* John Doggett, Jr. & Co., New York, NY. New York Public Library Digital Collections, New York, NY <https://digitalcollections.nypl.org/items/de9d5570-5291-0134-74fc-00505686a51c>.

Doherty, Thomas
1897   Notes on the Physique, Customs, and Superstitions of the Peasantry of Innishowen, Co. Donegal. *Folklore* 8(1):12–18.

Dolan, Jay P.
1975   *The Immigrant Church: New York's Irish and German Catholics, 1815–1865*. Johns Hopkins University Press, Baltimore, MD. Reprinted 1983 by Notre Dame University Press, Notre Dame, IN.

Donnelly, James S.
2001   *The Great Irish Potato Famine*. Sutton Publishing, Stroud, UK.

Doremus, H. Ogden
1854a   Poisonous Effects of Soda Water from Copper Fountains and Lead Pipes. *New York Daily Times* 7 July:1. New York, NY.
1854b   Soda-Water. *New York Daily Times* 16 August:3. New York, NY.

Dorian, Hugh
2000   *The Outer Edge of Ulster: A Memoir of Social Life in Nineteenth-Century Donegal*. Edited by Breandán Mac Suibhne and David Dickson. Liliput Press, Dublin, Ireland.

Dormandy, Thomas
1999   *The White Death: A History of Tuberculosis*. Hambledon Press, London, England.

Douglas, Mary
1966   *Purity and Danger: An Analysis of the Concepts of Pollution and Taboo*. Routledge, London, UK.

Dressler, William W.
1996   Culture, Stress, and Disease. In *Medical Anthropology: Contemporary Method and Theory*, Carolyn F. Sargent and Thomas M. Johnson, editors, pp. 252–271. Praeger, Westport, CT.

Drolet, Godias J., and Anthony M. Lowell
1952   *A Half a Century's Progress Against Tuberculosis in New York City 1900–1950*. New York Tuberculosis and Health Association, New York, NY.

Dublin Quarterly Journal of Medical Science
1849   Report on the Epidemic Fever in Ireland. *Dublin Quarterly Journal of Medical Science*. 7(8–9):64–125; 340–404. Dublin, Ireland.

Dublin University Magazine Advertiser
1840   Rowland's Macassar Oil: Advertisement. *Dublin University Magazine* November:64. Dublin, Ireland. Google Books <https://www.google.com/books/edition/Dublin_University_Magazine/uUEzAQAAMAAJ>.

Dubos, René J., and Jean Dubos
1952   *The White Plague: Tuberculosis, Man and Society*. Little, Brown and Company, Boston, MA.

Dúchas Project
2022   The National Folklore Collection (NFC) and Its Collections <https://www.duchas.ie/en/info/cbe>. Accessed 27 March 2023.

Duden, Barbara
1991 *The Woman Beneath the Skin: A Doctor's Patients in Eighteenth-Century Germany*, Thomas Dunlap, translator. Harvard University Press, Cambridge, MA.

Duffe, James
1853 Diary of a Male Nurse at Marine House, New York Hospital 1844–1853. Manuscript, *New-York Historical Society Manuscripts Collection*, The New-York Historical Society, New York, NY.

Duffy, John
1968 *A History of Public Health in New York City, 1625–1866*. Russell Sage Foundation, New York, NY.

Dupre, John
1993 *The Disorder of Things: Metaphysical Foundations of the Disunity of Science*. Harvard University Press, Cambridge, MA.

Dykstra, D. L.
1955 The Medical Profession and Patent and Proprietary Medicines during the Nineteenth Century. *Bulletin of the History of Medicine* 29(5):401–419.

Earle, Pliny
1845 Bloomingdale Asylum Report. In *State of the New-York Hospital and Bloomingdale Asylum for the Year 1844*. New York Hospital, pp. 21–51. Egbert, Hovey, & King, New York, NY.

Egan, F. W.
1887 Irish Folk-Lore. Medicinal Plants. *Folk-Lore Journal* 5:11–13.

Eisenberg, Leon
1977 Disease and Illness: Distinctions Between Professional and Popular Ideas of Sickness. *Culture, Medicine and Psychiatry* 1(1):9–23.

Ellis, P. Berresford
1972 *A History of the Irish Working Class*. George Braziller, New York, NY.

Elmes, William
1812 Irish Bogtrotters. Print attributed to William Elmes. *The Caricature Magazine or Hudibrastic Mirror* 1(111). Thomas Tegg, Cheapside, London, UK. *Digital Commonwealth*, Massachusetts Collections Online, Boston Public Library, Boston, MA <https://ark.digitalcommonwealth.org/ark:/50959/x346dn36r>. Accessed 27 March 2023.

Engels, Frederick
1887 *Condition of the Working-Class in England in 1844*. John W. Lovell Company, New York, NY. Internet Archive <https://archive.org/details/conditionofworkio0enge_0>.

Erickson, Paul A.
1986   The Anthropology of Josiah Clark Not. *Kroeber Anthropological Society Papers* 65–66:103–120. <https://digitalassets.lib.berkeley.edu/anthpubs/ucb/text/kas065_066-013.pdf>. Accessed 10 March 2023.

Ernst, Robert
1949   *Immigrant Life in New York City, 1825–1863*. King's Crown Press, New York, NY.

Estes, J. Worth
1995   The European Reception of the First Drugs from the New World. *Pharmacy in History* 37(1):3–23.

Etkin, N. L., P. J. Ross, and I. Muazzamu
1990   The Indigenization of Pharmaceuticals: Therapeutic Transitions in Rural Hausaland. *Social Science and Medicine* 30:919–28.

Evans, Estyn E.
1957   *Irish Folk Ways*. Routledge & Paul, London, UK. Reprinted 1972 by Routledge, London, UK.
1973   *The Personality of Ireland: Habitat, Heritage, and History*. Cambridge University Press, Cambridge, UK.

Fairchild, Amy
2003   *Science at the Borders: Immigrant Medical Inspection and the Shaping of the Modern Industrial Labor Force*. Johns Hopkins University Press, Baltimore, MD.

Fallon, Emer
1994   Folk Medicine from the East Kildare Area. Diploma in Irish Folklore, Department of Irish Folklore, University College Dublin, Dublin, Ireland.

Farmar, Tony
2004   *Patients, Potions, and Physicians: A Social History of Medicine in Ireland 1654–2004*. A. and A. Farmar, Dublin, Ireland.

Farmer, Paul
1993   *Aids and Accusation: Haiti and the Geography of Blame*. University of California Press, Berkeley.
1996   On Suffering and Structural Violence: A View from Below. *Daedalus* 125(1):261–283.
1999   *Infections and Inequalities: The Modern Plagues*. University of California Press, Berkeley.

Farrelly, Caroline
1979   The Folk Medicine of North County Meath. 2nd Year Essay, Department of Irish Folklore, University College Dublin, Dublin, Ireland.

Fee, Elizabeth and Evelynn M. Hammonds
1995 Science, Politics, and the Art of Persuasion: Promoting the New Scientific Medicine in NYC. In *Hives of Sickness: Public Health and Epidemics in New York City*, David Rosner, editor, pp. 155–196. Rutgers University Press, New Brunswick, NJ.

Feerick, Jean
2002 Spenser, Race, and Ire-Land. *English Literary Renaissance* 32(1):85–117.

Feldberg, Georgina
1995 *Disease and Class: Tuberculosis and the Shaping of Modern North American Society*. Rutgers University Press, New Brunswick, NJ.

Fennell, Christopher C.
2000 Conjuring Boundaries: Inferring Past Identities from Religious Artifacts. *International Journal of Historical Archaeology* 4(4):281–313.

Fields, Barbara J.
2001 Whiteness, Racism, and Identity. *International Labor and Working-Class History* 60(Fall):48–56.

Fike, Richard E.
1987 *The Bottle Book: A Comprehensive Guide to Historic Embossed Medicine Bottles*. Peregrine Smith Books, Salt Lake City, UT.

Fitch, Samuel Sheldon
1854 *Almanac for 1855 and Guide to Invalids, Comprising Directions for the Treatment of Consumption and Asthma*. S. S. Fitch & Co., New York, NY.

Fitts, Robert K.
1999 The Archaeology of Middle-Class Domesticity and Gentility in Brooklyn. *Historical Archaeology* 33(1):39–62.
2000a The Five Points Reformed. In *Tales of Five Points: Working-Class Life in Nineteenth-Century New York, Vol. 1, A Narrative History and Archaeology of Block 160*, Rebecca Yamin, editor, pp. 67–90. John Milner Associates, West Chester, PA.
2000b The Rhetoric of Reform: The Five Points Missions and the Cult of Domesticity. In *Tales of Five Points: Working Class Life in Nineteenth-Century New York, Vol. 2, A Narrative History and Archaeology of Block 160*, Rebecca Yamin, editor, pp. 423–440. John Milner Associates, West Chester, PA.

Fitzgerald, Maureen
2006 *Habits of Compassion: Irish Catholic Nuns and the Origins of New York's Welfare System, 1830–1920*. University of Illinois Press, Chicago.

Fleetwood, John F.
1983   *The History of Medicine in Ireland.* Skellig Press, Dublin, Ireland.

Fleming, H. B.
1953   Folklore, Fact, and Legend. *Irish Journal of Medical Science* 326:49–63.

Foley, Ronan
2015   Indigenous Narratives of Health: (Re)Placing Folk-Medicine within Irish Health Histories. *Journal of Medical Humanities* 36(1):5–18.

Foner, Eric
1995   *Free Soil, Free Labor, Free Men: The Ideology of the Republican Party Before the Civil War.* Reprint of 1970 original with updated preface. Oxford University Press, New York, NY.

Foner, Nancy
1999   Immigrant Women and Work in New York City, Then and Now. *Journal of American Ethnic History* 18(3):95–113.
2005   *In a New Land: A Comparative View of Immigration.* New York University Press, New York, NY.

Ford, Benjamin
1994   The Health and Sanitation of Postbellum Harpers Ferry. *Historical Archaeology* 28(4):49–61.

Frank, Julia Bess
1976   Body Snatching: A Grave Medical Problem. *The Yale Journal of Biology and Medicine* 49:399–410.

Frank Leslie's Illustrated Newspaper
1858a   Our Exposure of the Swill Milk Trade. *Frank Leslie's Illustrated Newspaper*, 22 May:385.
1858b   Destruction of the Quarantine Buildings near Tompkinsville, Staten Island, by the Inhabitants of Tompkinsville, During the Telegraph Jubilee in New York, on the Evening of Sept. 1, 1858. *Frank Leslie's Illustrated Newspaper*, 18 September.

Froggatt, Peter
1999   Competing Philosophies: The Preparatory Medical Schools of the Royal Belfast Academical Institution and the Catholic University of Ireland. In *Medicine, Disease, and the State in Ireland 1650–1940*, Elizabeth Malcolm and Greta Jones, editors, pp. 59–84. Cork University Press, Cork, Ireland.

Funderburg, Anne
2003   *Sundae's Best: A History of Soda Fountains.* University of Wisconsin Press, Madison.

Furey, Brenda
1991   *The History of Oranmore Maree (Co. Galway).* McGrath, Galway, Ireland.

Furnivall, Frederick J., (editor)
1878   *Harrison's Description of England in Shakespeare's Youth*. The New Shakespeare Society, N. Trübner & Co., London, UK.

Gallagher, Melissa
2006   The Archaeology of Late Nineteenth-Century Health and Hygiene: A View from San Francisco. Master's thesis, Sonoma State University, Sonoma, CA.

Gallman, J. Matthew
2000   *Receiving Erin's Children: Philadelphia, Liverpool, and the Irish Famine Migration, 1845–1855*. University of North Carolina Press, Durham.

Garner, Steve
2015   The Simianization of the Irish: Racial Ape-ing and Its Contexts. In *Simianization: Apes, Gender, Class, and Race*, Wulf D. Hund, Charles W. Mills, and Silvia Sebastiani, editors, pp. 197–223. LIT Verlag, Zürich, Switzerland.

Gaynor, Matthew
1849   Letter. Matthew Gaynor Letters, MS 13,554. National Library of Ireland. Dublin, Ireland.

Geber, Jonny, and Barra O'Donnabhain
2020   "Against Shameless and Systematic Calumny": Strategies of Domination and Resistance and Their Impact on the Bodies of the Poor in Nineteenth-Century Ireland. *Historical Archaeology* 54(1):160–183.

Geertz, Clifford
1973   *The Interpretation of Cultures*. Basic Books, New York, NY.

Geismar, Joan H.
1989   History and Archaeology of the Greenwich Mews Site, Greenwich Village, New York. Report on file with the New York City Landmarks Preservation Committee. New York, NY.
1993   "Where Is the Night Soil?" Thoughts on an Urban Privy. *Historical Archaeology* 27(2):57–70.

Geltson, Arthur L., and Thomas C. Jones
1977   Typhus Fever: Report of an Epidemic in New York City in 1847. *The Journal of Infectious Diseases* 136(6):813–821.

Gibian, Peter
2001   *Oliver Wendell Holmes and the Culture of Conversation*. Cambridge University Press, Cambridge, MA.

Giles, Henry
1869   *Lectures and Essays on Irish and Other Subjects*. D. & J. Sadlier & Co., New York, NY.

Gilfoyle, Timothy J.
1992   *City of Eros: New York City, Prostitution, and the Commercialization of Sex, 1790–1920*. W. W. Norton, New York, NY.

Gillespie, Raymond
1998   Popular and Unpopular Religion: A View from Early Modern Ireland. In *Irish Popular Culture, 1650–1850*, Kerby A. Miller and James S. Donnelly, editors, pp. 30–49. Irish Academic Press, Portland, OR.

Gilroy, Paul
1993   *The Black Atlantic-Modernity and Double Consciousness*. Harvard University Press, Cambridge, MA.

Glasco, Lawrence
1977   Ethnicity and Occupation in the Mid-Nineteenth Century: Irish, Germans, and Native-Born Whites in Buffalo, New York. In *Immigrants in Industrial America 1850–1920*, Richard L. Ehrlich, editor, pp. 151–175. University of Virginia Press, Charlottesville.

Glassie, Henry
1982   *Passing the Time in Ballymenone: Culture and History of an Ulster Community*. University of Pennsylvania Press, Philadelphia.
1985   *Irish Folktales*. Pantheon Books, New York, NY.

Godkin, Edwin L.
1895   *Reflections and Comments: 1865–1895*. Charles Scribner's Sons, New York, NY.

Goffman, Erving
1959   *The Presentation of Self in Everyday Life*. Doubleday Anchor Books, New York, NY.

Goldman, Lee, and J. Claude Bennett (editors)
2000   *Cecil Textbook of Medicine*, 21st edition. W. B. Saunders Company, Philadelphia, PA.

Grad, Roni
2004   Cod and the Consumptive: A Brief History of Cod-Liver Oil in the Treatment of Pulmonary Tuberculosis. *Pharmacy in History* 46(3):106–120.

Gray, Peter
1993   Punch and the Great Famine. *History Ireland* 1(2): 26–33.

Greenwood, Roberta
1996   *Down by the Station: Los Angeles Chinatown, 1880–1933*. Monumenta Archaeologica 18, Institute of Archaeology, University of California, Los Angeles.

Gregory, Lady Isabella Augusta Persee
1920 *Visions and Beliefs in the West of Ireland: Collected and Arranged by Lady Gregory With Two Essays and Notes by W. B. Yeats*, Vol. 1. G. P. Putman's Sons, New York, NY. Reprinted 1976 by Colin Smythe Gerrands Cross, Buckinghamshire, UK.

Grenham, John
2015 Irish Roots: Home of Begrudgery. *Irish Times*. 21 Dec. Dublin, Ireland <https://www.irishtimes.com/culture/heritage/irish-roots-home-of-begrudgery-1.2474870>. Accessed 26 March 2023.

Griffenhagen, George B., and James Harvey Young
1959 *Old English Patent Medicines in America*. United States National Museum Bulletin 218. Smithsonian Institution, Washington, DC.

Griggs, Heather
2000 Emigrant Bank and Transfiguration Church Records as Supplementary Historical Sources: A Statistical Analysis. In *Tales of Five Points: Working-Class Life in Nineteenth-Century New York, Vol. 2, An Interpretive Approach to Understanding Working-Class Life*, Rebecca Yamin, editor, pp. 31–48. John Milner Associates, West Chester, PA.

Griscom, John H.
1845 *The Sanitary Condition of the Laboring Population of New York: With Suggestions for Its Improvement. Discourse (with Additions), Delivered on the 30th December, 1844, at the Repository of the American Institute*. Harper & Brothers, New York, NY.

Groneman [Pernicone], Carol
1973 The "Bloody Ould Sixth": A Social Analysis of a New York City Working-Class Community in the Mid-Nineteenth Century. Doctoral dissertation, University of Rochester, Rochester, NY.
1977 "She Earns as a Child—She Pays as a Man": Women Workers in a Mid-Nineteenth-Century New York City Community. In *Immigrants in Industrial America 1850–1920*, Richard L. Ehrlich, editor, pp. 33–46. University Press of Virginia, Charlottesville.

Gross, Samuel D.
1861 *A Manual of Military Surgery: Hints on the Emergencies of Field, Camp, and Hospital Practice*. J. B. Lippincott & Co., Philadelphia, PA.

Grossman, James R.
1989 *Land of Hope: Chicago, Black Southerners, and the Great Migration*. University of Chicago Press, Chicago, IL.

Grzybowski, Stefan, and Edward A. Allen
1995 History and Importance of Scrofula. *The Lancet* 346(8988):1472–1474.

Haines, Michael R.
2001   The Urban Mortality Transition in the United States, 1800–1940. Historical Paper 134, NBER Working Papers Series on Historical Factors in Long Run Growth, National Bureau of Economic Research, Cambridge, MA <https://www.nber.org/papers/h0134.pdf>. Accessed 27 March 2023.

Hall, Martin, and Stephen W. Silliman
2006   Introduction: Archaeology of the Modern World. In *Historical Archaeology*, Martin Hall and Stephen W. Silliman, editors, pp. 1–22. Blackwell Publishing, Malden, MA.

Hall, Stuart
1990   Cultural Identity and Diaspora. In *Identity: Community, Culture, Difference*, Jonathan Rutherford, editor, pp. 222–237. Lawrence and Wishart, London, UK.

Haller, John S.
1981a   *American Medicine in Transition 1840–1910*. University of Illinois Press, Urbana.
1981b   Hypodermic Medication, Early History. *New York State Journal of Medicine* 81(11):1671–1679.

Hamilton-Miller, J. M. T.
1995   Antimicrobial Properties of Tea (*Camellia sinensis* L.). *Antimicrobial Agents and Chemotherapy* 39(11):2375–2377.

Hamlin, Christopher
1992   Predisposing Causes and Public Health in Early Nineteenth-Century Medical Thought. *Social History of Medicine* 5(1):43–70.

Hand, Wayland D.
1981   European Fairy Lore in the New World. *Folklore* 92(2):141–148.

Handlin, Oscar
1941   *Boston's Immigrants, 1790–1865*. Harvard University Press, Cambridge, MA.

Hardesty, Donald L.
1994   Class, Gender Strategies, and Material Culture in the Mining West. In *Those of Little Note: Gender, Race, and Class in Historical Archaeology*, Elizabeth M. Scott, editor, pp. 129–145. University of Arizona Press, Tucson.

Hardy, Anne
1988   Urban Famine or Urban Crisis? Typhus in the Victorian City. *Medical History* 32(4):401–425.

Hardy, Philip Dixon
1840   *The Holy Wells of Ireland*. Hardy and Walker, Dublin, Ireland <http://www.geoffb.me.uk/wells/hardy/hardy.html>.

Harper's Weekly (HW)

1857	Saratoga Springs. *Harper's Weekly* 1 August:483. New York, NY.
1858	The Voting-Place: Illustration. *Harper's Weekly* 13 November:724. New York, NY.
1860	J. R. Stafford's Olive Tar: Advertisement. *Harper's Weekly* 19 May:318. New York, NY.
1861	Dr. Riggs Waterproof Trusses: Advertisement. *Harper's Weekly* 9 March:159. New York, NY.
1862	Hegeman & Co's Camphor Ice: Advertisement. *Harper's Weekly* 15 March:175. New York, NY.
1864	Advertisement for Hoyt's Imperial Coloring Cream. *Harper's Weekly* 26 March:208. New York, NY.
1865	Dr. Glover's Lever Truss: Advertisement. *Harper's Weekly* 30 December:830. New York, NY.
1867a	Young Hibernia: Cartoon. *Harper's Weekly* 18 May:320. New York, NY.
1867b	J. R. Stafford's Olive Tar: Advertisement. *Harper's Weekly* 27 July:479. New York, NY.
1867c	Hostetter's Bitters Advertisement. *Harper's Weekly* 10 August:511. New York, NY.
1868	Eva Eve. *Harper's Weekly* 14 November:725–726. New York, NY.
1871	A Saturday Night Scene in the Bowery, New York. *Harper's Weekly* 20 May:469. New York, NY.
1872	Pomeroy & Co.: Advertisement. *Harper's Weekly* 14 September:726. New York, NY.
1873a	An Irish Wake. *Harper's Weekly* 15 March:211. New York, NY.
1873b	Bartlett Truss: Advertisement. *Harper's Weekly* 11 October:902. New York, NY.
1874	What's Next?: Cartoon. *Harper's Weekly* 31 January:112. New York, NY.
1877	Home and Foreign Gossip. *Harper's Weekly* 19 May:387. New York, NY.
1879	Experiences of an Irish Doctor. *Harper's Weekly* 11 October:806. New York, NY.
1886	Some Poisonous Food and Drinks. *Harper's Weekly* 10 July:446. New York, NY.

Harris, Bernard, and Waltraud Ernst (editors)
1999   *Race, Science, and Medicine, 1700–1960*. Routledge, New York, NY.

Harris, K. M.
1960   Notes—Cures and Charms. *Ulster Folklife* 6:65–67.

Harris, Ruth-Ann Mellish
1989 Introduction. In *The Search for Missing Friends: Irish Immigrant Advertisements Placed in the Boston Pilot Vol. 1: 1831–1850*. Ruth-Ann Mellish Harris and Donald M. Jacobs, editors, pp. i–lxii. New England Historic Genealogical Society, Boston, MA.

Harris, Ruth-Ann Mellish, and Donald M. Jacobs
1989 *The Search for Missing Friends: Irish Immigrant Advertisements Placed in the Boston Pilot Vol. 1: 1831–1850*. New England Historic Genealogical Society, Boston, MA.

Harris, Stephen
2012 Non-Native Plants and Their Medicinal Uses. In *Plants, Health and Healing: On the Interface of Ethnobotany and Medical Anthropology*, Elisabeth Hsu and Stephen Harris, editors, pp. 53–82. Berghahn Books, Incorporated, New York, NY.

Hayes, J. N.
2009 *The Burdens of Disease: Epidemics and Human Response in Western History*, revised edition. Rutgers University Press, New Brunswick, NJ.

Hayward, George
1850 *Statistics of the Amputations of Large Limbs That Have Been Performed at the Massachusetts General Hospital from Its Establishment, to January 1, 1850*. David Clapp, Boston, MA.

Hayward, George and Thomas Wood
1845 New-York Hospital, illustration by George Hayward and lithographer Thomas Wood. Irma and Paul Milstein Division of United States History, Local History and Genealogy, The New York Public Library. New York Public Library Digital Collections <https://digitalcollections.nypl.org/items/e9c6bad0-8e10-0132-86b4-58d385a7bbd0>. Accessed 27 March 2023.

Hegyi, Juraj, Robert A. Schwartz, and Vladimír Hegyi
2004 Pellagra: Dermatitis, Dementia, and Diarrhea. *International Journal of Dermatology* 43(1):1–5.

Heywood, Audrey
1999 A Trial of the Bath Waters: The Treatment of Lead Poisoning. In *The Medical History of Waters and Spas*, Roy Porter, editor, pp. 82–101. The Wellcome Institute for the History of Medicine, London, UK.

Hilliard, Addie Suggs
1966 I Remember, I Remember. *Tennessee Folklore Society Bulletin* 32:121–128.

Hirota, Hidetaka
2017 *Expelling the Poor: Atlantic Seaboard States and the Nineteenth-Century Origins of American Immigration Policy.* Oxford University Press, New York, NY.

Hiss, A. Emil
1900 *Thesaurus of Proprietary Preparations and Pharmaceutical Specialties, Including "Patent" Medicines, Proprietary Pharmaceuticals, Open-Formula Specialties, Synthetic Remedies, Etc.* G.P. Engelhard & Co., Chicago, IL.

Ho, Wayne, and Brennan M. R. Spiegel
2008 The Relationship Between Obesity and Functional Gastrointestinal Disorders: Causation, Association, or Neither? *Gastroenterology & Hepatology* 4(8):572–578.

Hochschild, Arlie Russell, and Anne Machung
1989 *The Second Shift: Working Parents and the Revolution at Home.* Viking Adult, New York, NY.

Horsman, Reginald
1976 Origins of Racial Anglo-Saxonism in Great Britain before 1850. *Journal of the History of Ideas* 37(3):387–410.

Hospital for Special Surgery
2021 HSS Celebrates 150 Years. The History of the Hospital for Special Surgery. <https://www.hss.edu/history.asp>. Accessed 27 March 2023.

Howard-Jones, Norman
1947 A Critical Study of the Origins and Early Development of Hypodermic Medication. *Journal of the History of Medicine and Allied Sciences* 2(2):201–249.

Howes, David (editor)
1996 *Cross-Cultural Consumption: Global Markets, Local Realities.* Routledge, New York, NY.

Howson, Jean Ellen
1987 The Archaeology of Nineteenth-Century Health and Hygiene: A Case Study from Sullivan Street, Greenwich Village. Master's thesis, New York University, New York, NY.
1993 The Archaeology of 19th-Century Health and Hygiene at the Sullivan Street Site, New York City. *Northeast Historical Archaeology* 22(1):137–160.
2013 H.W. Epitaph for a Working Man. In *Tales of Gotham: Historical Archaeology, Ethnohistory and Microhistory of New York City*, Meta F. Janowitz and Diane Dallal, editors, pp. 159–178. Springer, New York, NY.

Hughes, Robert
1987   *The Fatal Shore*. Alfred A. Knopf, New York, NY.
Hull, Katharine L.
2004   Material Correlates of the Pre-Famine Agri-Social Hierarchy: Archaeological Evidence from County Roscommon, Republic of Ireland. Doctoral dissertation, University of Toronto, Toronto, Canada.
Humphreys, Margaret
2006   A Stranger to Our Camps: Typhus in American History. *Bulletin of the History of Medicine* 80(2):269–290.
Humphreys, Mary Gay
1891   The Evolution of the Soda Fountain. *Harper's Weekly*, 21 November:923. New York, NY.
Hund, Wulf D.
2015   Racist King Kong Fantasies: From Shakespeare's Monster to Stalin's Ape-Man. In *Simianization: Apes, Gender, Class, and Race*, Wulf D. Hund, Charles W. Mills, and Silvia Sebastiani, editors, pp. 43–73. LIT Verlag, Zürich, Switzerland.
Hutchings, John
1997   Folklore and the Symbolism of Green. *Folklore* 108:55–64.
Hyatt, Harry Middleton
1935   *Folk-Lore from Adams County, Illinois*. Memoirs of the Alma Egan Hyatt Foundation, New York. Alma Egan Hyatt Foundation, New York, NY.
Illustrated London News
1851   Emigration vessel—between decks. *Illustrated London News* 10 May 1851:387. London, UK. The Miriam and Ira D. Wallach Division of Art, Prints and Photographs: Picture Collection. New York Public Library Digital Collections <https://digitalcollections.nypl.org/items/510d47e1-3797-a3d9-e040-e00a18064a99>. Accessed 27 March 2023.
1859   Manners and Customs of the Irish Peasantry: The Fairy Doctor—From a Drawing by E. Fitzpatrick. *Illustrated London News* 31 Dec 1859:635, London, UK. HathiTrust Digital Library <https://babel.hathitrust.org/cgi/pt?id=mdp.39015007000857&view=1up&seq=627>. Accessed 27 March 2023.
Ingalls, William
1860   Record of Obstetrical Cases. *Boston Medical and Surgical Journal* LXII (19):373–376.

Irish American
1849 St. Vincent's Hospital: Advertisement. *Irish American* 18 November. New York, NY.

Irish American Weekly
1857 James McPeake: Obituary. *Irish American Weekly* 5 September:3. New York, NY.

Isaac, Benjamin
2006 *The Invention of Racism in Classical Antiquity*. Princeton University Press, Princeton, NJ.

J.P.
1872 Fevers. *Dublin University Magazine* 79:184–194.

Jacobson, Matthew Frye
1998 *Whiteness of a Different Color: European Immigrants and the Alchemy of Race*. Harvard University Press, Cambridge, MA.

Janowitz, Meta F., and Diane Dallal (editors)
2013 *Tales of Gotham, Historical Archaeology, Ethnohistory, and Microhistory of New York City*. Springer, New York, NY.

Jolly, Ellen Ryan
1927 *Nuns of the Battlefield*. Providence Visitor Press, Providence, RI.

Jones, Greta
2001 *"Captain of All These Men of Death": The History of Tuberculosis in Nineteenth and Twentieth Century Ireland*. Clio Medica 62: The Wellcome Series in the History of Medicine, Rodophi, Amsterdam, Netherlands.

2012 Women and Tuberculosis in Ireland. In *Gender and Medicine in Ireland 1700-1950*, Margaret H. Preston and Margaret Ó hÓgartaigh, editors, pp. 33–48. Syracuse University Press, Syracuse, NY.

Jones, Olive
1981 Essence of Peppermint, a History of the Medicine and Its Bottle. *Historical Archaeology* 15(1):1–57.

Jones, Olive, and Allen Vegotsky
2016 Turlington's Balsam of Life. *Northeast Historical Archaeology* 45:1–61.

Jordanova, Ludmilla
1980 Natural Facts: An Historical Perspective on Science and Sexuality. In *Nature, Culture, and Gender*, Carol P. MacCormack and Marilyn Strathern, editors, pp. 42–69. Cambridge University Press, Cambridge, UK.

Joyce, Rosemary. A.
2005 Archaeology of the Body. *Annual Review of Anthropology* 34:139–158.

Jung, Richard S., Jonathan R. Bennion, Frank Sorvillo, and Amy Bellomy
2010 Trends in Tuberculosis Mortality in the United States, 1990–2006: A Population-Based Case-Control Study. *Public Health Reports* 125(3):389–397.

Kasinitz, Philip, John H. Mollenkopf, and Mary C. Waters (editors)
2010 *Inheriting the City: The Children of Immigrants Come of Age*. Russell Sage Foundation Publications, New York, NY.

Kearns, Kevin
1994 *Dublin Tenement Life: An Oral History*. Gill and Macmillam, Dublin, Ireland.

Keeney, B. M.
1865 Report of the Third Sanitary Inspection District, Section B. In *Report of the Council of Hygiene and Public Health of the Citizens' Association of New York upon the Sanitary Condition of the City*, pp. 3–42. Citizens' Association of New York. D. Appleton & Co, New York, NY. Internet Archive <https://archive.org/details/reportcouncilhyoonygoog/page/n6>.

Kelly, Fergus
2001 Medicine and Early Irish Law. *Irish Journal of Medical Science* 170(1):73–76.

Kelly, Mary C.
2005 *The Shamrock and the Lily: The New York Irish and the Creation of a Transatlantic Identity, 1845–1921*. Peter Lang, New York, NY.

Kelly, Tamara
2000 Father Theobald Mathew. In *Tales of Five Points: Working-Class Life in Nineteenth Century New York, Vol. 2, An Interpretive Approach to Understanding Working-Class Life*, Rebecca Yamin, editor, pp. 265–271. John Milner Associates, West Chester, PA.

Keneally, Thomas
1998 *The Great Shame: A Story of the Irish in the Old World and the New*. Chatto and Windus, London, UK.

Kenny, Kevin
1998 *Making Sense of the Molly Maguires*. Oxford University Press, New York, NY.
2000 *The American Irish: A History*. Routledge, New York, NY.
2001 Race, Labor, and Nativism: A Response to Dale T. Knobel (Ernie O'Malley Lecture, New York University, November 2000). *Radharc* 2 (November):27–33.
2003 Diaspora and Comparison: The Global Irish as a Case Study. *The Journal of American History* 90(1):134–176.

2006 Race, Violence, and Anti-Irish Sentiment in the Nineteenth Century. In *Making the Irish American: History and Heritage of the Irish in the United States*, Joseph Lee and Marion R. Casey, editors, pp. 364–378. New York University Press, New York, NY.
2009 Twenty Years of Irish American Historiography. *Journal of American Ethnic History* 28(4):67–75.

Kinealy, Christine
2006 *This Great Calamity: The Irish Famine 1845–1852*, 2nd edition, revised from 1995 original publication. Gill & MacMillan, Dublin, Ireland.

Kleinman, Arthur
1986 *The Social Origins of Distress and Disease: Depression, Neurasthenia and Pain in Modern China*. Yale University Press, New Haven, CT.

Knobel, Dale T.
1986 *Paddy and the Republic*. Wesleyan University Press, Middletown, CT.
2001 "Celtic Exodus": The Famine Irish, Ethnic Stereotypes, and the Cultivation of American Racial Nationalism. *Radharc* 2:3–25.

Kraut, Alan
1994 *Silent Travelers, Germs, Genes, and the "Immigrant Menace."* Basic Books, New York, NY.
1995 Plagues and Prejudice: Nativism's Construction of Disease in Nineteenth- and Twentieth-Century New York City. In *Hives of Sickness: Public Health and Epidemics in New York City*, David Rosner, editor, pp. 65–90. Rutgers University Press, New Brunswick, NJ.
1996 Illness and Medical Care among Irish Immigrants in Antebellum New York. In *The New York Irish*, Ronald H. Bayor and Timothy J. Meagher, editors, pp. 153–168. Johns Hopkins University Press, Baltimore, MD.

Krieg, Joann P.
1992 *Epidemics in the Modern World*. Twayne, New York, NY.

Krochmal, A., R. S. Walters, and R. M. Doughty
1969 *A Guide to Medicinal Plants of Appalachia*. USDA Forest Service Research Paper NE-138. U.S. Forest Service <https://www.fs.usda.gov/nrs/pubs/rp/rp_ne138.pdf>. Accessed 27 March 2023.

Kunzle, David
1982 *Fashion and Fetishism: A Social History of the Corset, Tight-Lacing, and Other Forms of Body-Sculpture*. Rowman & Littlefield, Totowa, NJ.

Ladies of the Mission
1854   *The Old Brewery House and the New Mission House at the Five Points.* Stringer and Townsend, New York, NY.

Laird, Pamela Walker
1998   *Advertising Progress: American Business and the Rise of Consumer Marketing.* Johns Hopkins University Press, Baltimore, MD.

Lakoff, George, and Mark Johnson
1980   *Metaphors We Live By.* University of Chicago Press, Chicago, IL.

Larrabee, Eric
1971   *The Benevolent and Necessary Institution: An Informal History of a Great Teaching Hospital and the People Who Created It.* Doubleday and Co., Garden City, NY.

Larsen, Clark Spencer
2000   *Skeletons in Our Closet: Revealing Our Past Through Bioarchaeology.* Princeton University Press, Princeton, NJ.

Larsen, Eric
1994   A Boarding House Madonna—Beyond the Aesthetics of a Portrait Created through Medicine Bottles. *Historical Archaeology* 28(4):68–79.

Latour, Bruno
1992   Where Are the Missing Masses? The Sociology of a Few Mundane Artifacts. In *Shaping Technology/Building Society: Studies in Sociotechnical Change,* Wiebe E. Bijker and John Law, editors, pp. 225–258. MIT Press, Cambridge, MA.
1999   Give Me a Laboratory and I Will Raise the World. In *The Science Studies Reader,* Mario Biagioli, editor, pp. 258–275. Routledge, New York, NY.

Laurie, Bruce, Theodore Hershberg, and George Alter
1977   Immigrants and Industry: The Philadelphia Experience, 1850–1880. In *Immigrants in Industrial America 1850–1920,* Richard L. Ehrlich, editor, pp. 123–150. University Press of Virginia, Charlottesville.

Laxton, Edward
1996   *The Famine Ships: The Irish Exodus to America.* Bloomsbury, London, UK.

Leach, Maria (editor)
1949   *Funk and Wagnalls Standard Dictionary of Folklore, Mythology, and Legend,* Vol. 2. Funk and Wagnalls, New York, NY.

Leavitt, Judith W.
1992   "Typhoid Mary" Strikes Back: Bacteriological Theory and Practice in Early Twentieth-Century Public Health. *Isis* 83(4):608–629.

1999   Under the Shadow of Maternity: American Women's Responses to Death and Debility Fears in Nineteenth-Century Childbirth. In *Women and Health in America*, 2nd edition, Judith W. Leavitt, editor, pp. 328–346. University of Wisconsin Press, Madison.

Lee, J. J., and Marion Casey (editors)
2007   *Making the Irish American: History and Heritage of the Irish in the United States*. New York University Press, New York, NY.

Lees, Lynn Hollen
1979   *Exiles of Erin: Irish Migrants in Victorian London*. Cornell University Press, Ithaca, NY.

Leitman, I. M.
1991   The Evolution of Surgery at the New York Hospital. *Bulletin of the New York Academy of Medicine* 67(5):475–500.

Levin, Jed
1985   Drinking on the Job: How Effective Was Capitalist Work Discipline? *American Archaeology* 5(3):195–201.

Liem, E. B., T. V. Joiner, K. Tsueda, and D. I. Sessler
2005   Increased Sensitivity to Thermal Pain and Reduced Subcutaneous Lidocaine Efficacy in Redheads. *Anesthesiology* 102(3):509–14.

Lindsey, Bill
2020   Bottle/Glass Colors. In *Historic Glass Bottle Identification & Information Website*. Society for Historical Archaeology & Bureau of Land Management <https://sha.org/bottle/colors.htm>. Accessed 27 March 2023.
2021a   Bottle Typing/Diagnostic Shapes, Wine & Champagne Bottles. In *Historic Glass Bottle Identification & Information Website*. Society for Historical Archaeology & Bureau of Land Management <https://sha.org/bottle/wine.htm>. Accessed 27 March 2023.
2021b   Bottle Typing/Diagnostic Shapes, Soda & Mineral Water Bottles. In *Historic Glass Bottle Identification & Information Website*. Society for Historical Archaeology & Bureau of Land Management <https://sha.org/bottle/soda.htm>. Accessed 27 March 2023.
2021c   Bottle Typing/Diagnostic Shapes, Medicinal/Chemical/Druggist Bottles. In *Historic Glass Bottle Identification & Information Website*. Society for Historical Archaeology & Bureau of Land Management <https://sha.org/bottle/liquor.htm>. Accessed 27 March 2023.

Linn, Meredith B.
2008   *From Typhus to Tuberculosis and Fractures in Between: A Visceral Historical Archaeology of Irish Immigrant Life in New York City 1845–1870*. Doctoral Dissertation, Columbia University, New York, NY.

2010	Elixir of Emigration: Soda Water and the Making of Irish-Americans in Nineteenth-Century New York City. *Historical Archaeology* 44(4):69–109.
2014	Irish Immigrant Healing Magic in 19th-Century New York City. *Historical Archaeology* 48(3):144–165.
2019	The New York Irish: Fashioning Urban Identities in Nineteenth-Century New York City. In *Archaeology of Identity and Dissonance: Contexts for a Brave New World*, Diane F. George and Bernice Kurchin, editors, pp. 39–66. University Press of Florida, Gainesville, FL.
2022	Neither Snake Oils nor Miracle Cures: Interpreting Nineteenth-Century Patent Medicines. *Historical Archaeology* 56(4):681–702.

Little, David
2007	Hahnemann on Constitution and Temperament. *Homoeopathic Online Education* <http://www.simillimum.com/education/little-library/constitution-temperaments-and-miasms/hct/article04.php>. Accessed 27 March 2023.

Lobel, Cindy R.
2014	*Urban Appetites: Food and Culture in Nineteenth-Century New York*. University of Chicago Press, Chicago, IL.

Lock, Margaret M., and Judith Farquhar
2007	Introduction. In *Beyond the Body Proper: Reading the Anthropology of Material Life*, Margaret M. Lock and Judith Farquhar, editors, pp. 1–18. Duke University Press, Durham, NC.

Lock, Margaret M., and Vinh-Kim Nguyen
2018	*An Anthropology of Biomedicine*. Second. Wiley, Oxford, UK.

Logan, Michael H.
1973	Humoral Medicine in Guatemala and Peasant Acceptance of Modern Medicine. *Human Origins* 32(4):385–395.

Logan, Patrick
1963	Folk Medicine of the Cavan-Leitrim Area. *Ulster Folklife* 9:89–92.
1994	*Irish Country Cures*. Sterling Publishing Company, New York, NY. Reprinted from 1981 edition by Appletree Press, Belfast, UK.

Longworth's American Almanac (LAA)
1828	*Longworth's American Almanac, New York Register and City Directory, for the Fifty-Third Year of American Independence*. Thomas Longworth, New York, NY. New York Public Library Digital Collections, New York, NY <https://digitalcollections.nypl.org/items/1a60e720-3141-0136-677e-43204fe07e6c>. Accessed 27 March 2023.

1829   *Longworth's American Almanac, New York Register and City Directory, for the Fifty-Fourth Year of American Independence.* Thomas Longworth, New York, NY. New York Public Library Digital Collections, New York, NY <https://digitalcollections.nypl.org/items/a04bd020-973c-0136-7750-65cfeac8b95c>. Accessed 27 March 2023.

1830   *Longworth's American Almanac, New York Register and City Directory, for the Fifty-Fifth Year of American Independence.* Thomas Longworth, New York, NY. New York Public Library Digital Collections, New York, NY <https://digitalcollections.nypl.org/items/8c389d00-9a86-0136-f9d0-0514ab75291d>. Accessed 27 March 2023.

1841   *Longworth's American Almanac, New York Register and City Directory, for the Sixty-Sixth Year of American Independence.* Thomas Longworth, New York, NY. New York Public Library Digital Collections, New York, NY <https://digitalcollections.nypl.org/items/3d4349b0-4735-0136-39de-3584d3da32cb>. Accessed 27 March 2023.

Lönnroth, Knut, Brian G. Williams, Stephanie Stadlin, Ernesto Jaramillo, and Christopher Dye
2008   Alcohol Use as a Risk Factor for Tuberculosis: A Systematic Review. *BMC Public Health* 8(289):1–12.

Lupu, Jennifer A.
2022   "Cures after Doctors Fail": Marketing Pain Relief in 1900s Washington, DC. *Historical Archaeology* 56(4):703–721.

Lupu, Jennifer A. and Madeline Ryan (editors)
2022   Medicine and Bodily Care in 19th- and 20th-Century Contexts: Thematic Issue. *Historical Archaeology* 56(4):642–803.

Mac Cárthaigh, Crístóir
1988   Midwife to the Fairies: A Migratory Legend. Master's thesis, Department of Irish Folklore, National University of Ireland, University College Dublin, Dublin, Ireland.

MacLean, Mary
[1886–1900]   Manuscript, MS 11,428, Dr. E. E. R Green Letters, National Library of Ireland, Dublin, Ireland.

MacNamara, Donough Wheeler
1963   Do-It-Yourself Medicine in County Clare During the First Half of the Nineteenth Century. *Journal of the Irish Medical Association* LII:120–124.

MacNeven, Mary Jane
1842a   Biography of Dr. William James MacNeven. Manuscript, R. R. Maddon Papers, Special Collections, Trinity College, Dublin, Ireland.

1842b   What Dr. William James MacNeven Did for His Countrymen in
               America. Manuscript, R. R. Maddon Papers, Special Collections,
               Trinity College, Dublin, Ireland.

MacNish, Robert
1835   The Anatomy of Drunkenness. In *Curiosities of Literature*, Second
               Series, Isaac D'Israeli, editor, pp.57–96. William Pearson & Co.,
               New York, NY.

MacShane, Frank
1958   The Log of James Sutherland. *American Neptune* 18(4):306–14.

Maguire, John Francis
1864   *Father Mathew: A Biography*. D. & J. Sadlier and Company, Boston,
               MA.
1868   *The Irish in America*. D. & J. Sadlier, New York, NY. Reprinted
               1969 by Arno Press, New York, NY.

Mahon, Braid
1991   *Land of Milk and Honey: The Story of Traditional Irish Food and
               Drink*. Poolbeg Press, Dublin, Ireland.

Mahr, Susan
2022   Common Mullein, *Verbascum Thapsus*. Wisconsin Horticulture.
               University of Wisconsin, Madison <https://hort.extension.wisc
               .edu/articles/common-mullein-verbascum-thapsus/>. Accessed 27
               March 2023.

Majewski, Teresita, and David Gaimster (editors)
2009   *International Handbook of Historical Archaeology*. Springer, New
               York, NY.

Malaviya, A. N., and P. P. Kotwal
2003   Arthritis Associated with Tuberculosis. *Best Practice & Research
               Clinical Rheumatology* 17(2):319–343.

Malcolm, Elizabeth
1986   *Ireland Sober, Ireland Free: Drink and Temperance in Nineteenth-
               Century Ireland*. Gill and Macmillan, Dublin, Ireland.
1998   The Rise of the Pub: A Study in the Disciplining of Popular Culture.
               In *Irish Popular Culture, 1650–1850*, Kerby A. Miller and James S.
               Donnelly, editors, pp. 50–77. Irish Academic Press, Portland, OR.
1999   The House of Strident Shadows: The Asylum, the Family, and
               Emigration in Post-Famine Rural Ireland. In *Medicine, Disease,
               and the State in Ireland 1650-1940*, Elizabeth Malcolm and Greta
               Jones, editors, pp. 177–194. Cork University Press, Cork, Ireland.

Malcolm, Elizabeth, and Greta Jones (editors)
1999   *Medicine, Disease, and the State in Ireland 1650–1940*. Cork
               University Press, Cork, Ireland.

Maletnlema, T. N.
1992 Hunger and Malnutrition: The Determinant of Development: The Case for Africa and Its Food and Nutrition Workers. *East African Journal of Medicine* 69(8):424–427.

Maloney, Beatrice
1972 Traditional Herbal Cures in County Cavan. *Ulster Folklife* 18:66–79.

Manning, M. Chris
2014 The Material Culture of Ritual Concealments in the United States. *Historical Archaeology* 48(3):52–83.

Marsalic, Rafael Nicolas Cincu, Amit Agrawal, Nitin Dange, and Atul Goel
2007 Tincture Benzoin as an Antiseptic and Adhesive for Preoperative Surgical Preparation. *Neurology India* 55(1):88.

Matt, Susan J.
2007 You Can't Go Home Again: Homesickness and Nostalgia in U.S. History. *Journal of American History* 94(2):469–497.

Matthews, Christopher N.
2015 Whiteness and the Transformation of Home, Work, and Self in Early New York. In *The Archaeology of Race in the Northeast*, Christopher N. Matthews and Allison Manfra McGovern, editors, pp. 255–272. University Press of Florida, Tallahassee, FL.

Mayne, Alan, and Timothy Murray (editors)
2001 *The Archaeology of Urban Landscapes: Explorations in Slumland*. Cambridge University Press, Cambridge, UK.

Mayo Clinic Staff
2023 Fish Oil. Mayo Clinic. Mayo Foundation for Medical Education and Research <https://www.mayoclinic.org/drugs-supplements-fish-oil/art-20364810>. Accessed 27 March 2023.

McArthur, William P.
1956 The Medical History of the Famine. In *The Great Famine*, R. Dudley Edwards and T. Desmond Williams, editors, pp. 263–315. Browne & Nolan, Dublin, Ireland.

McCarthy Brown, Karen
1999 Staying Grounded in a High-Rise Building: Ecological Dissonance and Ritual Accommodation in Haitian Vodou. In *Gods of the City: Religion and the American Urban Landscape*, Robert A. Orsi, editor, pp. 79–102. Indiana University Press, Bloomington.

McCauley, Bernadette
2005 *Who Shall Take Care of Our Sick?* Johns Hopkins University Press, Baltimore, MD.

McClafferty, George
1979 The Folk Medicine of County Wicklow. Master's thesis, Department of Irish Folklore, University College Dublin, Dublin, Ireland.

McGowan, Gary
2000   Hidden Industries at Five Points. In *Tales of Five Points: Working-
              Class Life in Nineteenth Century New York, Vol. 2, An Interpretive
              Approach to Understanding Working-Class Life*, Rebecca Yamin,
              editor, pp. 305–313. John Milner Associates, West Chester, PA.

M'Clintock, Letitia
1912   Donegal Cures and Charms. *Folk-Lore Journal* 23:473–478.

McMahon, Cian T.
2015a   *The Global Dimensions of Irish Identity: Race, Nation, and the
              Popular Press 1840–1880*. University of North Carolina Press,
              Chapel Hill.
2015b   The Pages of Whiteness: Theory, Evidence, and the American
              Immigration Debate. *Race & Class* 56(4):40–55.
2021   *The Coffin Ship: Life and Death at Sea During the Great Irish
              Famine*. New York University Press, New York, NY.

McNeur, Catherine
2014   *Taming Manhattan: Environmental Battles in the Antebellum City*.
              Harvard University Press, Cambridge, MA.

Meehan, Andrew B.
1907   Balsam. *The Catholic Encyclopedia*, Vol. 2. Robert Appleton
              Company, New York, NY <http://www.newadvent.org/cathen
              /02226a.htm>. Accessed 27 March 2023.

Meskell, Lynn, editor,
2005   *Archaeologies of Materiality*. Wiley-Blackwell, Malden, MA.

Miller, Daniel, editor,
1998   *Material Cultures: Why Some Things Matter*. University of Chicago
              Press, Chicago, IL.

Miller, George L., Patricia Samford, Ellen Shlasko, and Andrew Madsen
2000   Telling Time for Archaeologists. *Northeast Historical Archaeology*
              29(1):1–22.

Miller, Kerby A.
1985   *Emigrants and Exiles: Ireland and the Irish Exodus to North
              America*. Oxford University Press, New York, NY.
1993   Paddy's Paradox: Emigration to America in Irish Imagination
              and Rhetoric. In *Distant Magnets: Expectations and Realities in
              the Immigrant Experience, 1840–1930*, Dirk Hoerder and Horst
              Roessler, editors, pp. 264–293. Holmes and Meyer, New York, NY.

Milne, Claudia
2000   Unhealthy New York: Sanitation and Health in the Tenements
              at Five Points. In *Tales of Five Points: Working-Class Life in
              Nineteenth-Century New York, Vol. 2, An Interpretive Approach
              to Understanding Working-Class Life*, Rebecca Yamin, editor, pp.
              341–370. John Milner Associates, West Chester, PA.

Milne, Claudia, and Pamela Crabtree
2000　　　　Revealing Meals: Ethnicity, Economic Status, and Diet at Five Points. In *Tales of Five Points: Working-Class Life in Nineteenth Century New York, Vol. 2, An Interpretive Approach to Understanding Working-Class Life*, Rebecca Yamin, editor, pp. 130–196. John Milner Associates, West Chester, PA.

Mitchell, Paul Wolff
2018　　　　The Fault in His Seeds: Lost Notes to the Case of Bias in Samuel George Morton's Cranial Race Science. *PLOS Biology* 16(10):e2007008 <https://doi.org/10.1371/journal.pbio.2007008>. Accessed 27 March 2023.

Mitchell, Samuel Augustus
1850　　　　*A New Universal Atlas Containing Maps of the Various Empires, Kingdoms, States and Republics of The World*. Thomas, Cowperthwait & Co., Philadelphia, PA. David Rumsey Map Collection, David Rumsey Map Center, Stanford Libraries, Creative Commons Attribution-Share Alike 3.0 Unported License <https://www.davidrumsey.com/luna/servlet/detail/RUMSEY~8~1~251292~5517507:City-of-New-York#>. Accessed 27 March 2023.

Mitchell, Silas Weir
1910　　　　*Works of S. Weir Mitchell: Characteristics*. The Century Company, New York, NY. Originally published in 1891.

Moerman, Daniel E.
2000　　　　Cultural Variations in the Placebo Effect: Ulcers, Anxiety, and Blood Pressure. *Medical Anthropology Quarterly* 14(1):51–72.
2002　　　　*Meaning, Medicine, and the "Placebo Effect."* Cambridge University Press, Cambridge, UK.

Mooney, James
1887　　　　The Medical Mythology of Ireland. *Proceedings of the American Philosophical Society* 24(125):136–166.

Mooney, Thomas
1850　　　　*Nine Years in America*. James McGlashan, Dublin, Ireland <https://books.google.com/books?id=TuBCAQAAMAAJ>.

Moran-Thomas, Amy
2013　　　　A Salvage Ethnography of the Guinea Worm: Witchcraft, Oracles, and Magic in a Disease Eradication Program. In *When People Come First: Critical Studies in Global Health*, João Biehl and Adriana Petryna, editors, pp. 207–239. Princeton University Press, Princeton, NJ.

Morris, Henry
1937   Features Common to Irish, Welsh, and Manx Folklore. *Beáloideas* 7:168–179.

Mott, Valentine
1862   *Pain and Anaesthetics: An Essay, Introductory to A Series of Surgical and Medical Monographs.* Sanitary Commission, Washington, DC. National Library of Medicine Digital Collections <http://collections.nlm.nih.gov/pdf/nlm:nlmuid-101202295-bk>.

Mrozowski, Stephen. A
2006   Environments of History: Biological Dimensions of Historical Archaeology. In *Historical Archaeology*, Martin Hall and Stephen Silliman, editors, pp. 23–41. Blackwell Publishing, Malden, MA.

Mrozowski, Stephen A., E.L. Bell, Mary C. Beaudry, D.B. Landon, and G.K. Kelso
1989   Living on the Boott: Health and Well-Being in a Boardinghouse Population. *World Archaeology* 21(2):298–319.

Mullins, Paul R.
1999   Race and the Genteel Customer: Class and African-American Consumption 1850–1930. *Historical Archaeology* 33(1):22–38.

Munson Chapman, Nancy
1997   Evidence for Spanish Influence on Activity-Induced Musculoskeletal Stress Markers at Pecos Pueblo. *International Journal of Osteoarchaeology* 7(5):498–509.

Murchison, Charles
1862   *A Treatise on the Continued Fevers of Great Britain.* Parker, Son, and Bourn, London, UK. Internet Archive <https://archive.org/details/treatiseoncontin1862murc>.

Murphy, Sherry L., Kenneth D. Kochanek, Jiaquan Xu, and Elizabeth Arias
2021   Mortality in the United States 2020. *National Center for Health Statistics Data Brief,* U.S. Department of Health and Human Services, Centers for Disease Control and Prevention <https://www.cdc.gov/nchs/data/databriefs/db427.pdf>. Accessed 27 March 2023.

Murray, John C.
1870   On the Nervous, Bilious, Lymphatic, and Sanguine Temperaments: Their Connection with Races in England, and Their Relative Longevity. *Anthropological Review* 8(28):14–28.

Murthy, J. M. K.
2010   Tuberculous Meningitis: The Challenges. *Neurology India* 58:716–722.

The National Cyclopedia of American Biography
1893   Barker, Fordyce. *The National Cyclopedia of American Biography, Vol. 4.* James T. White & Co., New York, NY. Google Books <https://www.google.com/books/edition/The_National_Cyclopedia_of_American_Biog/QsdKAAAAYAAJ>.

National Folklore Collection
2023   History of the National Folklore Collection <https://www.ucd.ie/irishfolklore/en/about/historyofnfc/>. Accessed 27 March 2023.

National Folklore Collection—Main Manuscripts Collection (NFC)
[ca. 1929]   Information reported in Baile Ádhaimh, County Laois, to Collector Áine bean Ní Ciarbaic. NFC 35, University College Dublin, Dublin, Ireland.
[ca. 1929]   Information reported in County Laois to Collector Áine bean Ní Ciarbaic. NFC 36, University College Dublin, Dublin, Ireland.
[1930s?]   Information reported in Kilworth, County Cork, to Collector L. Ó Floinn. NFC 128, University College Dublin, Dublin, Ireland.
[1930s?]   Information reported in Ceann Tuirc (Kanturk), County Cork, to Collector M. J. Bowman. NFC 132, University College Dublin, Dublin, Ireland.
1930   Information reported in County Longford to Collector Pádraig MacGréine. NFC 80, University College Dublin, Dublin, Ireland.
1935   Information reported in County Wexford to Collector Thomas O'Ciardha. NFC 54, University College Dublin, Dublin, Ireland.
1935   Information reported in County Wexford to Collector Caoimhín Ó Danachair. NFC 96, University College Dublin, Dublin, Ireland.
1935   Information reported in Cill Uird (Kilworth), County Cork, to Collector T. Ó Ciardha. NFC 107, University College Dublin, Dublin, Ireland. <https://www.duchas.ie/en/cbe/9001188>. Accessed 27 March 2023.
1935   Information reported in County Mayo to Collector S. P. Ó Piotáin. NFC 117, University College Dublin, Dublin, Ireland.
1935   Information reported in County Mayo to Collector S. P. Ó Piotáin. NFC 227, University College Dublin, Dublin, Ireland.
1935   Information reported in County Carlow to Collector Patrick O'Toole. NFC 265, University College Dublin, Dublin, Ireland.
1937   Information reported in Cappagh White/Cappawhite, County Tipperary, to Collector Peadar Mac Domhnaill. NFC 402, University College Dublin, Dublin, Ireland <https://www.duchas.ie/en/cbe/9000963>. Accessed 27 March 2023.
1937   Information reported in Cappagh White/Cappawhite, County Tipperary, to Collector Peadar Mac Domhnaill. NFC 407, University College Dublin, Dublin, Ireland <https://www.duchas.ie/en/cbe/9000963>. Accessed 27 March 2023.

1937	Information reported in County Sligo to Collector Brígid M. Ní Ghamhnáin. NFC 463, University College Dublin, Dublin, Ireland.
1938	Information reported in County Cork. NFC 514, University College Dublin, Dublin, Ireland.
1938	Information reported in Counties Tipperary and Limerick to Collector Peadar Mac Domhnaill. NFC 560, University College Dublin, Dublin, Ireland.
1941	Information reported in County Kerry to Collector P. J. O' Sullivan. NFC 782, University College Dublin, Dublin, Ireland.
1951	Information reported in County Tyrone to Collector Michael J. Murphy. NFC 1220, University College Dublin, Dublin, Ireland.
1953	Information reported in County Antrim to Collector Michael J. Murphy. NFC 1364, University College Dublin, Dublin, Ireland.
1955	Information reported in Glenariffe, County Antrim, to Collector Michael J. Murphy. NFC 1389, University College Dublin, Dublin, Ireland.
1974	Information reported in Counties Cavan, Armagh, and Fermanagh to Collector Michael J. Murphy. NFC 1837, University College Dublin, Dublin, Ireland.
1974	Information reported in Counties Cavan, Fermanagh, and Louth to Collector Michael J. Murphy. NFC 1838, University College Dublin, Dublin, Ireland.

National Folklore Collection—Folklore Photograph Collection

1930	Aran Boy on Rock, Inishmaan, Co. Galway. Folklore Photograph Collection, National Folklore Collection, E001.01.00001. UCD School of Irish, Celtic Studies, Irish Folklore and Linguistics. University College Dublin, Dublin, Ireland <https://digital.ucd.ie/view/ivrla:10395>. Accessed 27 March 2023.
1935	Interior of House of M. Breathnach, Maam Cross, Co. Galway. Folklore Photograph Collection, National Folklore Collection, A015.01.00686. UCD School of Irish, Celtic Studies, Irish Folklore and Linguistics. University College Dublin, Dublin, Ireland <https://digital.ucd.ie/view/ivrla:10247>. Accessed 27 March 2023.
1942	Seosamh Ó Dálaigh recording from Máire and Cáit Ruiséal. Ediphone, Dunquin, County Kerry. Folklore Photograph Collection, M001.18.00037. UCD School of Irish, Celtic Studies, Irish Folklore and Linguistics. University College Dublin, Dublin, Ireland <https://digital.ucd.ie/view/ivrla:10121>. Accessed 27 March 2023.

National Folklore Collection—Schools Manuscripts Collection (NFCS)

1937	Information reported in Bunralte Iocht, County Clare, to children from the Meelick B School in Meelick (Killeely) Parish, Teacher Eoghan Ó Néill, and to children from the Coradh Chaitlín School in

	Cora Chaitlín Parish, Teacher Eibhlín, Bean Mhic Conmara. NFCS 598, University College Dublin, Dublin, Ireland.
1937	Information reported in Ibrickan, County Clare, to children from the Cluain an Droma, Mullach School in Cill Mhuire Parish, Teacher Brian Ó Huiginn. NFCS 624, University College Dublin, Dublin, Ireland <https://www.duchas.ie/en/cbes/4922393>. Accessed 27 March 2023.
1937	Information reported in Upper Loughtee, County Cavan, to children from Laragh School B in Laragh Parish, Teacher P. Ó Briain. NFCS 981, University College Dublin, Dublin, Ireland <https://www.duchas.ie/en/cbes/5044849>. Accessed 27 March 2023.
1938	Information reported in Cill Críosta (Kilchrest), County Galway, to children from the Cill Críosta School in Cill Críosta Parish, Teacher Seán Ó Cléirigh. NFCS 35, University College Dublin, Dublin, Ireland.
1938	Information reported in Cill Chonaill (Woodlawn), Country Galway, to children from the Móta Ghráinne Óige School in Cnoc Breac Parish, Teacher Eibhlís Ní Innse. NFCS 45, University College Dublin, Dublin, Ireland.
1938	Information reported in Drumeela, County Leitrim, to children from Druim Míleadh School in Carraig Áluinn Parish, Teacher Ailbeard Mac an Ríogh. NFCS 229, University College Dublin, Dublin, Ireland <https://www.duchas.ie/en/cbes/4658463>. Accessed 27 March 2023.
1938	Information reported in Lismoyle, County Roscommon, to children from Lismoyle School in Kiltoome Parish, Teachers Seán Ó Súilleabháin and Eoghan Mac Seághain. NFCS 268, University College Dublin, Dublin, Ireland <https://www.duchas.ie/en/cbes/4811595>. Accessed 27 March 2023.
1938	Information reported in Lowertown, County Cork, to children from Lowertown Girls' School in An Goilín Parish, Teacher Maíre Bean Uí Mhathúna. NFCS 289, University College Dublin, Dublin, Ireland <https://www.duchas.ie/en/cbes/4921600>. 27 March 2023.
1938	Information reported in Múscraí Thoir (Muskerry East), County Cork, to children from Cluain Taiohg (Clontead) School in Achaoh Bolg (Magourney) Parish, Teacher Máire, Bean Uí Mhurchadha. NFCS 345, University College Dublin, Dublin, Ireland.
1938	Information reported in Dúithche Eala, County Cork, to children from Ceann Tuirc Convent School in Ceann Tuirc (Kanturk) Parish, Teachers An tSr. Seosamh and An tSr. Berchamans. NFCS 353,

	University College Dublin, Dublin, Ireland <https://www.duchas.ie/en/cbes/4921744>. Accessed 27 March 2023.
1938	Information reported in Dúithche Eala, County Cork, to children from Longueville Malla School in Baile na gCloch Parish, Teacher Caitlín Ní Dhonnchadha. NFCS 364, University College Dublin, Dublin, Ireland <https://www.duchas.ie/en/cbes/4921786>. Accessed 27 March 2023.
1938	Information reported in An Barrach Mór, County Cork, to children from Carraig Thuathail School in Carraig Thuathail Parish, Teacher John Bowdren. NFCS 385, University College Dublin, Dublin, Ireland <https://www.duchas.ie/en/cbes/4921870>. Accessed 27 March 2023.
1938	Information reported in Oighreacht Uí Chonchobhair, County Kerry, to children from Listowell School in Listowell Parish, Teacher Brian Mac Mathúna. NFCS 405, University College Dublin, Dublin, Ireland <https://www.duchas.ie/en/cbes/4613715> Accessed 27 March 2023.
1938	Information reported in Borrisokane, County Tipperary, to children from Buirgheas Uí Chatháin Convent School in Buirgheas Uí Chatháin Parish, Teacher Sr. M. Vincent. NFCS 532, University College Dublin, Dublin, Ireland <https://www.duchas.ie/en/cbes/4922129> Accessed 27 March 2023.
1938	Information reported in Bunraite Uacht, County Clare, to children from An Daingean (Dangan) School in An Cuinche (Quin) Parish, Teachers Stiofán Mac Clúin and Treasa Ní Chonmara. NFCS 596, University College Dublin, Dublin, Ireland <https://www.duchas.ie/en/cbes/5177641>. Accessed 27 March 2023.
1938	Information reported in Ibrickan, County Clare, to children from Mullach (Mullagh) School in Cill Mhuire Parish, Teachers Proinnsias Ó Sandair and Tomás Ó Conaill. NFCS 624, University College Dublin, Dublin, Ireland.
1938	Information reported in Lower Kells, County Meath, to children from Edengorra School in Kilmainham Parish, Teacher Michael Hetherton. NFCS 710, University College Dublin, Dublin, Ireland <https://www.duchas.ie/en/cbes/5008991>. Accessed 27 March 2023.
1938	Information reported in Slane, County Meath, to children from Slane C. School in Slane Parish, Teacher Josephine Cooney. NFCS 713, University College Dublin, Dublin, Ireland < https://www.duchas.ie/en/cbes/5009004>. Accessed 27 March 2023.

1938	Information reported in North Salt, County Kildare, to children from the Kildrought School in Kildrought (Celbridge) Parish, Teacher E. Ní Armhultaigh. NFCS 773, University College Dublin, Dublin, Ireland <https://www.duchas.ie/en/cbes/4742157>. Accessed 27 March 2023.
1938	Information reported in Robertstown, County Kildare, to children from Robertstown, Naas School in Kilmeague Parish, Teacher P. Ó Harachtáin. NFCS 775, University College Dublin, Dublin, Ireland < https://www.duchas.ie/en/cbes/4742168>. Accessed 27 March 2023.
1938	Information reported in Ferrybank, County Waterford, to children at Ferrybank, Waterford School in South Ida Parish, Teacher R. Ó Luinn. NFCS 844, University College Dublin, Dublin, Ireland < https://www.duchas.ie/en/cbes/4758496>. Accessed 27 March 2023.
1938	Information reported in Knocktopher, County Kilkenny, to children at Móin Ruadh School in Aghavillar Parish, Teacher Donnacha Ó Dochartaigh. NFCS 849, University College Dublin, Dublin, Ireland <https://www.duchas.ie/en/cbes/4758517>. Accessed 27 March 2023.
1938	Information reported in Upper Talbotstown, County Wicklow, to children from Knockanargon, Dunlavin School in Donaghmore Parish, Teacher Annie Draper. NFCS 916, University College Dublin, Dublin, Ireland <https://www.duchas.ie/en/cbes/5044718>. 27 March 2023.
1938	Information reported in Ballinacor North, County Wicklow, to children from Ballinacarrig Lower School in Rathdrum Parish, Teacher Bean Ní Dhubhghaill. NFCS 918, University College Dublin, Dublin, Ireland <https://www.duchas.ie/en/cbes/5044732>. Accessed 27 March 2023.
1938	Information reported in Ballinacor South, County Wicklow, to children from Rathcoyle Lower School in Baile Droichid (Kiltegan) Parish, Teacher Aodh Ó Broin. NFCS 920, University College Dublin, Dublin, Ireland.
1938	Information reported in Tír Aodha (Tullymore), County Donegal, to children from Carraig Na Heorna (Carricknahorna) School in Kilbarron Parish, Teacher Sibéal Nic Pháidín. NFCS 1028, University College Dublin, Dublin, Ireland <https://www.duchas.ie/en/cbes/4428256>. Accessed 27 March 2023.
1938	Information reported in Tír Aodha (Tullymore), County Donegal, to children from Tulach Mor School in Beal Atha Seanaigh (Kilbarron) Parish, Teachers Nora Nic an Ultaigh and Maighread

	Nic an Ultaigh. NFCS 1029, University College Dublin, Dublin, Ireland.
1939	Information reported in Upper Kells, County Meath, to children from the Woodpole School in Loughan Parish, Teacher Siobhán, Bean Uí Chonaill. NFCS 705, University College Dublin, Dublin, Ireland.
1939	Information reported in Talbotstown Lower, County Wicklow, to children from Valleymount School in Boystown Parish, Teacher Del. Ó Cochláin. NFCS 917, University College Dublin, Dublin, Ireland <https://www.duchas.ie/en/cbes/5044723>. Accessed 27 March 2023.
1939	Information reported in Kilmacrennan, County Donegal, to children from the Fothar (Faugher) School in Tuatha (Clondahorky) Parish, Teacher Bláthnaid Ní Fhannghaile. NFCS 1076, University College Dublin, Dublin, Ireland <https://www.duchas.ie/en/cbes/4493636>. Accessed 27 March 2023.

National Library of Medicine

1871	"New York Hospital Scene." Images from the History of Medicine, ID no. 101395240. National Library of Medicine, Bethesda, MD <http://resource.nlm.nih.gov/101395240>. Accessed 27 March 2023.
[1850–1900]	Advertisement for Mexican Mustang Liniment (trade card). Images from the History of Medicine, ID no. 101701641. National Library of Medicine, Bethesda, MD <http://resource.nlm.nih.gov/101701641>. Accessed 27 March 2023.

Neal, Frank

1998	*Black '47: Britain and the Famine Irish*. St. Martin's Press, New York, NY.

New York City Municipal Death Records

1861	Rachael McPeake. New York, *New York City Municipal Deaths, 1795–1949 Database*, film #447564, *FamilySearch* <https://www.familysearch.org/ark:/61903/1:1:2W4T-CZF>.

New York County Surrogate's Court

1910	In the Matter of Proving the Last Will and Testament of William L. Cole Deceased. *Record of Wills, 1665–1916*. Vol. 0887, Liber 193, pp. 224–225. Probate date Feb 7, 1910. Ancestry.com, Lehi, UT, 2015. <https://www.ancestry.com/sharing/2752161?mark=86faab47a2acb9747bac14ea59a28b1a871070c7c98ee513a8083221aa40649f>. Accessed 28 March 2023.

New-York Daily Times

1852a	Death of Dr. A. Sidney Doane. *New-York Daily Times* 28 January:2. New York, NY.

1852b	Metropolitan Perils. *New-York Daily Times* 28 September:4. New York, NY.
1852c	William Gee: Advertisement. *New-York Daily Times* 24 June:1. New York, NY.
1853	Lyon's Kathairon: Advertisement, *New-York Daily Times* 5 February:7. New York, NY.
1854	Rowland's Macassar Oil: Advertisement, *New-York Daily Times* 23 March:7. New York, NY.
1855	Hyatt's Life Balsam: Advertisement. *New-York Daily Times* 26 May:5. New York, NY.
1857a	Marsh's Radical Cure Truss: Advertisement. *New-York Daily Times* 9 May:5. New York, NY.
1857b	Lyon's Kathairon: Advertisement, *New-York Daily Times* 21 May:5. New York, NY.

New-York Daily Tribune
1844	Advertisement for Lubin Perfume at A. B. Sands & Co. *New-York Daily Tribune* 27 July:3. New York, NY.
1852	Work and Wages. *New-York Daily Tribune.* 15 October:4. New York, NY.

New York Dispensary Annual Reports (NYDAR)
1856	*The Annual Report of the Board of Trustees of the New York Dispensary.* Holman & Gray, New York, NY.
1857	*The Annual Report of the Board of Trustees of the New York Dispensary.* Miller and Holman, New York, NY.
1858	*The Annual Report of the Board of Trustees of The New-York Dispensary.* Dr. H. Gomez, editor. James Egbert, New York, NY.
1866	*The Annual Report of the Board of Trustees of The New-York Dispensary.* Dr. Godfrey Aigner, editor. John W. Amerman, New York.

New-York Evening Post
1830	Allay McPeake: Death Record. *New-York Evening Post* 27 July. New York, NY. *Newspaper Extractions from the Northeast, 1704-1930* [database online]. Ancestry.com. Provo, UT. Original data: Newspapers and Periodicals, American Antiquarian Society, Worcester, MA. <https://www.ancestry.com/sharing/2752251?mark=b4a1c6b3f470d9e17a47604c57cdf15c6ded5488d7b398565a748c2ad3e7d1ba>. Accessed 28 March 2012.
1844	Yellow Fever. *New-York Evening Post* 25 October:3. New York, NY.

[New York] Freeman's Journal and Catholic Register [NYFJ]
1854a	A. G. Bragg and Co.: Advertisement for Mexican Mustang Liniment. *Freeman's Journal and Catholic Register* 7 January:8. New York, NY.

1854b Udolpho Wolfe's Aromatic Schnapps: Advertisement. *Freeman's Journal and Catholic Register* 7 January:6. New York, NY.

1854c R. Dillon's Drugstore: Advertisement. *Freeman's Journal and Catholic Register* 1 July:6. New York, NY.

1854d Lyon's Magnetic Insect Powder: Advertisement. *Freeman's Journal and Catholic Register* 20 May:6. New York, NY.

1855 Gouraud's Liquid Hair Dye: Advertisement. *Freeman's Journal and Catholic Register* 12 May:8. New York, NY.

1860a Udolpho Wolfe's Aromatic Schnapps: Advertisement. *New York Freeman's Journal and Catholic Register* 3 November:5. New York, NY.

1860b Hegeman & Co. Cod Liver Oil: Advertisement. *New York Freeman's Journal and Catholic Register* 21 January:5. New York, NY.

New York Hospital (Annual Report) (NYHAR)

1835 *State of the New-York Hospital and Bloomingdale Asylum for the Year 1834.* Mahlon Day, Printer, New York, NY.

1836 *State of the New-York Hospital and Bloomingdale Asylum for the Year 1835.* Mahlon Day, Printer, New York, NY.

1837 *State of the New-York Hospital and Bloomingdale Asylum for the Year 1836.* Mahlon Day, Printer, New York, NY.

1838 *State of the New-York Hospital and Bloomingdale Asylum for the Year 1837.* Mahlon Day, Printer, New York, NY.

1839 *State of the New-York Hospital and Bloomingdale Asylum for the Year 1838.* Mahlon Day, Printer, New York, NY.

1840 *State of the New-York Hospital and Bloomingdale Asylum for the Year 1839.* Press of Mahlon Day & Co., New York, NY.

1841 *State of the New-York Hospital and Bloomingdale Asylum for the Year 1840.* Press of Mahlon Day & Co., New York, NY.

1842 *State of the New-York Hospital and Bloomingdale Asylum for the Year 1841.* Press of Mahlon Day & Co., New York, NY.

1843 *State of the New-York Hospital and Bloomingdale Asylum for the Year 1842.* Press of M. Day & Co., New York, NY.

1844 *State of the New-York Hospital and Bloomingdale Asylum for the Year 1843.* H. Ludwig, New York, NY.

1845 *State of the New-York Hospital and Bloomingdale Asylum for the Year 1844.* Egbert, Hovey, & King, New York, NY.

1846 *State of the New-York Hospital and Bloomingdale Asylum for the Year 1845.* Egbert, Hovey, & King, New York, NY.

1847 *State of the New-York Hospital and Bloomingdale Asylum for the Year 1846.* Egbert, Hovey, & King, New York, NY.

1848 *State of the New-York Hospital and Bloomingdale Asylum for the Year 1847.* Egbert, Hovey, & King, New York, NY.

1849   *State of the New-York Hospital and Bloomingdale Asylum for the Year 1848.* Egbert, Hovey, & King, New York, NY.
1850   *State of the New-York Hospital and Bloomingdale Asylum for the Year 1849.* Egbert & King, New York, NY.
1851   *State of the New-York Hospital and Bloomingdale Asylum for the Year 1850.* Egbert & King, New York, NY.
1852   *State of the New-York Hospital and Bloomingdale Asylum for the Year 1851.* Wm. C. Bryant & Co., New York, NY.
1853   *State of the New-York Hospital and Bloomingdale Asylum for the Year 1852.* Wm. C. Bryant & Co., New York, NY.
1854   *State of the New-York Hospital and Bloomingdale Asylum for the Year 1853.* Wm. C. Bryant & Co., New York, NY.
1855   *State of the New-York Hospital and Bloomingdale Asylum for the Year 1854.* Wm. C. Bryant & Co., New York, NY.
1856   *State of the New-York Hospital and Bloomingdale Asylum for the Year 1855.* Wm. C. Bryant & Co., New York, NY.
1857   *State of the New-York Hospital and Bloomingdale Asylum for the Year 1856.* Wm. C. Bryant & Co., New York, NY.
1858   *State of the New-York Hospital and Bloomingdale Asylum for the Year 1857.* Wm. C. Bryant & Co., New York, NY.
1859   *State of the New-York Hospital and Bloomingdale Asylum for the Year 1858.* Wm. C. Bryant & Co., New York, NY.
1860   *State of the New-York Hospital and Bloomingdale Asylum for the Year 1859.* Wm. C. Bryant & Co., New York, NY.
1861   *Report of the State of the New-York Hospital and Bloomingdale Asylum for the Year 1860.* Wm. C. Bryant & Co., New York, NY.
1862   *Report of the State of the New-York Hospital and Bloomingdale Asylum for the Year 1861.* Wm. C. Bryant & Co., New York, NY.
1863   *Report of the State of the New-York Hospital and Bloomingdale Asylum for the Year 1862.* Wm. C. Bryant & Co., New York, NY.
1864   *Report of the State of the New-York Hospital and Bloomingdale Asylum for the Year 1863.* Wm. C. Bryant & Co., New York, NY.
1865   *Report of the State of the New-York Hospital and Bloomingdale Asylum for the Year 1864.* Wm. C. Bryant & Co., New York, NY.
1866   *Report of the State of the New-York Hospital and Bloomingdale Asylum for the Year 1865.* Wm. C. Bryant & Co., New York, NY.

New York Hospital Medical Casebooks (NYHMCB)
1847–1853, 1865. Medical Casebooks. Medical Center Archives of New York-Presbyterian/Weill Cornell, New York, NY.

New York Hospital Surgical Casebooks (NYHSCB)
1848, 1851–1853, 1861–1862, 1865. Surgical Casebooks. Medical Center Archives of New York-Presbyterian/Weill Cornell, New York, NY.

New York Orthopaedic Dispensary Annual Reports (NYODAR)

1867 *Report of the Orthopaedic Dispensary.* Wm. C. Martin Printer, New York, NY.

1869 *First Annual Report of the New York Orthopaedic Dispensary, Located at 1299 Broadway.* Wm. C. Martin Printer, New York, NY.

1872 *Fourth Annual Report of the New York Orthopaedic Dispensary, Located at 1299 Broadway.* Wm. C. Martin Printer, New York, NY.

1876 *Eighth Annual Report of the New York Orthopaedic Dispensary, Located at 1299 Broadway.* Wm. C. Martin Printer, New York, NY.

New York Orthopaedic Dispensary Patient Records (NYODPR)
1870, 1871, 1872, 1873. Patient Records. Special Collections, Augustus C. Long Health Sciences Library, Columbia University Medical Center, New York, NY.

The New York Public Library

[1856–1870] St. Vincent's Hospital, (under the charge of the "Sisters of Charity,") corner of Eleventh Street and Seventh Avenue. Art and Picture Collection, The New York Public Library. New York Public Library Digital Collections <https://digitalcollections.nypl.org/items/510d47e0-d3d7-a3d9-e040-e00a18064a99>. Accessed 27 March 2023.

1868 The New York Dispensary, Northwest Corner of Centre and White Streets. Art and Picture Collection, The New York Public Library. New York Public Library Digital Collections <http://digitalcollections.nypl.org/items/510d47e0-d3c3-a3d9-e040-e00a18064a99>. Accessed 27 March 2023.

New York State Census (NYSC)

1855 Census Returns for the Sixth Ward of the City of New York in the County of New York. Manuscript, Department of Records and Information, Municipal Archives of the City of New York, New York, NY.

New York Times

1857 Hyatt's Life Balsam: Advertisement. *New York Times* 19 September:5. New York, NY.

1858a Radway's Ready Relief: Advertisement. *New York Times* 7 March:5. New York, NY.

1858b Hyatt's Life Balsam: Advertisement. *New York Times* 7 March:5. New York, NY.

1858c   The Physicians of New-York. *New York Times* 24 July:5. New York, NY.

1859   Hegeman & Co. Advertisement. *New York Times* 21 November:5. New York, NY.

1860   Rats at Bellevue Hospital—The Case of The New-Born Child Gnawed by Vermin—Investigation by The Commissioners of Public Charities—How the Hospital Is Overrun. *New York Times* 27 April:8. New York, NY.

1863   Hyatt's Life Balsam: Advertisement. *New York Times* 25 March:5. New York, NY.

1866a   Saratoga "A" Spring Water: Advertisement. *New York Times* 7 July:1. New York, NY.

1866b   Local Intelligence, Summer Drinks. What Soda Water is Made of. *New York Times* 7 July:2. New York, NY.

1868a   Advertisement for Lyon's Magnetic Insect Powder. *New York Times* 16 June:5. New York, NY.

1868b   Batchelor's Hair Dye: Advertisement. *New York Times* 16 June:5. New York, NY.

1870a   Lyon's Kathairon and Hagan's Magnolia Balm: Advertisement. *New York Times* 17 May:5. New York, NY.

1870b   The Drink of the Period. *New York Times* 29 August:6. New York, NY.

1871   Summer Drinks. *New York Times* 18 August, 1:2. New York, NY.

1877   The Grand Jury's Eyes Opened: The Necessity for a Small Lying-In Hospital—Bellevue Hospital in Deplorable Condition—Blackwell's Island Institutions a Public Disgrace. *New York Times* 30 March:8. New York, NY.

1878   More Illegal Whisky—A Still Seized in West Houston Street—Two Men and a Boy Captured. *New York Times* 26 June:8.

1879   A "Miracle" Accounted For. *New York Times* 7 September:12. New York, NY.

1883   Death of John Gelston. *New York Times* 20 January:3. New York, NY.

1893   In Honor of Dr. Fordyce Barker. *New York Times* 14 May:5. New York, NY.

1895   Not Witches, But Fairies. *New York Times* 22 April:4. New York, NY.

1908   Father Thomas Adams Dead; Attracted Attention by His Faith Cures—Once Removed from the Church. *New York Times* 23 November:9. New York, NY.

Ní Bhrádaigh, Cait

1936   Folklore from Co. Longford. *Béaloideas* 6:257–269.

Novak, Shannon A., and Alanna L. Warner-Smith
2020   Vital Data: Re/Introducing Historical Bioarchaeology. *Historical Archaeology* 54(1):1–16.

Numbers, Ronald, L.
1977   Do-It-Yourself the Sectarian Way. In *Medicine Without Doctors*, Guenter Risse, Ronald Numbers, and Judith Walzer Leavitt, editors, pp. 49–72. Science History Publications, New York, NY.

O'Brien, Eoin
1983   *Conscience and Conflict: A Biography of Sir Dominic Corrigan, 1802-1880*. The Glendale Press, Dublin, Ireland.

Ó Cadhla, Stiofan
2002   *The Holy Well Tradition: The Pattern of St. Declan, Ardmore, Co. Waterford, 1800-2000*. Four Courts Press, Dublin, Ireland.

O'Connell, Lucille
1980   Kealing Hurly's Scrip Book: An Irish Immigrant in America, 1847–48. *Éire-Ireland* 15(2):105–112.

O'Connor, Patrick
1943   Keogh's Blood. *Béaloideas* 13:278–279.

Ó Crualaoich, Gearóid
1998   The "Merry Wake" in Irish Popular Culture. In *Irish Popular Culture, 1650-1850*, Kerby A. Miller and James S. Donnelly, editors, pp. 173–200. Irish Academic Press, Portland, OR.
2003   *The Book of the Cailleach: Stories of the Wise-Woman Healer*. Reprinted 2021 by Cork University Press, Cork, Ireland.

Ó Danachair, Caoimhín
1955   The Holy Wells of County Limerick. *Journal of the Royal Society of Antiquaries of Ireland* 85:193–217 <https://archive.org/details/journalofroyalso1955roya/page/192/mode/2up>.

O'Donnell, L. A.
1997   *Irish Voice and Organized Labor in America*. Greenwood Press, Westport, CT.

O'Donovan, Jeremiah
1969   *Irish Immigration in the United States: Immigrant Interviews*. Arno Press and the New York Times, New York, NY. Original publication 1864.

Ó Giolláin, Diarmuid
1998   The Pattern. In *Irish Popular Culture 1650-1850*, James S. Donnelly and Kerby A. Miller, editors, pp. 201–221. Irish Academic Press, Portland, OR.

Ó Gráda, Cormac
1994   *Ireland: A New Economic History, 1780-1939*. Clarendon Press, Oxford, UK.

2000   *Black '47 and Beyond: The Great Irish Famine in History, Economy and Memory*. Princeton Economic History of the Western World. Princeton University Press, Princeton, NJ.
2005   The New York Irish in the 1850s: Locked in by Poverty? *New York Irish History* 19:5-13.

Ó Murchadha, Ciarán
2013   *The Great Famine: Ireland's Agony 1845-1852*. Bloomsbury Academic, London, UK.

Oleson, Charles
1896   *Secret Nostrums and Systems of Medicine*. Oleson & Co., Chicago, IL.

Online Archive of American Folk Medicine
2001   Online Archive of American Folk Medicine. University of California, Los Angeles <http://www.folkmed.ucla.edu/index.html>. Accessed 30 April 2012. (Website no longer exists, new version under renovation: See <https://humtech.ucla.edu/project/archive-of-ritual-healing-and-transformation/>). Accessed 5 May 2022.

O'Reilly, Thomas
1848   Letter. John M. Kelly Letters, MS 10,511. National Library of Ireland. Dublin, Ireland.

O'Regan, Paula
1997   *Healing Herbs in Ireland*. Primrose Press, Dublin, Ireland.

Orser, Charles E., Jr.
1996   *A Historical Archaeology of the Modern World*. Plenum Press, New York, NY.

Ortiz de Montellano, Bernard
1990   *Aztec Medicine, Health, and Nutrition*. Rutgers University Press, New Brunswick, NJ.

Oshinsky, David
2016   *Bellevue: Three Centuries of Medicine and Mayhem at America's Most Storied Hospital*. Anchor Books, New York, NY.

Ó Súilleabháin, Seán
1970   *A Handbook of Irish Folklore*. Spring Tree Press, Detroit, MI.
1977   *Legends from Ireland*. Rowman and Littlefield, Totowa, NJ <https://archive.org/details/legendsfromirelaoooosill/page/n5/mode/2up>.

Ott, Katherine
1996   *Fevered Lives: Tuberculosis in American Culture Since 1870*. Harvard University Press, Cambridge, MA.

Owen, Bruce
2004 Statistical Analysis of Bottle Data by General Categories. In *Putting the "There" There: Historical Archaeologies of West Oakland*, Adrian Praetzellis and Mary Praetzellis, editors, pp. G.1-G.32. Anthropological Studies Center, Sonoma State University, Rohnert Park, CA.

Owens, Gary
1998 Nationalism Without Words: Symbolism and Ritual Behavior in the Repeal "Monster Meetings" of 1843-5. In *Irish Popular Culture 1750-1850*, James S. Donnelly and Kerby A. Miller, editors, pp. 242-270. Irish Academic Press, Portland, OR.

Oxford English Dictionary
1989a Carron oil, n. *Oxford English Dictionary, 2nd edition*. Oxford University Press, Oxford, UK <https://www.oed.com/view/Entry/28244?redirectedFrom=carron+oil#eid>. Accessed 27 March 2023.
1989b Friar, n. *Oxford English Dictionary, 2nd edition*. Oxford University Press, Oxford, UK <https://www.oed.com/view/Entry/74600?redirectedFrom=friar%27s+balsam>. Accessed 27 March 2023.
2001a Miasma, n. *Oxford English Dictionary*, 3rd edition. Oxford University Press, Oxford, UK <http://www.oed.com/view/Entry/117825?redirectedFrom=miasma>. Accessed 27 March 2023.
2001b Merchant tailor, n. *Oxford English Dictionary*, 3rd edition. Oxford University Press, Oxford, UK <http://www.oed.com/view/Entry/116671?redirectedFrom=merchant+tailor>. Accessed 27 March 2023.
2017 Summer complaint, n. *Oxford English Dictionary*, 3rd edition. Oxford University Press, Oxford, UK <http://www.oed.com/view/Entry/193944?redirectedFrom=summer+complaint>. Accessed 27 March 2023.

New York Passenger Lists, 1820-1891
1827 *Ship Robert Fulton*. Arrived August 10, 1827, from Londonderry, Ireland. Records of the U.S. Customs Service, Record Group 36, Series M237, Roll 10, National Archives and Records Administration, Washington DC. "New York Passenger Lists, 1820-1891" database with images, *FamilySearch* <https://www.familysearch.org/ark:/61903/3:1:939V-KF9P-HQ?i=479&cc=1849782&personaUrl=%2Fark%3A%2F61903%2F1%3A1%3AQVPX-2NYG>. Accessed 28 March 2023.

Paster, Gail Kern
1998   Unbearable Coldness of Female Being: Women's Imperfection and the Humoral Economy. *English Literary Renaissance* 28(3):416–440.

Pavia, Charles S., Alexandra Pierre, and John Nowakowski
2000   Antimicrobial Activity of Nicotine against a Spectrum of Bacterial and Fungal Pathogens. *Journal of Medical Microbiology* 49:674–675.

Pearlstein, Kristen K.
2015   Health and the Huddled Masses: An Analysis of Immigrant and Euro-American Skeletal Health in 19th Century New York City. Doctoral Dissertation, American University, Washington DC.

Penny, Virginia
1863   *The Employments of Women: A Cyclopedia of Women's Work*. Walker, Wise, and Company, Boston, MA.

Pernick, Martin S.
1983   The Calculus of Suffering in Nineteenth-Century Surgery. *The Hastings Center Report* 13(2):26–36.
1985   *A Calculus of Suffering: Pain, Professionalism, and Anaesthesia in Nineteenth-Century America*. Columbia University Press, New York, NY.

Perris, William
1853   Plate 31: Map bounded by Spring Street, Mercer Street, Canal Street, Laurens Street. In *Maps of the City of New York*. William Perris, New York, NY. Lionel Pincus and Princess Firyal Map Division, The New York Public Library. New York Public Library Digital Collections <https://digitalcollections.nypl.org/items/510d47e0-c7e2-a3d9-e040-e00a18064a99>. Accessed 27 March 2023.

Pitts, Reginald H.
2000   "Suckers, Soap-Locks, Irishmen, and Plug-Uglies": Block 160, Municipal Politics, and Local Control. In *Tales of Five Points: Working-Class Life in Nineteenth-Century New York, Vol. 2, An Interpretive Approach to Understanding Working-Class Life*, Rebecca Yamin, editor, pp. 59–86. John Milner Associates, West Chester, PA.

Ponz, Jesse
2000   Bottle Embossments: The Trade and Industry. In *Tales of Five Points: Working-Class Life in Nineteenth-Century New York, Vol. 2, An Interpretive Approach to Understanding Working-Class Life*, Rebecca Yamin, editor, pp. 49–58. John Milner Associates, West Chester, PA.

Porter, Roy
1985   The Patient's View: Doing Medical History from Below. *Theory and Society* 14(2):175–198.
Porter, Roy (editor)
1990   *The Medical History of Waters and Spas.* Vol. Medical History, Supplement No. 10. The Wellcome Institute for the History of Medicine, London, UK.
Praetzellis, Adrian, and Mary Praetzellis
1998   Archaeologists as Storytellers. *Historical Archaeology* 32(1):94–96.
Praetzellis, Mary, and Adrian Praetzellis (editors)
2004   *Putting the "There" There: Historical Archaeologies of West Oakland.* Anthropological Studies Center, Sonoma State University, Rohnert Park, CA.
2009   South of Market: Historical Archaeology of 3 San Francisco Neighborhoods, The San Francisco-Oakland Bay Bridge West Approach Project. Report to California Department of Transportation, District 4, Oakland, CA, from Anthropological Studies Center, Sonoma State University, Rohnert Park, CA.
Preston, Margaret H., and Margaret ÓhÓgartaigh
2012   *Gender and Medicine in Ireland 1750–1900.* Syracuse University Press, Syracuse, NY.
Puck
1882   American Gold: Illustration by Frederick Burr Opper. *Puck* 24 May, 11(272):194. New York, NY.
1883   The Irish Declaration of Independence That We Are All Familiar With: Illustration by Frederick Burr Opper. *Puck* 19 May, 13(322):cover. New York, NY.
1889   The Mortar of Assimilation—and the One Element That Won't Mix. *Puck* 26 June. New York, NY.
1893   Looking Backward: They Would Close to the New-Comer the Bridge that Carried Them and their Father Over. *Puck.* 11 January. New York, NY.
Puckrein, Gary Alexander
1981   Humoralism and Social Development in Colonial America. *Journal of the American Medical Association* 245(17):1755–1757.
Pulling, Ezra R.
1865   Report of the Fourth Sanitary Inspection District. In *Report of the Council of Hygiene and Public Health of the Citizens' Association of New York upon the Sanitary Condition of the City*, Citizens' Association of New York, editor, pp. 43–65. D. Appleton & Co., New York, NY. Internet Archive <https://archive.org/details/reportcouncilhyoonygoog/page/n6>.

Punch
1867 The Fenian Guy Fawkes: Illustration by John Tenniel. *Punch* 28 December:263. London, UK.

Purdon, Dr. Henry S.
1895a Notes on Old Native Remedies. *Dublin Journal of Medical Science* C(3):214–218.
1895b Further Notes on Old Native Remedies. *Dublin Journal of Medical Science* C(3):293–296.
1898 Old Irish "Herbal" Skin Remedies. *Dublin Journal of Medical Science* 104:27–31.
1904 Cure for Consumption. *Ulster Journal of Archaeology* 10(1):41.

Pyne, Kate Lawless
1897 Folk-Medicine in County Cork. *Folklore* 8:179–180.

Quinlan, F. J. B.
1883 A Note upon the Use of the Mullein Plant in the Treatment of Pulmonary Consumption. *British Medical Journal* 1:149–150.

Quinlan, Marsha B.
2004 *From the Bush: The Front Line of Health Care in a Caribbean Village*. Wadsworth/Thomson Learning, Belmont, CA.

Quiroga, Virginia Anne Metaxes
1984 Poor Mothers and Poor Babies: A Social History of Childbirth and Childcare Institutions in Nineteenth Century New York City. Doctoral dissertation, State University of New York at Stonybrook, Stonybrook, NY.

Rabin, Bruce
1999 *Stress, Immune Function, and Health: The Connection*. Wiley-Liss, New York, NY.

Rajakumar, Kumaravel
2003 Vitamin D, Cod-Liver Oil, Sunlight, and Rickets: A Historical Perspective. *Pediatrics* 112:e132–e135.

Ravenstein, E. G.
1879 On the Celtic Languages of the British Isles: A Statistical Survey. *Journal of the Statistical Society of London* 42(3):579–643.

Ray, Celeste
2015 Paying the Rounds at Ireland's Holy Wells. *Anthropos* 110(2):415–432.

Raymer, Leslie E., Richard Fuss, and Cynthia Rhodes
2000 Macroplant Remains from the Five Points Neighborhood, New York City: A Study of Nineteenth-Century Urban Subsistence Patterns. In *Tales of Five Points: Working-Class Life in Nineteenth-Century New York, Vol. 2, An Interpretive Approach*

to Understanding Working-Class Life, Rebecca Yamin, editor, pp. 197–250. John Milner Associates, West Chester, PA.

Read, D. H. Moutray
1916 Some Characteristics of Irish Folklore. *Folklore* 27(3):250–278.

Real Estate Record and Builders Guide
1889 Mortgages and Assignments. *Real Estate Record and Builders Guide* 13 July (Vol. 44, No. 1113):996, New York, NY <https://www.google.com/books/edition/_/LZNRAAAAYAAJ>.
1899 Satisfied Mortgages—Manhattan. *Real Estate Record and Builders Guide* 2 Dec (Vol. 64, No.1655):859, New York, NY <https://www.google.com/books/edition/Real_Estate_Record_and_Builders_Guide/85RRAAAAYAAJ>.

Reckner, Paul
2000 Negotiating Patriotism at the Five Points: Clay Tobacco Pipes and Patriotic Imagery among Trade Unionists and Nativists in a Nineteenth-Century New York Neighborhood. In *Tales of Five Points: Working-Class Life in Nineteenth-Century New York, Vol. 2, An Interpretive Approach to Understanding Working-Class Life*, Rebecca Yamin, editor, pp. 99–110. John Milner Associates, West Chester, PA.
2002 Remembering Gotham: Urban Legends, Public History, and Representations of Poverty, Crime, and Race in New York City. *International Journal of Historical Archaeology* 6(2):95–112.

Reckner, Paul, and Stephen A. Brighton
1999 "Free From All Vicious Habits": Archaeological Perspectives on Class Conflict and the Rhetoric of Temperance. *Historical Archaeology* 33(1):63–86.
2000 "Free From All Vicious Habits": Archaeological Perspectives on Class Conflict and the Rhetoric of Temperance. In *Tales of Five Points: Working-Class Life in Nineteenth-Century New York, Vol. 2, An Interpretive Approach to Understanding Working-Class Life*, Rebecca Yamin, editor, pp. 441–459. John Milner Associates, West Chester, PA.

Reckner, Paul, and Diane Dallal
2000 The Long and the Short, Being a Compendium of Eighteenth and Nineteenth-Century Clay Tobacco Pipes from the Five Points Site, Block 160, New York. In *Tales of Five Points: Working Class Life in Nineteenth-Century New York, Vol. 6*, Rebecca Yamin, editor. John Milner Associates, West Chester, PA.

Rediker, Marcus
1987   *Between the Devil and the Deep Blue Sea: Merchant Seamen, Pirates, and the Anglo-American Maritime World, 1700–1750.* Cambridge University Press, New York, NY.

Reilly, Matthew C.
2019   *Archaeology Below the Cliff: Race, Class, and Redlegs in Barbadian Sugar Society.* University of Alabama Press, Tuscaloosa.

Reinhard, Karl J.
1994   Sanitation and Parasitism of Postbellum Harper's Ferry. *Historical Archaeology* 28(4):63–67.
2000   Parasitic Disease at Five Points: Parasitological Analysis of Sediments from the Courthouse Block. In *Tales of Five Points: Working-Class Life in Nineteenth-Century New York, Vol. 2, An Interpretive Approach to Understanding Working-Class Life,* Rebecca Yamin, editor, pp. 391–404. John Milner Associates, West Chester, PA.

Remington, Joseph P., and Horatio C. Wood
1918   *The Dispensatory of the United States of America,* 20th edition. Lippincott, Philadelphia, PA.

Risse, Guenter, Ronald L. Numbers, and Judith Walzer Leavitt (editors)
1977   *Medicine Without Doctors: Home Health Care in American History.* Science History Publications, New York, NY.

Roberts, Frederick
1884   *The Theory and Practice of Medicine.* Blakiston and Sons, Philadelphia, PA.

Robins, Joseph
1986   *Fools and Mad: A History of the Insane in Ireland.* Institute of Public Administration, Dublin, Ireland.
1995   *The Miasma: Epidemic and Panic in 19th Century Ireland.* Institute of Public Administration, Dublin, Ireland.

Robinson, Henry R.
1849   Mose, Lize & Little Mose Going to California. Print, ca. 1849. The Edward W. C. Arnold Collection of New York Prints, Maps and Pictures, Bequest of Edward W. C. Arnold, 1954. The Metropolitan Museum of Art, Accession Number: 54.90.1360 <https://www.metmuseum.org/art/collection/search/388715>. Accessed 27 March 2023.

Robinson, Victor
1946   *Victory Over Pain: A History of Anesthesia.* Henry Schuman, New York, NY.

Rode, Charles R.
1854   *The New-York City Directory, for 1853-1854*. Charles R. Rode, New York, NY. New York Historical Society, Patricia D. Kingenstein Library.

Roney, Frank
1931   *Frank Roney, Irish Rebel and California Labor Leader: An Autobiography*. University of California Press, Berkeley.

Roosa, D. B. St. John
1900   The Old New York Hospital. *The Post-Graduate* January 1900(1):6-21.

Rorabaugh, W. J.
1979   *The Alcoholic Republic: An American Tradition*. Oxford University Press, Oxford, UK.

Rosenberg, Charles E.
1974a   The Bitter Fruit: Heredity, Disease, and Social Thought in Nineteenth-Century America. In *From Consumption to Tuberculosis: A Documentary History*, Barbara Rosenkrantz, editor, pp. 154-194. Garland Press, New York.
1974b   Social Class and Medical Care in America: The Rise and Fall of the Dispensary. *Journal of the History of Medicine and Allied Sciences* 29:32-54.
1977   The Therapeutic Revolution: Medicine, Meaning, and Social Change in Nineteenth-Century America. *Perspectives in Biology and Medicine* 20(4):485-506.
1987a   *The Cholera Years: The United States in 1832, 1849, and 1866*. University of Chicago Press, Chicago, IL.
1987b   *The Care of Strangers: The Rise of America's Hospital System*. Basic Books, New York, NY.

Rosenwaike, Ira
1972   *Population History of New York City*. Syracuse University Press, Syracuse, NY.

Rosenzweig, Roy
1983   *"Eight Hours for What We Will": Workers and Leisure in an Industrial City, 1870-1920*. Cambridge University Press, New York, NY.

Rosner, David
1979   Business at the Bedside: Health Care in Brooklyn, 1890-1915. In *Health Care in America: Essays in Social Health*, Susan Reverby and David Rosner, editors, pp. 117-131. Temple University Press, Philadelphia, PA.

Rosner, David (editor)
1995　　　*Hives of Sickness: Public Health and Epidemics in New York City.* Rutgers University Press, New Brunswick, NJ.

Rothschild, Nan A.
2003　　　*Colonial Encounters in a Native American Landscape: The Dutch and Spanish in the New World.* Smithsonian Institution Press, Washington, DC.

Rothschild, Nan A., and Cynthia Robin
2002　　　Archaeological Ethnographies: Social Dynamics of Outdoor Space. *Journal of Social Archaeology* 2(2):159–172.

Rothschild, Nan A., and Diana diZerega Wall
2014　　　*The Archaeology of American Cities.* University Press of Florida, Gainesville.

Rowlands, Michael
1993　　　The Role of Memory in the Transmission of Culture. *World Archaeology* 25(2):141–151.

Rutto, Laban K., Yixyiang Xu, Elizabeth Ramirez, and Michael Brandt
2013　　　Mineral Properties and Dietary Value of Raw and Processed Stinging Nettle (*Urtica dioica* L.). *International Journal of Food Science* 2013, Article ID 857120, 9 pages <https://doi.org/10.1155/2013/857120>.

Sahlins, Marshall
2000　　　*Historical Metaphors and Mythical Realities: Structure in the Early History of the Sandwich Island Kingdom.* ASAO Special Publications No. 1. University of Michigan Press, Ann Arbor.

Said, Edward
1978　　　*Orientalism.* Pantheon Books, New York, NY.

Saint Vincent's Hospital Annual Reports (SVHAR)
1861　　　*Annual Reports of Saint Vincent's Hospital, under the Charge of The Sisters of Charity for the Years 1859–60*, William O'Meagher, editor. D. & J. Sadlier and Company, New York, NY.

1864　　　*Fourteenth Annual Report of Saint Vincent's Hospital Corner of 11th Street and 7th Ave under the Charge of The Sisters of Charity for the Year 1863.* John Lynch, editor. D. & J. Sadlier and Company, New York, NY.

1875　　　*Twenty-Fifth Annual Report of Saint Vincent's Hospital of the City of New York Corner of 11th Street and 7th Ave under the Charge of The Sisters of Charity for the Year Ending September 30th, 1874.* The NY Catholic Protectory Printing Dept., New York, NY.

1882　　　*Thirty-Second Annual Report of the Saint Vincent's Hospital of the City of New York for the Year Ending September 30, 1881.* John F. Luby, editor. The NY Catholic Protectory, New York, NY.

Salazar, James B.
2010   *Bodies of Reform: The Rhetoric of Character in Gilded Age America.*
        New York University Press, New York, NY.
Salwen, Bert, and Rebecca Yamin
1990   The Archaeology and History of Six Nineteenth Century Lots:
        Sullivan Street, Greenwich Village, New York City. Report to New
        York University Law School, New York, NY, from Department of
        Anthropology, New York University, New York, NY.
Scally, Robert
1995   *The End of Hidden Ireland.* Oxford University Press, New York, NY.
Schablitsky, Julie
2006   Genetic Archaeology: The Recovery and Interpretation of Nuclear
        DNA from a Nineteenth-Century Hypodermic Syringe. *Historical
        Archaeology* 40(3):8–19.
Scheper-Hughes, Nancy
2001   *Saints, Scholars, and Schizophrenics: Mental Illness in Rural
        Ireland, 20th anniversary edition,* updated and expanded.
        University of California Press, Berkeley.
Scheper-Hughes, Nancy, and Margaret M. Lock
1987   The Mindful Body: A Prolegomenon to Future Work in Medical
        Anthropology. *Medical Anthropology Quarterly New Series* 1(1):
        6–41.
Schmidt, Robert A., and Barbara L. Voss (editors)
2000   *Archaeologies of Sexuality.* Routledge, London, UK.
Schrire, Carmel
1995   *Digging Through Darkness: Chronicles of an Archaeologist.*
        University Press of Virginia, Charlottesville.
Schroeder-Lein, Glenna R.
2008   *The Encyclopedia of Civil War Medicine.* Routledge, New York, NY.
Schütz, Katrin, Carle Reinhold, and Andreas Schieber
2006   Taraxacum: A Review on Its Phytochemical and Pharmacological
        Profile. *Journal of Ethnopharmacology* 107(3):313–323.
Science
1885   The Consumptive Period. *Science* 6(127) July 10:35.
Scientific American
1847   Typhus Fever. *Scientific American* 25 September:43.
The Select Committee of the Senate of the United States
1854   Report of the Select Committee of the Senate of the United States
        on the Sickness and Mortality on Board Emigrant Ships.
        Washington, DC. Internet Archive <https://archive.org/details
        /101092405.nlm.nih.gov/page/n1>.

Sexton, Sean
1994   *Ireland in Old Photographs.* Bulfinch Press, New York, NY.
Sharp, Lesley
2000   The Commodification of the Body and Its Parts. *Annual Review of Anthropology* 29:287–328.
Shaw, Douglas V.
1977   Political Leadership in the Industrial City: Irish Development and Nativist Response in Jersey City. In *Immigrants in Industrial America 1850–1920*, Richard L. Ehrlich, editor, pp. 85–95. University Press of Virginia, Charlottesville.
Shumsky, Neil L. (editor)
1976   Frank Roney's San Francisco: His Diary, April, 1875–March, 1875. *Labor History* 17(2):245–264.
Singer, Merrill, Hans Baer, Debbi Long, and Alex Pavlotski
2020   *Introducing Medical Anthropology: A Discipline in Action*, 3rd edition. Roman & Littlefield, Lanham, MD.
Singh, M., M. L. Mynak, L. Kumar, J. L. Mathew, and S. K. Jindal
2005   Prevalence and Risk Factors for Transmission of Infection among Children in Household Contact with Adults Having Pulmonary Tuberculosis. *Archives of Disease in Childhood* 90(6):624-628.
Smith, Nicole L.
2008   *The Problem of Excess Female Mortality: Tuberculosis in Western Massachusetts, 1850–1910.* University of Massachusetts Amherst, Amherst.
Smith, William
1850   *An Emigrant's Narrative; or A Voice from the Steerage.* William Smith, New York, NY.
Snively, J. H.
1872   Soda-Water: What It Is, and How It Is Made. *Harper's New Monthly Magazine.* 45(267):341–346. New York, NY.
Sofaer, Joanna R.
2006   *The Body as Material Culture: A Theoretical Osteoarchaeology.* Cambridge University Press, Cambridge, UK.
Sontag, Susan
2001   *Illness as Metaphor and AIDS and Its Metaphors.* Picador USA, New York, NY.
Southworth, Albert Sands and Josiah Johnson Hawes
1847   Use of Ether for Anesthesia, daguerreotype. The J. Paul Getty Museum, 84.XT.958, Getty Open Content Program, Los Angeles, CA <https://www.getty.edu/art/collection/object/1040HZ>. Accessed 27 March 2023.

Spillers, Hortense
1987   Mama's Baby, Papa's Maybe: An American Grammar Book. *Diacritics* 17(2):64–81.

Stallybrass, Peter, and Allon White
1986   *The Politics and Poetics of Transgression.* Cornell University Press, Ithaca, NY.

Stansell, [Mary] Christine
1986   *City of Women: Sex and Class in New York, 1789–1860.* Alfred A. Knopf, New York, NY.

Stelmack, Robert M., and Anastasios Stalikas
1991   Galen and the Humour Theory of Temperaments. *Personality and Individual Differences* 12(3):255–263.

Stewart, James
1846   *A Practical Treatise on the Diseases of Children*, 3rd edition. Harper, New York, NY. HathiTrust Digitial Library, Original from University of Chicago <https://babel.hathitrust.org/cgi/pt?id=chi.69880891>.
1854   *A Practical Treatise on the Diseases of Children: Including an Introductory Chapter on the Management of Infants in Health.* Harper & Bros., New York, NY. HathiTrust Digital Library, Original from The Ohio State University <https://babel.hathitrust.org/cgi/pt?id=osu.32436001921228>.

Stillé, Alfred
1861   Reviews [of Four Current Books on Phthisis Pulmonalis and Scrofula]. *The American Journal of the Medical Sciences* 42(83):137–181.

Stivers, Richard
2000   *Hair of the Dog: Irish Drinking and Its American Stereotype.* Continuum, New York, NY. Revised from 1976 edition published by Penn State University Press, University Park.

Stott, Richard B.
1990   *Workers in the Metropolis: Class, Ethnicity, and Youth in Antebellum New York City.* Cornell University Press, Ithaca, NY.

Stowe, Harriet Beecher
1852   *Uncle Tom's Cabin.* Clark & Co., London, UK. Smithsonian Libraries <https://library.si.edu/digital-library/book/uncletomsoostow>.

Strang, Veronica
2005   Common Senses: Water, Sensory Experience and the Generation of Meaning. *Journal of Material Culture* 10(1):92–120.

Strauss, Erwin
1966   Upright Posture. In *Phenomenological Psychology: The Selected Papers of Erwin W. Strauss*, 137–165. Basic Books, New York, NY.

Stuart, George Reilley
1938   *A History of St. Vincent's Hospital in New York City*. Alumnae Association of the St. Vincent's Hospital School of Nursing, New York, NY.

Sugg, Richard
2015   *Mummies, Cannibals and Vampires: The History of Corpse Medicine from the Renaissance to the Victorians*, 2nd edition. Routledge, New York, NY.

Sugrue, Thomas J.
2014   *The Origins of the Urban Crisis: Race and Inequality in Postwar Detroit: With a New Preface by the Author*, updated from the original 1996 edition. Princeton University Press, Princeton, NJ.

Sullivan, Stephen Jude
2013   A Social History of the Brooklyn Irish, 1850–1900. Doctoral dissertation, Department of History, Columbia University, New York, NY. University Microfilms International, Ann Arbor, MI.

Sundar, Shyam, and Jaya Chakravarty
2010   Antimony Toxicity. *International Journal of Environmental Research and Public Health* 7(12): 4267–4277.

Taussig, Michael
1993   *Mimesis and Alterity: A Particular History of the Senses*. Routledge, New York, NY.

Tetherston, Maryann
1864   Letter dated 20 December, MS 4824-32, Purdon Papers, Special Collections, Trinity College, Dublin, Ireland.

Thomas, F.
1830   On Temperament. *The Medico-Chirurgical Review and Journal of Practical Medicine* 13:1–23.

Thomas, Nicholas
1991   *Entangled Objects: Exchange, Material Culture and Colonialism in the Pacific*. Harvard University Press, Cambridge, MA.

Thompson, E. P.
1967   Time, Work, Discipline, and Industrial Capitalism. *Past and Present* 38:56–97.

Thoms, William F.
1865   Report of the Sixth Sanitary Inspection District. In *Report of the Council of Hygiene and Public Health of the Citizens' Association of New York upon the Sanitary Condition of the City,*

pp. 73–84. Citizens' Association of New York. D. Appleton & Co., New York, NY. Internet Archive <https://archive.org/details/reportcouncilhyoonygoog/page/n6>.

Tomlins, Christopher L.
1988   A Mysterious Power: Industrial Accidents and the Legal Construction of Employment Relations in Massachusetts, 1800–1850. *Law and History Review* 6(2):375–438.

Townsend, Peter S.
1847   Daily Register of the Medical and Surgical Practice of P. S. Townsend M.D. of New York. Archives & Special Collections, Augustus C. Long Health Sciences Library, Columbia University, New York, NY.

Trow's New-York City Directory
1859   *Trow's New-York City Directory for the Year Ending May 1, 1860*. Compiled by H. Wilson. John F. Trow, New York, NY. New York Public Library Digital Collections, New York, NY <https://digitalcollections.nypl.org/items/4f239540-52bb-0134-5039-00505686a51c>.

Turker, Arzu Ucar, and N. D. Camper
2002   Biological Activity of Common Mullein, a Medicinal Plant. *Journal of Ethnopharmacology* 82(2–3):117–125.

United States Bureau of the Census (USBC)
1830   *Population Schedules of the City of New York in the County of New York of the Fifth Census of the United States, 1830*. U.S. Bureau of the Census, Washington, DC.
1840   *Population Schedules of the City of New York in the County of New York of the Sixth Census of the United States, 1840*. U.S. Bureau of the Census, Washington, DC.
1850   *Population Schedules of the City of New York in the County of New York of the Seventh Census of the United States, 1850*. U.S. Bureau of the Census, Washington, DC.
1860   *Population Schedules of the City of New York in the County of New York of the Eighth Census of the United States, 1860*. U.S. Bureau of the Census, Washington, DC.
1870   *Population Schedules of the City of New York in the County of New York of the Ninth Census of the United States, 1870*. U.S. Bureau of the Census, Washington, DC.

Valentine, David Thomas
1860   *Manual of the Corporation of the City of New York for 1860*. McSpedon & Baker, New York, NY. Columbia University Libraries via Internet Archive <https://archive.org/details/ldpd_6864652_011>.

Van der Geest, Sjaak, and Susan Reynolds Whyte
1989 The Charm of Medicines: Metaphors and Metonyms. *Medical Anthropology Quarterly, New Series* 3(4):345–367.
Van der Geest, Sjaak, Susan Reynolds Whyte, and Anita Hardon
1996 The Anthropology of Pharmaceuticals. *Annual Review of Anthropology* 25:153–178.
Verling, Martin (editor)
2003 *Beara Women Talking: Folklore from the Beara Peninsula*. Mercer Press, Douglas Village, Ireland.
Virginia Tech
2022 Virginia Tech Weed Identification Guide. College of Agriculture and Life Sciences <https://weedid.cals.vt.edu/profile/346>. Accessed 27 March 2023.
Vogel, Morris J.
1979 The Transformation of the American Hospital, 1850–1920. In *Health Care in America: Essays in Social Health*, Susan Reverby and David Rosner, editors, 105–116. Temple University Press, Philadelphia, PA.
1985 Patrons, Practitioners, and Patients: The Voluntary Hospital in Mid-Victorian Boston. In *Sickness and Health in America: Readings in the History of Medicine and Public Health*, Judith W. Leavitt and Ronald L. Numbers, editors, pp. 323–333. University of Wisconsin Press, Madison.
Vogel, Morris J., and Charles Rosenberg
1979 *The Therapeutic Revolution: Essays in the Social History of American Medicine*. University of Pennsylvania Press, Philadelphia.
Wailoo, Keith
2001 *Dying in the City of the Blues: Sickle Cell Anemia and the Politics of Race and Health*. University of North Carolina Press, Chapel Hill.
Wall, Barbara Mann
2005 *Unlikely Entrepreneurs: Catholic Sisters in the Hospital Marketplace*. Ohio State University Press, Columbus, OH.
Wall, Diana di Zerega
1994 *The Archaeology of Gender: Separating the Spheres in Urban America*. Plenum, New York, NY.
Walsh, Sister Marie de Lourdes
1965 *With a Great Heart: The Story of St. Vincent's Hospital and Medical Center of New York 1849–1964*. St. Vincent's Hospital and Medical Center of New York, New York, NY.
Walter, Frederick A.
[1895–1905] City Home, Two women with wooden pails scrub the entry to South Pavilion, Blackwell's Island, Photograph. Department

of Public Charities (DPC): Charities & Hospitals Collection, dpc_0468, Municipal Archives, City of New York <https://nycma.lunaimaging.com/luna/servlet/detail/RECORDSPHOTOUNIT ARC~20~20~561624~111726>. Accessed 27 March 2023.

Warner-Smith, Alanna
2022 Working Hands, Indebted Bodies: Embodiment of Labor and Inequality in an Era of Progress. Doctoral dissertation, Department of Anthropology, Syracuse University, Syracuse, NY.

Watkins, Rachel J.
2012 Biohistorical Narratives of Racial Difference in the American Negro: Notes toward a Nuanced History of American Physical Anthropology. *Current Anthropology* 53(Supplement 5):S196–S209.

Waugh, Samuel Bell
[1855] *The Bay and Harbor of New York*. Oil on canvas. Gift of Mrs. Robert M. Littlejohn, 1933. 33.169.1. Museum of the City of New York, New York, NY.

Weiner, Mark
2002 Consumer Culture and Participatory Democracy: The Story of Coca-Cola During World War II. In *Food in the USA: A Reader*, Carole Counihan, editor, pp. 123–141. Routledge, New York, NY.

Weir, Robert Fulton.
1917 *Personal Reminiscences of the New York Hospital from 1856 to 1900*. New York Hospital, New York, NY.

Wells, Samuel R.
1866 *New Physiognomy*. Fowler and Wells, New York, NY.

Westropp, Thomas J.
2000 *Folklore of Clare*. Clasp Press, Ennis, Ireland.

White, John
1870 *Sketches from America*. Sampson Low, Son, and Marston, London, UK.

White, Luise
2000 *Speaking With Vampires: Rumor and History in East and Central Africa*. University of California, Berkeley, CA.

White, Richard
1991 *The Middle Ground: Indians, Empires, and Republics in the Great Lakes Region, 1650–1815*. Cambridge University Press, Cambridge, UK.

Whyte, Robert
1848 *The Ocean Plague: Or, A Voyage to Quebec in an Irish Emigrant Vessel : Embracing a Quarantine at Grosse Isle in 1847: With Notes Illustrative of the Ship-Pestilence of That Fatal Year*. Coolidge and Wiley, Boston, MA <https://books.google.co.uk/books?id=aJ5s6a DoekIC>.

Wilczak, Cynthia, Rachel Watkins, Michael L. Blakey, Christopher C. Null, and Lesley M. Rankin-Hill
2004 Skeletal Indicators of Work: Musculoskeletal, Arthritic, and Traumatic Effects. In *The New York African Burial Ground Project*, Vol. 1, Part 1, Michael L. Blakey, editor, pp.199–226. Howard University Press for US General Services Administration, Washington, DC <https://www.gsa.gov/about-us/regions/welcome-to-the-northeast-caribbean-region-2/about-region-2/african-burial-ground/introduction-to-african-burial-ground-fina-reports>. Accessed 27 March 2023.

Wilde, Lady [Jane Francesca Agnes]
1887a *Legends, Mystic Charms, and Superstitions of Ireland*. Vol. 1. Tickenor & Co, Boston, MA.
1887b *Ancient Legends, Mystic Charms, and Superstitions of Ireland*. Vol. 2. Ticknor & Co., Boston, MA.
1890 *Ancient Cures, Charms, and Usages of Ireland: Contributions to Irish Lore*. Ward and Downey, London, UK <https://archive.org/details/cu31924098811023>.

Wilde, William R.
1849 A Short Account of the Superstitions and Popular Practices Relating to Midwifery and Some of the Diseases of Women and Children in Ireland. *Monthly Journal of Medical Science* 9(5):713.
1852 *Irish Popular Superstitions*. Irish University Press, Dublin, Ireland. Reprinted 1973 by Roman and Littlefield, Totowa, NJ <https://archive.org/details/irishpopularsupeooooowild>.
1856 *The Census of Ireland for the Year 1851. Part V. The Tables of Death: Dublin*. Alexander Thom for HMSO, Dublin, Ireland.

Wilkie, Laurie
1996 Medicinal Teas and Patent Medicines: African-American Women's Consumer Choices and Ethnomedical Traditions at a Louisiana Plantation. *Southeastern Archaeology* 15(2):119–31.
2000 Magical Passions: Sexuality and African-American Archaeology. In *Archaeologies of Sexuality*, Robert A. Schmidt and Barbara L. Voss, editors, pp. 129–142. Routledge, New York, NY.
2003 *The Archaeology of Mothering: An African American Midwife's Tale*. Routledge, New York, NY.
2009 Interpretive Historical Archaeologies. In *International Handbook of Historical Archaeology*, Teresita Majewski and David Gaimster, editors, pp. 333–345. Springer, New York, NY.

Williams, Susan
1985 *Savory Suppers and Fashionable Feasts: Dining in Victorian America*. Pantheon Books, New York, NY.

Wilson, Leonard G.
2005   Commentary: Medicine, Population, and Tuberculosis. *International Journal of Epidemiology* 34(1):521–24.

Wilson, Thomas George
1943   Some Irish Folklore Remedies for Diseases of the Ear, Nose, and Throat. *Irish Journal of Medical Science* 18(6):180–184.

Wirth, Louis
1938   Urbanism as a Way of Life. *The American Journal of Sociology* 44(1):1–24.

Wood Hill, Marilyn
1993   *Their Sisters Keepers: Prostitution in New York City, 1830–1870.* University of California Press, Berkeley.

Woodham-Smith, Cecil
1962   *The Great Hunger: Ireland 1845–1849.* Harper & Row, New York, NY.

Woods-Panzaru, Simon, David Nelson, Graham McCollum, Linda M. Ballard, B. Cherie Millar, Yasunori Maeda, Colin E. Goldsmith, Paul J. Rooney, Anne Loughrey, Juluri R. Rao, and John E. Moore
2009   An Examination of Antibacterial and Antifungal Properties of Constituents Described in Traditional Ulster Cures and Remedies. *Ulster Medical Journal* 78(1):13–15.

Yamin, Rebecca
1998   Lurid Tales and Homely Stories of New York's Notorious Five Points. *Historical Archaeology* 32(1):74–85.
2001   Alternative Narratives: Respectability at New York's Five Points. In *The Archaeology of Urban Landscapes: Explorations in Slumland*, Alan Mayne and Timothy Murray, editors, pp. 154–170. Cambridge University Press, London, UK.
2005   Wealthy, Free, and Female: Prostitution in Nineteenth-Century New York. *Historical Archaeology* 39(1):4–18.

Yamin, Rebecca (editor)
1999   *With Hope and Labor: Everyday Life in Paterson's Dublin Neighborhood, Vol. 1–4, Data Recovery on Blocks 863 and 866 within the Route 19 Connector Corridor in Paterson, New Jersey.* John Milner Associates, West Chester, PA.
2000[1]   *Tales of Five Points: Working-Class Life in Nineteenth-Century New York, Vol. 1, A Narrative History and Archaeology of Block 160*, Rebecca Yamin, editor, John Milner Associates, West Chester, PA.
2000[2]   *Tales of Five Points: Working-Class Life in Nineteenth-Century New York, Vol. 2, An Interpretive Approach to Understanding Working-Class Life*, Rebecca Yamin, editor, John Milner Associates, West Chester, PA.

2000[3]   *Tales of Five Points: Working-Class Life in Nineteenth-Century New York, Vol. 3, Documentary Data*, Rebecca Yamin, editor, John Milner Associates, West Chester, PA.

2000[4]   *Tales of Five Points: Working-Class Life in Nineteenth-Century New York, Vol. 4, Basic Artifact Inventory, the Courthouse Block (Block 160)*, Parts One and Two, Rebecca Yamin, editor, John Milner Associates, West Chester, PA.

2000[5]   *Tales of Five Points: Working-Class Life in Nineteenth-Century New York, Vol. 5, Conservation of Materials from the Courthouse Block (Block 160)*, Rebecca Yamin, editor, John Milner Associates, West Chester, PA.

2000[6]   *Tales of Five Points: Working-Class Life in Nineteenth-Century New York, Vol. 6, The Long and the Short, Being a Compendium of Eighteenth- and Nineteenth-Century Clay Tobacco Pipes from the Five Points Site, Block 160, New York City*, Rebecca Yamin, editor, John Milner Associates, West Chester, PA.

Yen, Y. F., M. Y. Yen, Y. S. Lin, Y. P. Lin, H. C. Shih, L. H. Li, P. Chou, and C. Y. Deng
2014   Smoking Increases Risk of Recurrence after Successful Anti-Tuberculosis Treatment: A Population-Based Study. *The International Journal of Tuberculosis and Lung Disease* 18(4):492–498.

Young, James Harvey
1961   *The Toadstool Millionaire: A Social History of Patent Medicines in America before Regulation*. Princeton University Press, Princeton, NJ.

Zausner, Philip
1941   *Unvarnished: The Autobiography of a Union Leader*. Brotherhood, New York, NY.

INDEX

Page numbers in **boldface** refer to illustrations.

Adams, Thomas [Father], 40, 127–28, 346n21. *See also* priests

advertisements, 166, **167**, 177, **199**, 201–3, 213–21, **216**, **218**, 224–28, 231, 297–304, **299**, 315–16, 320, 333, 363n24, 370nn54–55, 371n66, 372nn68–70. See also *Citizen, The*; *Harper's Weekly*; *New York [Daily] Times*; *New York Freeman's Journal (and Catholic Register)*

African Americans, 15, 69, 219, 348n29; medical practices, 194, 201, 295; presence in New York City, 15, 47, 135, 295, 325, 336, 339n2, 348n29, 378n44; racism against, 70–71, 94–95, 135, 173–74, 325, 341n7, 350n16, 351n19, 352n25, 377n41, 377n44, 386n57; terminology, 339n2; use of brand-name goods, 201, 219

age, 49, 59, 72, 74, 143, 226, 232, 316, 321, 353n33, 359n31, 386n2; and Irish healers 32, 123–26, 342n11; and labor-related injuries 134–36, 148, 164, 360n2; and physicians' treatments, 21–30, 86, 361n13; and tuberculosis 234, 250–57, 260–62, 375nn28–29, 376n36; and typhus fever 352n33, 356n16

alcohol, 65, 95, 111, 112–18, 121, 128, 198, 207, 248, 306–7, 313, 318, 323, 372n68, 377n40, 382nn26–27; and anesthesia, 170, 174–75, 269, 332, 363n24; in Irish popular medicine, 34, 97, 104–5, 112, 126, 164, 211, 345n16; Irish social uses of, 114–17, 126, 128, 258; physicians' uses of, 81, 105; withdrawal, 80, 149, 151–52, 317. *See also* liquor bottles; whiskey

alcoholism, 80, 82, 94, 174, 317, 321, 323, 363n24; and anti-Irish prejudice, 80, 82, 89, 94, 113, 174, 269, 317, 331–32. *See also* whiskey

Alcott, Louisa May, 270

almshouses, 83, 155, 165

American individualism, 258, 334

American professional medicine, 22–31. *See also* ethnomedicine

"American wake," 321. *See also* wakes

amputations, 149–52, 212, 217, 371n62; infections of, 156–58; mortality rates, 158, 176, 363n21; surgical procedures, 132, 157–58, 168, 172–73, 362n19, 363n20; use of anesthesia, 132, 172–76

anemia, 149, 162, 191, 250, 323, 351n19, 380n10, 383n38, 385n48

anesthesia, 158, 169–70, **171**, 172–79, 222, 331; debates about use, 132, 170–80, 363n25; poisoning, 170, 173; reactions with alcohol, 174, 363n26

Anglo-Saxon myth, 65, 78, 94, 335; "race" and British identification with, 75–77, 351n23. *See also* Celtic anti-Irish sentiment: in caricatures and cartoons, 54, **66**, 67–68, 82, 91, **92**, 93, 140, **141**, 229, **230**, 275–77, 294, 325, 335, 350n17, 352n26, 353n37, 378n45; in comparisons to animals, 68, 91, 94, 140–42, 173; in hospitals, 8, 54, 55, 89, 129, 170, 173–75, 322, 331, 353n34. *See also* Anglo-Saxon myth; Celtic; Keppler, Joseph; Nast, Thomas; nativism, American; Opper, Frederick Burr; political cartoons; *Puck*; *Punch*; race "science"

antimony, 23, 29, 35–36, 45, 236

apothecaries. *See* pharmacists

appearance, physical, 9, 11, 13, 26, 29, 65, 69, 72, 145, 154, 160, 266, 269, 278, 337, 367n21; in American reactions to Irish immigrants, 6, 67, 69, 82, 89, 132, 140, 144, 168–69, 224, 268, 271–72, 328–31; in humoral theory, 77, 82, 93, 140; in urban environments, 132, 168, 229, **230**; ways Irish immigrants altered theirs, 10, 223–31, 271, 278, 334. *See also* corsets; cosmetics; clothing; fashion

assimilation, 55, 224–25, 276, 335

Astor House, 21, 29, 46; injuries to Irish servants employed at, 28, 150

Australia, 4, 144, 217, 285, 336, 361n10

balsams, 19, 197–98, 202–6, 213, 217–18, 297–300, 382n28; in the Catholic Church, 209–10; 282–86, 299, 379n5; Friar's Balsam, 209–10, 298; Hyatt's Infallible Life Balsam, 204, 206, 209, 217–18, 297–300; Turlington's Balsam of Life, 197–98, 204–6, 209, 217

baptism, 282–86, 299, 379

Barker, Benjamin Fordyce, 371n61

Barrington, Jonah, 123

Batchelor's Hair Dye, 224, 226, 371n65, 372n69

beer, 81, 115, 149, 258, 386n56; bottles, 112, **118**, **122**

Belfast (city), 6, 100, 224, 320, 368n41

Bellevue Hospital, 13, 63, 64, 83, 88, 148, 152, 172, 212, 235–36, 264, 335, 357n21;

364n32, 371n61, 373n11; Irish immigrant admissions to, 131, **149–52**, 159–60, 162, 164, 178, 181, 195, 226, 241, 250, 251–55, 291, 320, 352n28; reputation of, 53, 352n28

bewitchment, 34, 40, 103, 280–87, 298–99, 345n14, 359n34, 372n72, 379n8

bioarchaeology, 15, 132, 143–45, 155, 165, 330, 353n34

bitters, 201–11, 222, 297, 382n26; Hostetter's Stomach Bitters, 198, 204, 206, 211, 219, 370n60, 382n26

Black Americans. *See* African Americans

blood, 8, 26, 31, 41–43, 52, 60, 76, 77, 90, 120, 149, 156, 168, 211, 235, 268, 269, 275, 315, 327, 347n25, 353n35, 354n3, 365n7, 366n16, 368n42, 369n46, 371n62; in humoral theory, 27, 73, 80, 82, 140; purification of, 184, 190, 211, 289, 293, 297–98, 345n17, 382nn26–27; used in Irish popular cures, 185, 187, 191, 290, 371n62, 382n18

boarders, 21, 30–33, 42, 46–51, 121, 135, 148, 245, 252, 256, 288, 303, 359n32, 374n16

boarding houses, 19–21, **24**, 31, 33, 35, 46–49, 53, 56–57, 64, 98, 102, 136, 329, 348n30

bogtrotter, **66**, 91, 175

bone (human), changes to, 15, 143–47, 155, 165, 187–88, 234, 241, 363n20, 367nn20–21

"Bone Bill," 145, 353n34

bonesetters, 20, 122, 187–89, 197, 366n20; families of, 42, 187–88, 366n20

Boston Pilot, 285, 363n24, 371n63

braces. *See* hernias

brandy, 2, 30, 32, 34, 37, 90, 104, 120, 170, 177, 345n16, 363n27

Bridget (stereotype), 91, 140, 223, 230, 250, 269, 272, 275, 331, 353n37. *See also* Pat (stereotype)

British government, 1, 66, 115

broken bones. *See* fractures

bronchitis, 22, 51–52, 149, 152, 377n39, 380n10

bruises, 99, 155, 362n16, 379n6, 384n45; treatment of, 38, 182, 184, 190, 196, 314

burns, 9, 52, **147**, 151, 154, 168, 181, 191, 207, 209; rates in New York Hospital, 155, 196; treatment of, 38, 42, 183, 187, 190, 192–93, 195–96, 209, 359n36, 364n2, 365nn8–9, 368n42, 369n43, 369n50, 379n6. *See also* carron oil; injuries

bursitis, 144, 149, 151, 165, 364n7; treatment of, 164, 184

Cabrini Medical Center. *See* Columbus Hospital

calomel, 35, 90

camphorated oil, 34, 291, 345n16

Canada, 4, 57, 79, 217, 336, 359n35, 386n2; Quebec, 1, 11, 21, 58, 59, 317, 354n2, 363n27

capitalism, 138–39, 258, 268, 347n25

carron oil, 154–55, 196, 369n50

Castle Garden, **5**, 64

Catholic: healing practices, 40, 127–28, 179, 209–10, 241, 310, **311**, 312, 346n21; hospitals, 10, 128; leaders, 8, 127, 259, 313; rituals, 40, 120, 210, 241, 285–86, 299, 310, **311**; values, 179, 258–59, 304, 362n18. *See also* baptism; Hughes, Angela [Sister]; Hughes, John [Archbishop]; MacNeven, William; Mathew, Theobald [Father]; Sisters of Charity; St. Vincent's Hospital; wakes

Catholicism, 55, 120; feast days, 39, 185, 191, 284, 310; Irish immigrant participation in, 6, 34, 127, 286, 342n13. *See also* Transfiguration Church

Catholics, prejudice against, 4, 65–67, 71, 93, 127, 140, 177, 319, 340n5, 354n3, 356n13. *See also* Penal Laws

Celtic, 14, 39, 43, 75–78, 124, 275, 310, 335, 351n23, 352n27; race and Irish identification with, 76–77, 275

Ceylon (ship), 59, 98

changeling, 39, 281–85, 379n7, 385n53. *See also* fairies: capture by

charm cures, 40, 42–43, 52, 123, 187, 345n19, 358n30, 360n3; fever charms, 105–6, 345n19; sign of the cross, 32, 39, 185, 282, 284, 344n8, 379n5, 385n53

chemists. *See* pharmacists

children: education of, 47, 119, 136, 223; illnesses and injuries suffered by, 51, 156, 158, 163, 242, 248, 254–55, 345n14, 375n24, 379n3; of Irish immigrants, 239, 255–56, 274–75, 278; labor, 47, 133, 136; mortality, 254, 282; toys, 119, 136; trouble fitting in, 226. *See also* age; fairies; orphans

chloroform. *See* anesthesia

cholera, 1–2, 21, 27, 28, 50, 58–59, 72, 99, 101, 104, 160, 225, 234, 246, 260–61, 263, 343n5, 359n35, 378n44; *infantum*, 336, 375n24

choleric temperament, 27, 73, 351n23, 352n27

chronic injury/pain. *See* injuries

Citizen, The, 221, 350n11, 362n16, 371n66

citizenship, 65, 70; American notions of, 6, 68–70; Irish eligibility for, 6, 65–72, 93–94, 140

City Hall, 46, 83

Civil War (American): hospitals in New York, 84, 128, 359n35, 374n11; Irish soldiers 275, 336, 341n7, 378n46

class: middle, 54, 68–69, 92, 107, 112, 118, 119, 142, 211, 225, 227–28, 245, 259, 272, 274, 306–18, 321, 324, 330, 339n2, 341n9, 347n25, 371n66; upper, 59, 67, 92, 136, 142, 144, 173, 198, 252, 267, 286, 341n9, 347n25, 386n56; working, 3, 5, 12, 15, 20, 26, 54, 58, 65, 77, 90, 93, 95, 107, 113–19, 123, 132, 136, 140–48, 156, 163–64, 170, 221–28, 248–49, 252–56, 260–61, 271, 275, 302, 309, 334, 337, 339n2, 340n5, 347n25, 350n15, 352n33, 356n16, 374n14, 386n56

climate, of New York, 137, 159, 360n4. *See also* frostbite; sunstroke

cloth: red flannel, 185, 366n16, 382n29; St. Brigid's (*Brath Bridhe*), 185; used in Irish popular medicine, 38, 105, 184, 191, 345n16, 356n18 clothing, 10, 40, 43, 69, 195, 247, 271, 273, 278, 334, 377n40; aboard ships, 6, 60–61, 67, 355n7; immigrant advice about, 223–24, 350n14, 355n7; and typhus, 60–61, 355n7; working-class, 159, 224–27, 229–30, 248, 252, 360n6. *See also* fashion

cod liver oil, 19, 202–6, 218, 220, 280, 303–5, 383n34, 383n35; Hegeman's Cod Liver Oil, 203–4, 206, 210, 218, 220, 303, 305; popular uses in Europe, 36, 183, 210, 266; for tuberculosis, 210, 236, 266

College of Physicians and Surgeons, 21, 83, 343n1

colors in Irish healing: green, 299–300; red, 120, 185, 345n16, 366n16, 382n29

Columbia-Presbyterian Medical Center, 167

Commissioners of Emigration, 57, 62–64, 83, 85, 90, 263, 348n2, 349n3

community, 1, 10, 44, 48, 98, 102, 114, 137, 220, 239, 277, 286–88, 310, 314, 317, 323, 324, 334, 347n25. *See also* Irish communities

consumption. *See* phthisis; tuberculosis

consumptive diathesis, 263–72, 278, 377n41

contusions, **147**, 163, 168, 374n12. *See also* injuries

Cork (city), 59, 100, 209, 313, 355n9

Cornell University Medical College. *See* New York Hospital

corsets, 228. *See also* clothing; fashion

cosmetics, 10, 19, 223, 231; face powders, 226, 271; hair preparations and oils, 224–29, 334, 371nn65–66, 372nn68–70, 372n73; perfumes, 224, 229, 371nn65–66. *See also* appearance

cough medicine: Irish popular remedies, 34, 41, 122, 190–91, 290–91, 345n16, 364n1, 368n40, 380n10, 381n22, 382n29; patent medicines, 202, 204–6, 293, 297–98, **299**. *See also* J. R. Stafford's Olive Tar

Coyle, Jug, 123. *See also* wisewomen

Darwin, Charles, 68, 264

debility, 150, 160, 164, 168, 212, 298, 307, 373n8

delirium tremens. *See* alcohol: withdrawal

Democratic Party, Irish support for, 46, 49, 67, **114**, 140

diaspora, 76, 309, 321, 322, 340n6; Irish, 4, 217, 275, 334. *See also* Irish communities

dispensaries, 13, 100, 125–27, 148, 152, 166–67, 179, 197, 222, 229, 235, **237**, 239, 242, 260, 264, 331, 333, 343n2, 355n10, 356n11, 362n14, 373n10; German Dispensary, 146, 334; New York Dispensary, 13, 53, 235, 237, 239, **240**, 242, 293; New York Orthopaedic Dispensary, 13, 125, 148, 152, 166–67, 222, 229, 264, 375n23, 376n36; shortage of bottles, 222

Doane, Sidney, 348n3, 349n10

domesticity, 69–70, 118–19, 306

domestic servants, 69, **92,** 70, 140, 169, 225, 227, 294, **295,** 330–31, 367n24; illnesses and injuries sustained by, 148, **149,** 155, 165, 252, 255; wages, 135, 252–53; working conditions, 135, 137, 159–60, **165,** 178, 252

donnybrooks, 163, 313

Draft Riots, 275, 331, 377n44, 378n44, 386n57

Draper, John 353n34

druggists. *See* pharmacists

Dublin (city) 6, 139, 159, 209, 252, 265, 291, 305, 342n10, 347n27, 355n9, 356n14, 371n63, 384n42; Dublin (city), medical care in, 35, 100–101, 220–21, 302, 355n10. *See also* Ireland, counties

Dublin Quarterly Journal of Medical Science, 120, 353n33

Duffe, James, 137, 177 *See also* nurses; Sisters of Charity

dysentery, 27, 50, 56, 99, 151

Early, Biddy, 123, 300. *See also* wisewomen

education, 70, 74, 76, 119, 161, 177, 223, 302, 386n57; Irish attitudes towards, 43, 199, 136; role in humoral theory, 378n44. *See also under* children

eel oil, 183, 191, 364n2
Emerald Isle, 33, 318
Emigrant Savings Bank, 17, 134, 164, 189, 342n13, 347n27, 348n32, 385n50
emigration from Ireland to America: assisted, 67, 68, 102, 331, 348n33, 350n15, 355n7; conditions of, 6, 63, 67, 85, 96–97, **98**, 99–100, 314, 354nn1–4, 355nn5–7; expectations of America, 99, 129, 133, 176–77, 223, 355n8
enchantment. *See* bewitchment
England, 4, 15, 47, 57, 59, 75–78, 81, 97–98, 119, 127, 134, 170, 197, 207, 209, 265–66, 270, 304, 313, 332, 336, 348n2, 353n33, 356n17, 370n53, 374n14, 376n34, 377n38, 381n17, 382n26, 385n48. *See also* Liverpool; London Hospitals
Erie Canal, 137, 360n4
Erie Railroad, 146, 154, 161, 367n23
erysipelas, 150, 156–57, 169; treatment for, 39, 187, 191
ether. *See* anesthesia
ethical medicine bottles. *See* prescription medicine bottles
ethnomedicine, 21, 33–34, 37, 329. *See also* heroic medicine; humoral theory; Irish popular medicine
Eva Eve, 272, **273**, 274, 278
evil eye. *See* bewitchment

faction fights. *See* donnybrooks
fairies, 33–34, 103, 123, 280–87, 298, 312, 359n34, 366n16, 379n2, 382n29; beliefs about in the U.S., 33, 40, 285, 344n8,10; capture by, 40–42, **43**, 280, 281–84, 287, 299, 379n7; protection from, 39–40, **43**, 281–85, 344n8, 344n10, 385n53, 378n8, 384n42. *See also* bewitchment; changeling; fairy doctors; Irish popular medicine; wisewomen
fairy doctors, 42, 282, **283**. *See also* healers, Irish popular; wisewomen
fashion, 6, 93, 223, 226, 228–29, 247, 278, 350n14, 377n40; middle class, 67, **92**, 271;

working class, 67, 226, **227**, 229, **230**. *See also* clothing
Fenians, 68, 275
fever: camp/gaol/ship/hospital, 56–57, 349n3, 358n25; and Great Famine, 57; heart, 187, 289, 290; intermittent, 150–52, 161; Irish popular cures, 35, 37, 39, 42, 104–7, 110, 112–13, 120–22, 126–28; remittent, 87, 90, 352n32; simple, 86–88, 90. *See also* charm cures; Irish fever; malaria; typhoid fever; typhus fever
Fitch, Samuel Sheldon, 301–2
Five Points: excavation of, 12, 15, **16–17**, 107–8, **109–111**, 112, 117–18, 126, 180, 190–96, 200–211, **212**, 213–18, 226–305, **306**, 313–14, 318, 357n20, 367nn23–24, 368n31, 368n33, 369n44, 370n57, 370n61, 371n65, 382nn26–27, 383n36, 385n49, 385n51; population of, 17, 47, 254–55, 342n10, 342n13; reputation of, 15
folklore, 9, 12, 33–35, 40, 96, 103–4, 182–84, 207, 256, 279–80, 283–90, 312, 329, 333, 341nn9–10, 342nn10–11, 344n14, 345n18, 347n25, 359n34, 364n7, 365n9, 366nn15–16, 366n19, 379n2, 379n5
food markets, 133, 191–92, **249**, 295, 358n23; dangers of, 248
fractures (broken bones), 9, 144–45, 148–52, 154–55, 163–64, 168, 212, 362n16, 373n8, 374n12; rates in New York Hospital, **147**, 236, 361n12; treatment of by Irish bonesetters, 42, 187–88. *See also* bonesetters; injuries
France, 15, 158, 170, 270, 381n17, 386n56
Frank Leslie's Illustrated Newspaper, 51, **64**
Friar's Balsam. *See under* balsams
friendship, Irish conception of, 114, 142, 294, **295**, 324, 362n18. *See also* throughother; rural: Irish views
frostbite, 149, 158–59, 169
funeral rites. *See* wakes

Gaelic speakers. *See* Irish language
Galway (city), 100, 209

462 Index

gangrene, 149–50, 156–58, 365n9. *See also* hospitalism
gender, 261, 268; and medical care, 86, 170, 173, 256; demographics of Irish immigrants, 86, 253, 256, 260; discrimination, 69, 77, 135, 253; racial nationalism, 77–78; rates of tuberculosis by, 253–56; roles, 124, 253
German Dispensary. *See under* dispensaries
German immigrants, 64, 85, 87–88, 90, 112, 115, 145–46, 159, 168, 175, 192, 202–3, 210, 222, 236, **238**, 245, 318, 334, 336–37, 349n8, 353n32, 368n40, 369n44
Germany/German States, 15, 56, 177, 305
germ theory, 3, 8, 156, 235, 263, 336
Godfrey's Cordial, 198, 204, 206, 211–13, 297, 370n53
goose grease: and Christmas, 38–39, 183; in healing in Ireland, 34, 38–39, 105, 183, 345n16, 356n18, 364n3; in healing in New York City, 32, 36–37, 110, 191, 291; material properties, 38–39, 364n3
Graves, Robert, 35, 353n36
Great Famine, the, 1–2, 4, 35, 45, 54, 57, 77, 144–45, 236, 340n4, 354n4, 385n48
Greenwich Mews, 318, 370n58, 371n66
Griscom, John, 59, 98, 172

hair, red, 82, 91, 140, 174–75, 226, 268, 284, 372n70, 372n72
Harper's Weekly, 68, 101, **114**, 123, 166, 214, 228–29, **230**, **249**, **257**, 272, **273**, 294, **295**, **308**, 316, 319, 350n17, 378n44, 384n47, 386n56; advertisements in, **167**, 218–19, 298, **299**, 300, 371n66; readership of, 274, 303
Hawthorne, Nathaniel, 68
healers, Irish popular, 26, 41–45, 112, 189, 197, 290. *See also* bonesetters; fairy doctors; herb doctors; midwives; posthumous children; priests; seventh son/daughter; wisewomen
heat stroke. *See* sunstroke
Hegeman and Co. drugstores, 206, 218–19, 220, 302–3, 305, 384n40

Hegeman's Cod Liver Oil. *See under* cod liver oil
herb doctors, 32, 42, 122. *See also* healers, Irish popular
herbs used medicinally. *See* plants used medicinally
heredity, 9, 25, 73, 79, 103, 143, 264, 267, 277
hernias, 150, 164–66; braces for, **167**, 228
heroic medicine, 26, 172, 306
historical archaeology, 11–12
holy places, 11, 39, 106, 182; St. Bridget's Chair, **186**. *See also* holy wells
holy water, 39, 120, 282, 354n3, 379n5, 380n8
holy wells, 284, 316–23, 333, 379n5, 384nn42–43, 385n53; fairs, 310, 312, 319–20; healing associated with, 39, 106, 186, 282, 290, 310, 312, 314–15, 379n5, 381n18, 384n42, 385n53; patterns (religious rituals), 310, **311**, 312–13
homeopathists. *See* sectarian doctors
hospital, conditions in, 8, 156, **157**, 160, 331. *See also* hospitalism
hospital case records, information typically contained, 86, 148
Hospital for Special Surgery, 167. *See also* New York Hospital
Hospital for the Relief of the Ruptured and Crippled, 166–67
hospitalism, 156, 222
Hostetter's Stomach Bitters. *See under* bitters
housemaid's knee, 149, 164. *See also* bursitis
housing, 7, 8, 47, 50, 58, 107, **124**, 139, 245–47, 252, 286, 324, 337, 386n57. *See also* tenements
Hughes, Angela [Sister], 177
Hughes, John [Archbishop], 62, 177, 217, 234, 266, 280, 305, 323, 364n31, 375n20, 376n20
humoral theory, 8, 23, 27, 28, 34, 58, 72–82, 93–94, 144, 275, 330, 332, 343n4
Huntington Collection. *See* "Bone Bill"
Huxley, Mrs., 21–23, **24**, 25–56, 102, 125, 288–92, 303, 329, 344n8, 345n1
Hyatt's Infallible Life Balsam. *See under* balsams

Illustrated London News, **98**, 283
Indigenous people of America. *See* Native Americans
injuries, 2–13, 19–20, 30, 41, 49, 52, 53, 97–101, 112, 131–32, 137–234, 277, 293, 296, 317, 326–37, 342n11, 352n29, 370n59, 371n61, 372n1, 373n4; acute, 144, 146, **147**, **149–52**, 153–64; and chronic pain, 150, 152, 164–67, 202, 223, 230, 293, 370n59. *See also* Astor House; bruises; burns; bursitis; contusions; fractures; hernias; lacerations; sprains; wounds
intestinal worms, 32–37, 42, 54, 105, 190, 194, 289–90, 295, 315, 345n15, 357n19
Ireland, colonization of, 75–76
Ireland, counties: Antrim, 183, 354n2, 381n16; Carlow, 184, 187, 365n8; Cavan, 46, 105, 343n13, 345n19, 347n27, 356n11, 366n15, 367n20, 381n18; Clare, 17, 106, 123, 187, 188, 265, 281, 342n10, 343n13, 365n9; Cork, 7, 17, 37, 38, 43, 47, 48, 104–5, 133, 265, 311, 340n5, 342n10, 343n13, 344n13, 345n19, 347n27, 367n20, 368n42, 375n19; Donegal, 48, 105, 110, 121, 139, **186**, 289, 312, 345n19, 346n19, 364n3; Down, 342n10; Dublin, 187, 265, 347n27; Fermanagh, 46; Galway, 17, 43, 124, 183, 208, 291, 342n10, 343n13, 347n27, 363n29, 367n20; Kerry, **14**, 17, 47, 48, 105, 106, 127, 183, 265, 282, 289, 340n5, 342n10, 343n13, 347n27, 348n33, 371n62, 375n19, 380n13, 384n42; Kildare, 17, 187, 343n13; Kilkenny, **153**, 342n10, 343n13, 347n27, 356n12; King's, 342n10, 343n13; Leitrim, 1, 46, 342n10, 347n27, 366n15, 367n20; Limerick, 188, 347n27, 384n43; Longford, 187, 367n20, 372n71; Louth, 188; Mayo, 17, 105, 217, 303, 343n13, 345n19, 367n20; Meath, 312, 343n13; Monaghan, 342n10, 347n27; Roscommon, 17, 105, 345n19, 384n41; Sligo, 17, 47, 265, 343n13, 354n2, 355n5, 358n29, 371n64; Tipperary, 17, 47, 347n27, 356n12, 366n12, 379n7; Tyrone, 48, 290, 347n27, 379n5; Waterford, 342n10, 343n13, 356n12; Westmeath, 105, 158, 223, 342n10, 345n19, 367n20; Wexford, 106, 183–84, 186, 343n13; Wicklow, 187

Ireland, regions: Connaught, 6, 46, 100, 347n27; Leinster, 5, 100; Munster 6, 100, 347n27; Ulster 5, 46, 48, 100, 115, 347n27, 347n28
Irish American Weekly, 233, 243, 250, 254, 274, 296, 326
Irish communities, 102, 115, 123–27, 138, 221, 228, 233–34, 241–42, 253–60, 277, 280, 292–93, 320, 323, 325, 335, 376n33
Irish Emigrant Society, 62, 286
Irish female heads of house, 117–19, 256. *See also* gender roles
Irish fever, 9, 57–58, 69, 234, 260, 330–31. *See also* typhus fever
Irish healers. *See* healers, Irish popular
Irish language, 6, 14, 17, **18**, 75, 342n10
Irish popular medicine, 13, 33–45. *See also* alcohol; cloth; cod liver oil; colors in Irish healing; eel oil; ethnomedicine; goose grease; healers, Irish popular; holy water; holy wells; plants used medicinally; potatoes; whiskey
Irish Potato Famine. *See* Great Famine, the
Irish prejudice. *See* anti-Irish sentiment
Irish speakers. *See* Irish language

jaundice, 27, 33, 38, 149, 191, 206, 314, 368n41, 384n45
Jewish immigrants, and tuberculosis, 10, 266
Jews' Hospital, 146, 334
J. R. Stafford's Olive Tar, 204–6, 218–19, 298, **299**, 300

Keeney, B. M., 51, 246, 375n24
Keppler, Joseph, **338**
Knox, John, 76–77, 351n23
Koch, Robert, 262–64, 344n5

lacerations, 150, 154–56, 217. *See also* injuries; wounds
laudanum. *See* opium
lead poisoning. *See* poisoning, lead

Lenox Hill. *See* dispensaries: German Dispensary
lice, 60–61, 225, 371n67, 372n68
liniments, 19, 182–83, 196, 203–10, 213–15, **216**, 222, 296, 298, 375n28; advertisements for, **199**, 207, **216**, 218–19; bottles, 204–5, 207–8, 215–16; Mexican Mustang Liniment, **199**, 204, 206, 214–15, 217; Radway's Ready Relief, 204–6, 215, **216**, 218–19, 296
liquor bottles, **118**, 293, 358nn26–27, 370n59. *See also* alcohol; brandy; whiskey
literacy, among Irish immigrants, 213, 243, 245, 359n31
Liverpool, 56–59, 62, 68, 81, 96, 98, 348n2, 354n2, 355nn5–6
London hospitals, 86, 88, 158, 373n11; Irish immigrants in, 176, 353n33; rates of tuberculosis in, 242
Long Island Railroad, 154
Ludlam, George, 362n19
Lyon's Kathairon, 224–28, 371n65, 372nn68–69, 372n73

MacLean, Mary, 1–2, 4, 11, 19, 21, 28, 46, 59, 304, 317, 339n1, 354n2, 363n27, 386n2
MacNeven, William, 177, 223, 363n29
Maguire, John Francis, 7, 51, 57, 64, 69, 154, 258, 287, 318, 350n12, 354n3, 359n35
malaria, 58, 150–52, 161, 198, 370n52, 374n12. *See also* fever, intermittent
malingering, 149–51, 160
malnutrition, 7, 35, 85, 97, 144, 147, 160, 162, 247–50, 260, 315, 349n5, 373n4, 385n48. *See also* starvation
Marine Hospital. *See* Staten Island Quarantine Hospital
markets. *See* food markets
Massachusetts General Hospital, 154, 173
Mathew, Theobald [Father], 259, 313, 318. *See also* temperance
McGuire, Huxley, 21–56, 193, 196, 287–91, 329, 344n8, 348n31, 387
McLoughlin, Peter and Michael, 286, 357n20, 358n29

McPeake family, 232, **233**, **237**, 243, **244**, 245–47, 250–51, 253–56, 258–59, 261–65, 274, 278, 280, 296, 325–26, 374n15, 374nn17–18, 376n32, 386n2. *See also* Van Peake, Ella Louise
meaning response, 29, 41, 196, 199, 342n12, 344n6
medical anthropology, 11–14, 29, 41, 142–43, 329, 333
melancholic temperament, 27, 73, 80, 267
mental illnesses: bipolar disorder, 81, 384n42; insanity, **149**, 312, 384n42; mania, 80–82, 94; melancholy, 159; schizophrenia, 81
Mexican Mustang Liniment. *See under* liniments
miasma, 8, 23, 28, 60, 79, 103
midwives, 42, 52, 124, 336, 376n33
mineral water, **111**, 305–7, 315, **316**, 317–19, 384n36, 385n51. *See also* soda water
misdiagnosis, 58, 82–83, 87–91, 94, 331
Morton, Samuel, 70, 76, 350n18
Mose the Bowery B'hoy, 226, **227**
Mott, Valentine, 172, 175, 179–80, 363n25, 364n32
Mrs. Winslow's Soothing Syrup. *See under* opium
Mt. Sinai. *See* Jews' Hospital

Nast, Thomas, 68, 350n17
Nation, The, 139
National Folklore Collection [Irish], 12, **14**, 37, **43**, 103, **124**, 341nn9–10
nationalism: American, 7, 76, 95, 319; British, 74–78, 94, 341n7; Irish, 6, 58, 67, 76–77, 115, 275–77, 286, 300, 312–13, 319, 323, 334, 335, 341n7, 351n23, 376n31. *See also* Celtic; citizenship; Fenians; O'Connell, Daniel; race; race "science"
Native Americans, 71, 94, 194, 295
nativism, American, 58, 65–71, 93, 96, 101, 127–28, 277–78, 323, 325, 340n2; Know-Nothings, 67, 378n44. *See also* anti-Irish sentiment; race; race "science"
newspapers, 13, 32, 52, 122, 136, 166, 189, 198–99, 214–24, 291, 300, 319, 370n55

Index   465

New York [Daily] Times (New York), 40, 127, 134, 320, 349n3, 352n28, 363n23, 377n44, 383n40; advertisements in, 166, **218,** 219, 302–3, 321
New York Daily Tribune, 134–35, 137, 224, 371n66, 378n44
New York Dispensary. *See under* dispensaries
New York Freeman's Journal (and Catholic Register) (New York), 178, 217–18, 275, 303, 364n31, 371n63, 371n66
New York Hospital, 13, 28, 46, 52–53, 59, 64, 81–90, **84,** 101, 129, 137, 146–56, **157,** 158–78, 189, 192–98, 207, 212, 235–37, **238,** 239–41, 248, 255, 272, 292, 315, 319, 348n3, 349n9, 352n32, 356n16, 357n21, 361n12, 362n17, 362n19, 364n32, 370n59, 373n6, 373n8, 373n11, 374n13, 376n36, 381n23
New York Orthopaedic Dispensary. *See under* dispensaries
Normal College of the City of New York, 326
Nott, Josiah, 70, 76, 350n18
nurses, 85, 99, 135, **157,** 263, 333–36, 352n28, 373n11; Irish, 10, 132, 137, 177, 179, 180, 304, 334, 359n35. *See also* Duffe, James; Sisters of Charity

Oakland, CA, 117–18
O'Connell, Daniel, 313
ointments, 32–41, 182–85, 197, 201–2, 222, 345n16, 364n3; patent medicine, 203, 204–8, 210, 297, 367n28
opium, 170, 270, 354n2, 375n28; dependency, 198, 212, 297, 373n8; Mrs. Winslow's Soothing Syrup, 198, 204–6, 211, 219; overdose, 177, 198, 382n25; in patent medicines, 90, 198, 211, 212, 297; prescribed by physicians, 25, 212, 236, 297, 373n8
Opper, Frederick Burr, 91, **92,** 140, **141**
Orange Riot, 275
orphans, 50, 252, 286, 343n2, 348n31, 377nn43–44, 378n44
overlooking. *See* bewitchment

passenger laws, 61–62
Pat (stereotype), 91, **141,** 142, 223, 229, **230,** 250, 269, 272, 275, 331, **338,** 350n17
patent medicines: advertisement techniques, 199–200, 214–19, 300–301, 370n55, 371n66; bottles, 111, 199, 202, **216, 299,** 370n57; definition, 197, 369n51; interpretations of, 20, 112, 200–223, 231, 296–301, 333; popularity in U.S., 53, 197–200, 382nn27–28, 382n30
Paterson, NJ, 203–5, 209–10, 217, 220, 285, 298, 305, 318, 323, 344n11, 358n25, 385n51
Paterson Evening News, 285, 344n11
Pearl Street, New York, 17, 20, 102–3, 107–8, **109,** 110, 111, 112–17, **118,** 119–21, **122,** 123–26, 129, 135–36, 161, 182, 189–90, 195–97, 202–3, 207–24, 231, 245, 251–55, 286–87, 293–303, **306,** 309, 313, 316–20, 328, 333, 342n13, 348n31, 357n20, 358n29, 361n11, 362nn16–17, 367nn22–24, 370nn57–58, 371n61, 371n65, 382nn26–27, 383n36, 385n49. *See also* Five Points
Penal Laws (in Ireland), 177, 286, 340n5, 356n13, 366n20
Pennsylvania Hospital, 173, 175
perfumes. *See under* cosmetics
Peruvian bark *(cinchona)*, 198, 211, 236, 370n52
pharmacists, 201, 206, 210, 277, 307, 309, 315, 382n27; female, 221, 371n64; in Ireland, 53, 220, 302, 368n41, 383n33; in New York City, 10, 20, 52, 120, 210, 220–21, 277, 292–93, 296, 302–5, 325, 333, 371n64; in relation to patent medicines, 197–98, 220–22, 293, 302–3, 315–16
phlegmatic temperament, 9, 27, 72, **73,** 74–75, 130, 267–69, 278, 335, 351n24, 352n26
phrenology, 28, 140, 343n4
phthisis, 9, 10, 27, 38, 39, 52, 54, 113, 115, 120, 137, 149, 160, 178, 191, 195, 200–201, 212, 232–37, **238,** 239–307, 312–15, 321–28, 345n14, 356n15, 364n1, 372n1, 373nn5–7, 373n9, 375nn25–26, 376n35, 377n39, 377n41, 378n1, 381n21, 384n45. *See also* consumptive diathesis; tuberculosis

466   Index

physicians: American, 8, 20–31, 34, 38, 40, 43, 45, 52–54, 60, 88, 94, **157**, 159, **171**, 269, 292, 305, 353n34, 364n32; Irish, 10, 35, 103, 123, 177, 223, 236, 353, 354n36, 356n13, 363n29. *See also* Doane, Sidney; Draper, John; Fitch, Samuel Sheldon; Graves, Robert; Griscom, John; Keeney, B. M.; Ludlam, George; MacNeven, William; Mott, Valentine; Pulling, Ezra R.; Stimson, Lewis Atterbury; Thoms, William F.; Townsend, Peter S.

pipes, smoking, 66, **110**, 123, **124**, 195, 229, **230**, 231, 256, **257**, **283**, 365n11. *See also* smoking

placebo. *See* meaning response

plants used medicinally: chickweed, 38, 184, 192, **193**, 288, 368n42, 380n9; dandelion, 34, 38, 288–89, 345n16, 380nn9–11, 380n14; dock, 184, 190–92, 289, 290, 295, 365n9, 367n27, 380n14; foxglove, 123, 282, **283**, 284, 290, 379n6, 381n20; jimsonweed, 194, 295, 369nn44–45; mullein, 290–91, 295, 302, 381nn20–21; nettle, 35–36, 38, 184, 192, 288–90, 345n17, 365n9, 366n15, 380n9; oats, 34, 184, 187, 289, 345n16, 372n71, 381n18; plantain ("St. Patrick's leaf" or *slánlus*), 38–39, 184–85, 288, 364n6, 380n11; pokeweed, 194, 369n44, 369n46; ragweed (ragwort or *buachalán*), 184–85, 191–92, 365n9, 368n41; willow ("sally"), 184, 187, 365n9

pneumonia, 22, 27, 149, 151–52, 194, 235

Poe, Edgar Allen, 269

poisoning, 101, 161–62, 195, 260, 315, 381n18; blood, 8, 34–35, 103–5, 126, 184, 211, 289, 365n7; lead, 151–52, 162–63, 168, 226, 251, 315, 323, 383n38, 385n48; mercury, 90, 150, 162–63, 168; phosphorus, 150, 161, 363n22. *See also* anesthesia, poisoning; opium: overdose

poitín. *See* whiskey

political cartoons, 54, 66, 68, 91–**92**, 140, **141**, 275, **276**, 277, 335, **338**, 350n17, 353n37, 378n45. *See also* anti-Irish sentiment; Keppler, Joseph; Nast, Thomas; Opper, Frederick Burr; *Puck*; *Punch*

posthumous children, 42, 346n22

potatoes, 4, 30, 32, 66, 117, 121, 160, 289, 294, 340n5, 356n15, 358n22, 361n11; in Irish popular medicine, 34, 36–37, 54, 184–85, 193, 345n16, 356n15; reputation of among Americans, 30, 54–55, 175

poultices, 37–38, 41, 155, 169, 182, 184, 190–92, **193**, 194, 257, 290, 292, 295, 314, 364nn5–7, 365n9, 369n42, 371n62

Presbyterian Hospital. *See* dispensaries: New York Orthopaedic Dispensary

prescription medicine bottles, 112, 197–202, 222, 293, 370n58

priests, 6, 39–40, 42, 52, 67, 94, 96, 106, 120, 122, 127–29, 186, 241, 259, 285, 286, 310, 313, 333, 335, 346nn21–22, 354n1, 359nn34–35, 363n30, 366n17. *See also* Adams, Thomas [Father]; Hughes, John [Archbishop]; Mathew, Theobald [Father]

priest's bottle, 115, 119

prisons, 47, 57, 138, 144, 177, 354n3, 355n6, 378n46

prostitution, 113, 121, 136, 148

Protestantism, 69, 71, 75, 95, 128, 258

pub/saloon, 47, 49, 113, **114**, 115, 121, **151–52**, 163, 207, 223, 258, 317, 319, 368n40

Puck, 91, **92**, 140, **141**, **276**, **338**, 378n45

Pulling, Ezra R., 247–48

pulmonary tuberculosis. *See* phthisis

Punch, 68, 350n17

quarantine, 8, 59, 62–64, 72, 85, 94, 99, 102, 128–29, 278, 348n2, 350n11, 359n35

race, 25–26, 74–76, 79, 330; among Europeans and European Americans, 9, 75–78, 94, 268–69, 275, 335, 341n7, 351n23, 352n27, 378n44; and enslavement, 70–71, 95, 350n13, 350n16

race "science," 58, 70–72, 275, 330; as related to humoral theory, 73–79, 94–95, 268–69. *See also* phrenology

Radway's Ready Relief. *See under* liniments

railroad pace of labor, 52, 138, 195

railroads, 132, 140, 150–54, 161, 163, 172, 196, 301, 360nn7–8, 361n8, 370n54

reciprocity. *See* throughother
rheumatism, 104, 149, 152, 161, 184–85, 190–94, 207, 217, 266, 298, 307, 360n36, 365nn9–10, 366nn15–16, 369n43, 374n12, 380n10, 382n29
rickets, 37, 144, 210, 266, 384n46
Roney, Frank, 49, 52, 134, 138, 223–24, 247, 287, 313, 360n3
Rowland's Macassar Oil, 224–26, 371n65
Ruane, Bridget, 288, 380n11. *See also* wisewomen
rural: areas in Ireland, 6, 48, 100–102, 121, 123, 137, 182, 214, 221, 228, 289, 302, 310, 334, 347n27; Irish views, 44, 101, 115, 129, 137–38, 247, 280, 287, 384n44. *See also* friendship, Irish conception of; healers, Irish popular; Irish popular medicine; throughother

sailors. *See* seamen
San Francisco, 12, 247, 305, 323, 360n3
sanguine temperament, 9, 19, 27–28, 55, 58, 72–75, 79–82, 88–97, 126–32, 140, 142, 159, 169, 225–26, 230, 268, 269, 275, 330, 335, 351n22, 352n26
sanitary inspectors, 246–48, 254, 258. *See also* Griscom, John; Keeney, B. M.; Pulling, Ezra R.; Thoms, William F.
Saratoga Springs, 306–7, 315, 317, 319–20
sarsaparillas, 203, 204–6, 211, 219, 297, 358n25, 382n27, 383n40
scars, 3, 9, 143, 152, 154, 168–69, 180, 226, 363n24
Scotland, 15, 47, 170, 174, 196, 207, 210, 284, 348n2
scrofula, 235, 241, 248, 266, 281, 289–90, 297–300, 307, 312, 372n3, 377n36, 379n3, 381nn16–18, 382n27, 384n32
seamen, **84**, 98, 117, 146, 152–53, 155, 161, 166, 173, 352n29, 354n33, 362n16, 367n24, 375n26
sectarian doctors, 26, 28, 52, 175, 197, 343n4
seventh son/daughter, 32, 42, 106, 122, 290, 346n22, 381n16
shebeens, 121
Sisters of Charity, 53, 173, 177, **178**, 179–80,
241, 304, 334, 359n35, 363n30, 374n11. *See also* Hughes, Angela [Sister]; St. Vincent's Hospital
Sixth Ward, **24**, 46–53, 107, 113, **114**, 125, 134–35, 189, 221, **237**, 246, 254, 265, 286, 348n34, 371n64. *See also* Five Points; Pearl Street, New York
smallpox, 58, 266, 359n35, 361n13, 375n22
Smith, William, 56, 57, 62, 96–97, 99–100, 107, 129, 348n29, 354n1, 387n2
smoking, **66**, 93, 105, 110, 123–24, 194–95, 229, 256–60, 277, 290, 295, 365n11. *See also* pipes, smoking
soda water, 10, 19, 20, **111**, 120, 152, 162, 280, 285, 296, 302, 305, **306**, 307–25, 328, 333, 334, 336, 367n24, 370n57, 383nn36–40, 384n41, 385n48, 385nn51–52, 386nn55–56. *See also* mineral water
soda water fountains, 307, **308**, 310, 319–20, 322, 383n40, 385n48, 386n55
sprains, 38, 42, 150, 182–85, 191, 193, 196, 208, 314, 365nn9–10, 366n15, 369n43, 382n29, 384n45
St. Anthony's fire. *See* erysipelas
St. Luke's Hospital, 146
St. Patrick's Day Riot, 275
St. Peter's Church, 46
St. Vincent's Hospital, 10, 13, 53, 63, 146, 157, 161–62, 172–73, 177, **178**, 179, 212, 235, 239, 241–42, 270, 304, 334, 355n10, 359n35, 374nn11–13. *See also* Hughes, Angela [Sister]; Sisters of Charity
starvation, 4, 35, 69, 354n4. *See also* malnutrition
Staten Island Quarantine Hospital, 56, 62, 63, **64**, 88, 99, 261, 348n3. *See also* Doane, Sidney; quarantine
stereotypes, 9, 55, 58, 65, 72, 75, 81–82, 89–97, 113, 130–33, 145, 169, 174–75, 223–33, 264, 266–68, 272–78, 317, 325, 331–32, 337–38, 377n41, 378n46. *See also* anti-Irish sentiment; Bridget (stereotype); Pat (stereotype); race; race "science"
Stimson, Lewis Atterbury, 362n19
Sullivan Street, 318

sunstroke, 9, 52, 131, 147, 158–59, 181, 307
surgery, 132, 146, 149–52, 156–58, 167–76, 179, 212, 217, 220, 236, 302, 331, 361n13, 364n32, 381n23
swill milk, 51, 248
syphilis, 351n19, 352n31, 382n27
syringes, hypodermic, **212**, 213, 297, 370n61

tea, 22–23, 32, 105, 115, 117, 183, 190, 194–96, 248, 258, 294, 319, 356n18, 361n11, 368n40, 379n6; cups, 118–19, 136, 195, 222, 231, 313, 318–19
temperance, 71, 74, 81, 119, 121, 259, 307, 309, 313, 317, 318–19. *See also* Mathew, Theobald [Father]
tenements, 17, 20, 52, 107, 109, **118**, 120, 125, 129, 189, 190, 192, 206, 214, 220, 222, 245–46, 251, 253, 293, 298, 305, 375n20. *See also* housing
Thoms, William F., 51, 254
throughother, 44, 48, 102, 126, 258, 312, 323, 347n25, 362n13. *See also* friendship, Irish conception of; rural: Irish views
Townsend, Peter S., 21–23, 28–37, 40–55, 148, 152, 175, 193, 196, 206, 288, 329, 343n2, 344n8, 345n17, 358n25
toys. *See under* children
Transfiguration Church, 17, 49, 286, 342
tuberculosis, 2–3, 8–10, 19, 27, 104, 137, 149, 209, 212, 228–29, 279, 325, 328, 332–33, 336, 343n1, 351n19, 363n30, 367n21, 379n3; American understandings of, 232, 261–64, 266–78, 296, 307, 321, 377n39, 378n1; causes of, 51–52, 160, 234–35, 243–60, 376n33, 376n35; Irish ideas about, 279–92, 345n14, 360n6, 372n3, 375n24, 377n36, 377n40; Irish popular medicine for, 37–39, 191, 195, 282–305, 312, 314–17, 323–24, 356n15, 360n36, 364n1, 381nn21–22, 384n42, 384n45; mortality and hospital admissions rates, 50–51, 234–43, **265**, 266, 372n1, 373nn5–6, 374n14, 375n22, 375n29, 376n34, 377n38; physicians' treatment for 37, 210, 236, 266, 307, 373n7; rates of in Dublin, 252, 265–66. *See also* age; consumptive diathesis; phthisis
tuberculosis, various forms of: bovine, 51, 248, 372n3; *morbus coxarius*, 234–36, 241–42, 255, 297, 373n6, 374n13, 375n28; Pott's Disease, 234, 372n3, 377n36; pulmonary; strumous ophthalmia, 234, 241; tubercular meningitis, 235, 241, 242. *See also* phthisis
Turlington's Balsam of Life. *See under* balsams
turpentine, 38, 183–84, 207–8, 236, 296, 345n18, 370n59, 381n18
Twoomy, Mary, 125
typhoid fever, 61, 106, 160, 194, 246, 349n5, 372n2, 373n22, 374n12, 375n22, 378n46
typhus fever, 2–10, 19, 50, 56–65, 72, 79–130, 140, 195, 225, 234, 260–62, 269, 272, 277, 317, 328–32, 349n3, 349n5, 353n33; causes of, 60, 80, 86, 103–4; Irish cures for, 36, 378n46; mortality rates, 61, 87–88; murine, 348n1; symptoms of, 56, 58, 60, 79–83, 87. *See also* age; clothing; fever; Irish fever

Udolpho Wolfe's Aromatic Schnapps, 204–6, 217
ulcers, 149, 151, 156, 184, 190–91, 194, 217, 298, 360n36, 365n9, 379n6
upright posture, 142, 151, 168–69, 177, 228–29
U.S. Sanitary Commission, 179, 343n4

Van Peake, Ella Louise, 326–27, 386n58, 386n2
Vaseline, 201–2, 205–6, 208
Vick's Vapo Rub, 208
violence, 142, 325, 386n57; in anti-Irish stereotypes, 6, **66**, 75, 78, 82, 92, 94, 169, 378n44; domestic, 148, 163, 164; on the job, 148, 152, 163; riots, 68, 163, 378n44. *See also* African Americans; racism against;

donnybrooks; Draft Riots; Orange Day Riots; St. Patrick's Day Riots

visceral historical archaeology, 1, 11–15

wages, 47–48, 67, 114, 136–37, 164, 213, 223, 248, 317, 352n29, 360n7, 375n20; cost of living, 134–35; in New York City, 134, 252

wakes, 32, 71, 95, 99, 115, 127–28, 137, 229, 256, **257**, 287, 294, 344n10, 359n36, 362n18. *See also* "American wake"

Ward, Catherine, 102, 348n31

Ward, John, 102, 287, 357n20

Ward's Island, 53, 63, 85, 99, 335, 349n10, 350n10, 357n21, 359n35

whiskey, 111–22, 126–31, 136, 223, 229, 256, 258–60, 317–18, 382n26; bottles, 112, 115, 117, 121, 126, 195, 319; distilling, 122, 281; in hospitals, 196, 304; in Irish popular medicine, 34–35, 38, 104–5, 111–12, 115, 117, 120–21, 126–27, 131, 162, 181–84, 194–96, 211, 281, 289–93, 297, 324, 345n16, 356n18, 364n1, 369n47, 376n31; reputation of, 55, 112, 126, 230, 317–18, 331. *See also* priest's bottle

wine, 74, 81, 104, 112, 127, 155, 294, 358n27, 386n56; associations with gentility, 115; bottles, 19, 112, 117, **118**, 119–20, **122**, 126, 293, 333, 385n52; elderberry, 34, 105, 345n16; and Irish women, 117–22, 195

wisewomen, 32, 35, 42, 52, 106, 122–29, 282–83, 288, 300, 358n30. *See also* Coyle, Jug; Early, Biddy; Ruane, Bridget

witchcraft. *See* bewitchment

worms. *See* intestinal worms

wounds, 9, 147, 150–57, 161, 163; treatment of, 183–85, 189–94, 208–210, 217, 257, 295, 297, 324, 364n7, 365n8, 369n50, 371n62, 376n30, 379n6, 381n17, 382n28. *See also* injuries; lacerations

yellow fever, 21, 42, 58, 59, 83, 343n1

www.ingramcontent.com/pod-product-compliance
Lightning Source LLC
LaVergne TN
LVHW041957060526
838200LV00002B/49